Protecting Personnel at Hazardous Waste Sites

Second Edition

Edited by

William F. Martin
Steven P. Levine

Butterworth-Heinemann
Boston London Oxford Singapore Sydney Toronto Wellington

Library of Congress Cataloging-in-Publication Data

Martin, William F.
        Protecting personnel at hazardous waste sites / [edited by] William F. Martin,
Steven P. Levine -- 2nd ed.
        p. cm.
Includes bibliographical references and index.
ISBN 0-7506-9457-2
1. Hazardous wastes--Safety measures--United States. 2. Hazardous
wastes--Health aspects--United States.   I. Martin, William F. II. Levine,
Steven P.
TD1050.S24P76 1994   93-28510
628.4'2'0289--dc20   CIP

British Library Cataloguing-in-Publication Data

A catalogue record for this book is available from the British Library.

Butterworth-Heinemann
80 Montvale Avenue
Stoneham, MA 02180

10 9 8 7 6 5 4 3 2

Printed in the United States of America

CONTENTS

Chapter

Page

PREFACE

Professionals in environmental health, occupational health and engineering have often noted the need for a well referenced health and safety textbook to prepare new workers for hazardous materials and hazardous waste cleanup activities.

This need is addressed in this second edition by the two editors, Steven P. Levine, Ph.D., C.I.H., and William F. Martin, P.E. by uniting twenty-plus contributing authors from federal agencies, academia and industry. These authors average over fifteen years each in professional experience in teaching, regulating, consulting and handling of hazardous materials. The first edition of this book was published in 1985 with excellent acceptance by academic, industrial and governmental colleagues.

Additional field experience and new regulations have prompted the editors to assemble this second edition. Two new chapters have been added to address the 1990's effort to cleanup and convert to civilian use major Department of Defense (DoD) and Department of Energy (DoE) lands and facilities. These chapters introduce radiation, unexploded ordnance, and explosive waste health and safety for site investigators, managers, supervisors and workers. A chapter to review occupational health and toxicology has been added because class room experience at educational centers all across the United States indicated that many professional people were being cross trained for hazardous waste occupations with very limited backgrounds in applied occupation health.

The final new chapter is a real life example of a site health and safety plan. Many users of the first edition had requested that the editors make available for classroom use a site safety plan that had been used for a complex site clean up.

The second edition has expanded and updated material in every chapter. References have been revised to reflect current sources. The main objective of this textbook continues to be its use as a resource book for training professionals in the practice of occupational safety and health in hazardous materials and waste activities. It is the strong feeling of the editors that anyone teaching or training hazardous waste workers should have thoroughly covered at least the content of this second edition in an academic setting and have had considerable field experience under close supervision.

This edition is considered a minimum of academic exposure for trainers of the hazardous work course commonly referred to as the Occupational Safety and Health Administration (OSHA) 40 hour or Hazardous Waste Operation and Emergency Response (HAZWOPER) training. The Environmental Protection Agency (EPA), DoD, DoE and OSHA regulations and contracts usually require this training for all on-site personnel.

Hazardous waste management is a challenging endeavor in our national effort to protect the quality of our environment. The authors of this book feel that this challenge can be met without sacrificing the health of those individuals and companies called upon to accomplish the task.

ACKNOWLEDGEMENTS

Recognition is given to the U.S. Public Health Service, the Occupational Safety and Health Administration (OSHA), the U.S. Environmental Protection Agency (EPA), and the U.S. Coast Guard for their efforts under Superfund to gather, develop and make publicly available health and safety publications and contractor reports.

The authors would like to thank Vicki Santoro for providing information and suggestions for Chapter 1. Thanks and recognition is given to Dr. Paul Jonmaire, Ph.D., Corporate Director of Health and Safety, and Steven J. Sherman, C.I.H. of Ecology and Environment, Inc., 368 Pleasantview Drive, Lancaster, New York, 14086, for all support and technical insight provided in the preparation of Chapter 3.

James P. Kirk, Director of Training, Ecological Safety Services, Houston; and Joseph A. Gispanski, Jr., and William R. Gourdie, III, Hygiene Safety and Training, Inc., Pittsburgh made many excellent recommendations for the second edition of the "Hazardous Waste Handbook for Health and Safety" which were also incorporated in this textbook.

This practical hazardous waste health and safety textbook would not be possible without the previous work of many individuals, companies and government agencies. During the past ten years, the authors have worked with a host of highly qualified professionals in the nation's efforts to contain hazardous waste spills, clean up abandoned landfills and control hazardous chemical threats to the environment and public health.

Outside reviewers contributed substantially to the quality and focus of this edition. An extensive review by William Keffer, Senior Engineering Advisor, Emergency Planning and Response, Region 7, EPA was very helpful for this edition, and also provided some excellent options for further editions. A review by Ray Bock and Larry Dunning of Rust International, Inc., Westchester, Florida helped to keep the textbook practical. Dr. Thomas Binder and his National Institute for Occupational Safety and Health (NIOSH) staff, especially Stephen P. Berardinelli, Ph.D., Aaron W. Schoppee, Ph.D., Jim Spahr, and Dr. Belard in the Division of Safety Research, Morgantown, West Virginia identified the current technology relating to Personal Protective Equipment.

Special thanks to Jeffrey A. Loy and Stephen L. Gurba, Ph.D., Environmental Systems & Services, Inc., for technical contributions and administrative support during the production of this edition.

The editors wish to thank Lynn A. Reid for her desktop publishing skills in the layout, design and editing of this second edition.

EDITORS

William F. Martin holds a Masters degree in Environmental Health Engineering from the University of Texas, and has been a Commissioned Officer of the U.S. Public Health Service for over 20 years. He has held positions with the Indian Health Service, U.S. Coast Guard, Federal Water Pollution Control Administration, and National Institute for Occupational Safety and Health. A registered professional engineer in Texas and Kentucky, he has presented and published numerous technical papers both foreign and domestic. He served on the Superfund steering committee made up of EPA, OSHA, NIOSH, and the U.S. Coast Guard. He served as the NIOSH Hazardous Waste Program Director with primary responsibility for coordinating all Institute Superfund activities including research projects and the production of comprehensive health and safety guidelines, worker bulletins and training materials. Mr. Martin has consulted on environmental engineering and hazardous waste health and safety with Valentec International Corporation and, most recently with Environmental Systems & Services, Inc.

Steven P. Levine, Ph.D. is an Associate Professor of Industrial Hygiene at the University of Michigan, School of Public Health. Prior to his present position, Dr. Levine held positions on the Research Staffs of Stauffer Chemical and of Ford Motor Company, as well as having worked with O.H. Materials Company in the field of hazardous waste site and contaminated structure evaluation and remediation. Dr. Levine earned his doctoral degree in Analytical Chemistry from the University of Colorado in 1972. He is the author of numerous publications on the subjects of analytical and environmental chemistry.

AUTHORS

Barrett E. Benson has been with the USEPA National Enforcement Investigations Center (NEIC) in Denver, Colorado, since 1972, except for 1981 when he was an associate in the Denver office of Fred C. Hart Associates. Before joining the NEIC, he was the Chief, Division of Industrial Waste, Pollution Control Department, city of Kansas City, Missouri, and a sanitary engineer with the U.S. Public Health Service, Arctic Health Research Center in Alaska. He is a registered engineer in Missouri and Colorado and has published technical papers in ASCE, AWWA, WPCF, and other technical journals. Currently, he serves as a principal sanitary engineer for the NEIC Technical Evaluation Staff with responsibilities in the areas of water pollution and hazardous waste management. In 1980, he was awarded the EPA Silver Medal for developing the EPA methods for conducting hazardous waste site investigations.

Edward Bishop, Ph.D., C.I.H. has over twenty-one years experience in the industrial hygiene field. He is currently a Senior Project Manager and Federal Programs Department Manager for the Fairfax, Virginia, office of Engineering-Science, Inc. In this position he develops and reviews health and safety plans and performs health and safety audits for CERCLA and RCRA hazardous waste operations. He has taught professional development courses on instrument selection and use at the American Industrial Hygiene Conferences since 1985. Prior to his present position, he was a Bioenvironmental Engineer in the United States Air Force.

Leslie W. Cole is a Certified Health Physicist and works as a Senior Scientist with Auxier & Associates in Knoxville, TN. He has a M.S. degree from the U.S. Naval Postgraduate School in Monterey, CA. He spent twenty-one years as a commissioned officer in the U.S. Army. Some of his assignments were: Senior Instructor, U.S. Command and General Staff College with responsibility for all instruction in Radiological Safety and Defense and preparation of Army publications related to Nuclear Weapons employment and defense; Nuclear Effects Officer at Continental Army Command; and Nuclear Accident/Incident Control Officer and Radiation Safety Officer at various Army installations in the United States, Germany and Korea. Before coming to Auxier & Associates, he was Director of Environmental, Health and Safety and Radiation Safety Officer with Aerojet

Ordnance Tennessee. At Aerojet, he was the technical manager for three major radiological decontamination and decommissioning projects. Mr. Cole is a member of an NCRP Committee that is preparing a guideline publication on Uranium and Chairman, Committee on Government Agency Issues in the American Academy of Health Physics.

David L. Dahlstrom is Corporate Director of Safety and Health for Ecology and Environment, Inc. (E&E), a firm specializing in environmental evaluation and design especially as applied to hazardous materials and waste site investigation, remediation, and personnel health and safety. Previously, he developed and presented several training programs for the USEPA and U.S. Coast Guard covering response to hazardous materials incidents, including: personnel protection and safety; field monitoring and analysis; incident mitigation and treatment; hazard evaluations; and damage assessment. He has had over 10 years experience in chemistry, microbiology, and occupational safety and health. This includes developing and managing E&E's employee medical monitoring, respiratory training, and field operations programs, and assisting in the design of similar programs for both governmental and industrial clients. He is the author of numerous papers on employee medical surveillance, personnel protection, health and safety program development, and hazardous materials incident response techniques.

Margo R. Dusenbury is currently employed as an Environmental Engineer with the U.S. Environmental Protection Agency, National Enforcement Investigations Center in Denver, Colorado. She coordinates and provides technical support to multi-media civil and criminal field investigations at commercial, industrial, and federal facilities. She also participated in the national Hazardous Waste Groundwater Task Force investigations. Previously, she was part of the RCRA Enforcement Section in EPA, Region V in Chicago, where she evaluated RCRA groundwater monitoring and assessment programs and prepared hazardous waste enforcement cases. Additionally, she conducted solid waste, RCRA hazardous waste, groundwater monitoring, and Underground Injection Control inspections for the Illinois EPA in Collinsville, Illinois. She earned a B.S. degree in Geological Engineering (with an emphasis in hydrogeology and hazardous waste management) from the University of Missouri-Rolla in 1983.

Michael Gochfeld, M.D., Ph.D. is Director of Occupational Health at New Jersey's Environmental and Occupational Health Sciences Institute (EOHSI) and Clinical Professor of Occupational Medicine at the UMDNJ-Robert Wood Johnson Medical School. He was formerly director of Environmental and Occupational Health Services at the New Jersey Department of Health. Dr. Gochfeld received his undergraduate training in ecology at Oberlin College and his medical degree at Albert Einstein College of Medicine. He served as a staff pediatrician in the U.S. Navy and spent a year as a Provincial Public Environmental Health Department of Columbia School of Public Health and obtained a Ph.D. in Environmental Biology at the City University of New York with post-doctoral research in behavioral sciences at Rockefeller University. His areas of interest include medical surveillance in relation to hazardous chemical wastes, clinical exposure and environmental risk assessment, and clinical and laboratory studies of heavy metals and neurobehavioral development. He has co-edited a book on Medical Surveillance of Hazardous Waste Workers and an Environmental Health Perspectives issue on Chromium. He serves as an editor of Industrial Hygiene and Occupational Health for the Mosby-Yearbook Series.

Ralph F. Goldman has a B.S. degree in Chemistry from the University of Denver, and M.S. and Ph.D. degrees in Physiology from Boston University. There, he worked on resistance to stress through endocrine mechanisms following irradiation of the adrenal glands in animals. He then worked for the U.S. Army at the Natick, Massachusetts, Quartermaster R/D Laboratories. Dr. Goldman then became the Director of a program he established in Military Ergonomics in the Army Institute of Environmental Medicine. He received numerous awards including the highest medal the Army can give to a civilian, and was appointed to the Senior Executive Service. He resigned in 1982 to form Comfort Technology, Inc. and as Senior Vice President and Chief Scientist, and is continuing his work on evaluation of human tolerance limits to heat and cold. He is working to extend human hot and cold tolerance limits by modified clothing, equipment and physical conditioning. Prediction models which accurately projects the physiological responses of workers wearing a given clothing ensemble in any work setting are current projects. He is Chairman of the NATO Research Study Group-7 on Biomedical Effects of Clothing, and has faculty appointments at Boston University, MIT and the University of Rhode Island.

Virginia T. Kiefert, M.A. has an A.A. degree from Mount Mary College, Wisconsin and B.A. and M.A. degrees in Applied Medical Anthropology from the University of South Florida, Tampa, Florida. Her health experience has been in three major areas: 1) implementation of medical research concerning fetal stress/maternal blood oxygen levels during labor and comparative evaluations of Dynamap, Finapress and arterial line blood pressure monitoring during surgery; 2) development of toxicology training materials for hazardous waste courses and technical publications, including development and presentation of the health efforts and toxicology sessions of the OSHA 40 hour HAZWOPER Course; and 3) extensive experience with computer assisted Electromyography for muscle tension, migraine headache and neuro-muscular re-education.

John M. Lippitt is a Registered Sanitarian with the Ohio State Board of Sanitation Registration. He is currently employed as a Project Scientist for SCS Engineers, a consulting engineering firm specializing in hazardous and solid waste management. Mr. Lippitt provides expertise in health and safety management for SCS projects and has prepared several documents concerning methods of worker protection and costs of worker safety and health for NIOSH and the USEPA. His professional experience prior to joining SCS involved five years as a Public Health Sanitarian, a year conducting carcinogen testing research and development with the USEPA Health Effects Research Laboratory, and nine months as an on-site coordinator for the Ohio EPA to monitor the activities of a licensed hazardous waste landfill.

James M. Melius received his B.A. from Brown University in 1970, followed by a M.M.S. in 1972. In 1974, he received his M.D. from the University of Illinois in Chicago, followed by a residency in family practice and occupational medicine. He received his Dr. P.H. degree in Epidemiology in 1984 from the University of Illinois School of Public Health. He is board certified in Family Practice and Occupational Medicine.

Since 1980, he has been Chief of the NIOSH Health Hazard Evaluation Program, Cincinnati, Ohio. This program conducts approximately 500 occupational health field evaluations each year throughout the country. For the past two years, Dr. Melius has been involved in evaluations at hazardous waste cleanup sites and in advising EPA on occupational health matters related to Superfund. His other research interests include occupational health problems for fire fighters, PCB combustion products, neurotoxicity, and indoor air quality.

Richard C. Montgomery is a graduate of California Polytechnical Institute with management and business experience in environmental training. He is currently the Director of the Environmental Training Center, U.S. Army, Fort Sill, Oklahoma. His DoD program is developing and conducting an extensive array of environmental courses that are targeted to military facility cleanup and/or base closure.

Christopher C. O'Leary, C.I.H., C.S.P. is a senior consultant and manager of Arthur D. Little's Occupational Health and Safety consulting activities. His professional interests lie in the area of occupational health and safety management, exposure and risk assessment and control, program development and implementation, and industrial respiratory protection. He has served as the Chair of the Respiratory Protection Technical Committee of the American Industrial Hygiene Association, and is currently the Vice-Chair of that organization's Management Committee. He holds a M.S. in Environmental Health Sciences (Industrial Hygiene and Safety) from Harvard University, and a B.S. in Chemistry from Bates College. Mr. O'Leary is certified in the Comprehensive Practice of Industrial Hygiene as well as in Safety.

James P. Pastorick is a graduate of the U.S. Naval School of Explosive Ordnance Disposal and has a B.A. degree in Journalism from the University of South Carolina. He has served in the U.S. Navy on active duty as an Explosive Ordnance Disposal Officer and is currently serving in the U.S. Navy Reserve assigned to the Explosive Ordnance Disposal Technology Center in Indian Head, Maryland.

Mr. Pastorick is employed by IT Corporation in Edison, New Jersey as Manager of Unexploded Ordnance Projects. In this position he manages unexploded ordnance investigation and remediation projects at active and formerly used defense sites.

Timothy G. Prothero has had extensive field experience performing remedial investigations and cleanups of several abandoned hazardous waste dump sites. Mr. Prothero has both planning experience and the practical "hands-on" experience of implementing those plans. His responsibilities and duties ranged from initial site investigations, remedial action planning, health and safety planning and reviews, to plan implementations, waste handling and direction of site cleanup activities. Mr. Prothero participated in and directed activities at several Superfund sites including Chem-Dyne, Pristine and Summit National in Ohio.

Mr. Prothero has also toured the continental United States on behalf of USEPA to instruct Federal, State and Local government officials on the hazards of abandoned chemical wastes, the methods and techniques used for control of those hazards, and ultimately, the proper cleanup of the orphaned sites.

Mr. Prothero has been an independent consultant since 1980, and his clients have included Federal and State agencies, and several consulting engineering firms.

Mark A. Puskar currently is manager of the industrial hygiene laboratory at Abbot Pharmaceutical Laboratories. He received his M.S. and Ph.D. in industrial hygiene from the University of Michigan where the focus of his research was in developing a FTIR-AIR method for compatibility testing. While completing his graduate studies, Mr. Puskar was awarded an American Industrial Hygiene Foundation fellowship for the 1983-1984 academic year. In January 1981, he began working at hazardous waste sites for O.H. Materials, Findlay, Ohio, as an on-site field chemist. He took part in numerous remedial action programs. The majority of his time was spent performing instrumental analysis and compatibility testing.

Charles J. Sawyer is Manager, Environmental Affairs for Syntex Inc., a west coast based pharmaceutical manufacturer. His responsibilities include management of domestic and international programs of environmental engineering, industrial hygiene, and safety/fire protection. He is a registered professional engineer (Ohio and California), and a certified industrial hygienist (comprehensive practice). Prior to working at Syntex, Mr. Sawyer spent five years in various aspects of environmental health and safety consulting, and before that was with Proctor and Gamble for six years. He has a Bachelors degree in chemical engineering from the University of Michigan (1965), and a Masters degree in chemical engineering from the University of Toledo (1967). He is an adjunct professor at the University of California--Hayward in the Environmental Health Studies program. He has published and spoken at many professional meetings on uncontrolled hazardous waste site remediation activities dealing specifically with dioxin-contaminated wastes.

Arthur D. Schwope is manager of the Applied Polymer Science Unit at Arthur D. Little, Inc. His professional activities have focused on the study of permeation through polymeric materials including the testing, analysis and specification of protective clothing. His interest in the subject began with a program for NIOSH entitled "Development of Performance Criteria for Protective Clothing Used Against Carcinogenic Liquids." He is lead author on the recent American Conference of Governmental Industrial Hygienists

(ACGIH) publication *Guidelines for the Selection of Chemical Protective Clothing.* Mr. Schwope has conducted clothing studies for the U.S. Coast Guard, NASA, the Army, the Navy, the Federal Drug Administration (FDA) and several commercial organizations. He is chairman of American Society for Testing and Materials (ASTM) subcommittee F23.30 to develop standardized test methods for assessing protective clothing materials. Mr. Schwope did his undergraduate work at Cornell University and obtained a Masters degree from MIT, both in chemical engineering.

Rodney D. Turpin is currently Safety and Occupational Health Manager, EPA, Environmental Response Team, Edison, New Jersey. In 1973, he received a B.S. in Food Industry from Delaware Valley College, Doylestown, Pennsylvania, and in 1978, a M.S. in Environmental Science from Rutgers University, New Brunswick, New Jersey. Rod's primary responsibilities are developing/implementing hazardous waste site occupational health and safety protocols, air monitoring plans and waste compatibility tests.

Lynn P. Wallace, Ph.D. is an Associate Professor of Civil Engineering at Brigham Young University, Provo, Utah, and a Diplomate of the AAEE. Prior to his present position, he served with NIOSH in Cincinnati, Ohio, compiling comprehensive guidelines for the protection of workers at hazardous waste sites and with the USEPA in charge of the initial hazardous waste research activities of that agency. He earned his doctoral degree in Environmental Engineering from West Virginia University in 1970 quantifying and categorizing hospital solid wastes, including pathogenic wastes. He is the author of several publications on the protection of workers at hazardous waste sites.

Wm. Bryon Witmer has a B.S., M.S. and Ph.D. in chemistry from Texas A&M University. He is currently a training specialist with the Occupational and Environmental Safety Training Division, Texas Engineering Extension Service, Texas A&M University, College Station, Texas.

Dr. Witmer has held several industrial positions in management, environmental health and safety and quality assurance with the Monsanto Companies in West Germany and the United States. He also served active duty as a Chemical Corps Instructor, CBR Agents for the Chemical Corps School. He has published numerous articles over the past twenty years on chemical, industrial and occupational health related issues.

Kenna Roberson Yarbrough has a B.S. degree from the University of Missouri-Rolla in Geological Engineering with an emphasis in hazardous waste management. She is currently employed at the USEPA's National Enforcement Investigations Center in Denver, Colorado where she coordinates complex, multi-media field investigations. Ms. Yarbrough plans and conducts civil compliance investigations to identify pollution problems and necessary remedial actions. Additionally, she is responsible for providing technical support and expert testimony in nationally significant criminal investigations and has been involved in several precedent setting environmental enforcement cases. Ms. Yarbrough was previously employed by Ecology & Environmental, Inc. where she performed pre-remedial field investigations and coordinated the EPA Region VII Hazard Ranking System model in support of the Superfund program.

INTRODUCTION AND OVERVIEW

PROTECTING PERSONNEL AT HAZARDOUS WASTE SITES: CURRENT ISSUES[1]

Steven P. Levine, Ph.D., C.I.H.
Rodney D. Turpin, M.S.
Michael Gochfeld, M.D., Ph.D.

HISTORY

"The problem of protecting personnel at a hazardous waste site may be viewed as being fundamentally the same as the problems encountered at traditional workplaces... Certainly, if the traditional industrial hygiene triad of recognition, evaluation and control can be applied to... [diverse] workplaces, those principles can also be applied to hazardous waste sites..."[1]. Those words are as true today as when they were written in 1984. However, from the perspective of over a decade of practice at hazardous waste sites, the industrial hygiene profession now has more tools with which to protect the worker [2].

Our perspective dates back to April 21, 1980, when a fire broke out at an abandoned waste treatment facility called, ironically, "Chemical Control Corporation", in Elizabeth, New Jersey. The tens of thousands of leaking and burning drums at the site obviously posed a real industrial hygiene problem to the fire fighters and other emergency responders, and subsequently to site cleanup personnel. From this incident, and others of the same type, the EPA and NIOSH developed two important guidance documents for environmental and industrial hygiene [3, 4].

While these documents were very important from the perspective of training and general practice of good hygiene at hazardous waste remediation

---

[1] Feature Article, December, 1991 issue of *Applied Occupational and Environmental Hygiene Journal*. Only minor changes have been made in format so that it may be uniformally maintained in this textbook.

and emergency response sites, these documents had a more important impact.

On February 26, 1980, President Jimmy Carter signed Presidential Executive Order (EO) 12196 requiring the federal government to comply with the General Industry Standards in Section 6 of the Occupational Health and Safety Act [5]. EPA Order 1440 [6], published on July 12, 1981 (to comply with EO 12196), required all EPA employees engaged in field operations to have 24-40 hours of related training prior to field activities. For those employees engaged in hazardous waste activities, EPA Order 1440 requires EPA employees to have 40 hours of hazardous waste health and safety training, which is essentially equivalent to following the guidelines set forth in the Standard Operating Safety Guides (SOSG)[7].

Since EPA felt that 29 Code of Federal Regulations (CFR) 1910 and 29 CFR 1926 did not address all the specific health and safety needs for hazardous waste site workers, EPA required all public and private site workers involved in EPA Superfund activities to follow, as a minimum, the EPA Office of Emergency and Remedial Response (OERR) Standard Operating Safety Guides. These SOSGs became the de-facto federal "regulation" for industrial hygiene practice by contractors engaged in emergency response or remedial action at hazardous waste sites. The regulatory authority for extending these SOSGs from federal employees to contractors was inherent in the EPA's power to write site contract specifications. Implementation of the SOSGs rested with the On-Scene Coordinators (OSCs) who were either EPA employees posted to hazardous waste sites, or Resident Engineers from the U.S. Army Corps of Engineers under contract to the EPA.

The SOSG defacto "regulations" stood virtually unchanged for about ten years. The SOSGs contained specifications, for example, for worker training, air monitoring, personal protective equipment, site control, decontamination, and medical surveillance. They were an example of the use of a "guidance" document to produce de-facto rule-making.

In October, 1985, a joint NIOSH, OSHA, EPA and Coast Guard guidance manual was published as a complement to the EPA SOSGs [8]. In addition, a number of text books [1,9,10] and conference proceedings [11] on this subject were published in this period. Many case studies were presented in those conference proceedings.

CURRENT REGULATORY ACTIVITY

We are presently in a period of maturation of regulations and procedures for protecting personnel at hazardous waste sites. These regulations and procedures are important in the context of Superfund remedial actions, Resource Conservation and Recovery Act (RCRA) activities and emergency response activities. While EPA is the lead Federal agency, other Federal and State agencies, such as the Department of Energy (DOE) and Department of Defense (DOD), are involved in hazardous waste site activities.

Under the authority of Section 126 of the Superfund Amendments and Reauthorization Act of 1986 (SARA), EPA and OSHA promulgated identical health and safety standards to protect workers engaged in hazardous waste operations and emergency response. The OSHA standard became effective March 6, 1990. These worker protection standards affect employers whose employees are engaged in hazardous waste operations and emergency response during:

- Clean-up operations at uncontrolled hazardous waste sites;
- RCRA corrective actions;
- Voluntary clean-up operations at sites recognized by Federal, State or Local governments;
- Hazardous waste operations at RCRA Treatment, Storage and Disposal (TSD) facilities, and;
- Emergency response operations without regard to location.

The OSHA standard (29 CFR 1910.120)[12], or equivalent state standards, protect all private employees, federal employees, and state and local government employees in states with delegated OSHA programs. The EPA standard (40 CFR 311)[13] covers state and local government employees engaged in hazardous waste operations and emergency response in states that do not have an OSHA-approved state plan. 40 CFR 311 defines "employee" as a compensated or non-compensated worker who is controlled directly by a State or Local government (including, for example, a volunteer fire fighter).

The OSHA standard addresses requirements for medical surveillance, training, planning, and several important site-specific activities, including site safety plans. One written health and safety plan (HASP) must be developed for each site to cover all contractors and all aspects of site operations. Chapter 9 of EPA 1440 requires the On-Scene Coordinator (OSC) to be responsible for all health and safety requirements on a site. The standard can be divided into three primary parts: operations at hazardous waste sites; operations at RCRA TSD facilities, and; emergency response operations conducted without regard to location. Strategies invoked for protecting hazardous waste workers include: education and training, site health and safety plans, personal protection, environmental monitoring, and medical surveillance. (For more information, see Chapter 2, Federal Government Programs and Information Gathering.)

Additional regulatory action during this period includes:

- Rule Making for Accreditation of Training Programs for Hazardous Waste Operations [14]. Public hearings in early 1991 were held in order to address the question of "what constitutes an adequate training program." This is a difficult problem that involves questions of credentials and experience of instructors, adequacy and relevance of course materials, and the equivalency of programs administered by industry, unions, consultants, governments and academia.
- Letters of "clarification" and "guidance" from OSHA to field personnel and various interested parties [15, 16]. These letters and memos define important concepts so that the full intent of 29 CFR 1910.120 can be understood and enforced. For example, "emergency response", "uncontrolled" and "incidental releases" are defined, "de minimis" criteria are spelled out, and scenarios are addressed.
- The Hazard Ranking System Final Rule was published [17]. While this rule does not directly affect the issue of personal protection, it does provide a tool with which hazardous waste remedial action sites are placed on the National Priorities List, and thereby prioritized for clean-up. Thus, this document is important to occupational and environmental health professionals.

IN-DEPTH ANALYSIS

Although the general principles of industrial hygiene apply to hazardous waste workers as well as to those in more traditional industrial jobs, there are important differences in emphasis. Education and training are mandated for hazardous waste workers. Personal protection, an interim or temporary strategy in the industrial workplace, becomes a requisite strategy at the hazardous waste site. The results of air monitoring play a pivotal role in the selection of personal protection. Medical surveillance, a secondary prevention strategy, plays a more prominent role in the quality assurance of the primary prevention strategies [18]. Conversely, engineering approaches such as substitution/process modification and ventilation have more limited application in hazardous waste work.

Following is an in-depth discussion of two specific subject areas of industrial hygiene concern when dealing with the hazardous waste area:

(1) Air monitoring and its relationship to decisions regarding personal protection equipment; and

(2) Medical screening and surveillance, and its relationship to decisions such as fitness for duty, ability to wear respiratory protection equipment, detection of adverse health effects from chemical exposure, and sensitivity and specificity of screening protocols.

(1)   Air monitoring and personal protection:

The selection of the appropriate level of protective equipment is basic to all site activities. Over protection (e.g., wearing Level B when C would suffice) is not just costly in terms of equipment and reduced productivity, but requires increased training and practice, increases the risk of heat stress, is associated with significant ergonomic factors [19] and, in rare instances, can seriously jeopardize health. At Chemical Control, a worker in Level A was on a barge when his air ran out. He was too impeded to leave the barge or even to remove his clothing. Only heroic measures by a co-worker who leapt (inadequately protected) onto the barge, prevented a fatality caused by "over protection".

An example of one of the features of the original Standard Operating Safety Guides (SOSGs) was the section on criteria for choice of Levels of Protection [4]. If a reading taken on a hazardous waste site with a portable total hydrocarbon (THC) air monitor read greater than 5 ppm over the background air value, then workers had to use Level B protection.

Level B protection requires supplied air respiratory protection (usually self-contained breathing apparatus {SCBA}). If the reading on the THC was less than 5 ppm above background, and if conditions immediately dangerous to life and health (IDLH) would not occur, then air purifying respirators (APR) could be used. This was called Level C protection. The APR of choice usually, but not always, utilized an organic vapor-acid gas- high efficiency particulate absorber (HEPA) stacked canister.

(For additional information on Levels of Protection and on PPE for Hazardous Chemical Emergencies, the NIOSH Selection Guide [20], EPA guidelines [21, 22], and the National Fire Protection Association Guides [23-25] can be consulted.) (For more information, see Chapter 9, Personal Protective Equipment.)

The NIOSH selection criteria for air purifying respirators states that the following criteria have to be met prior to the use of APR for personal protection [26]:

(a) All air contaminants must be both identified and quantified;
(b) An APR canister must be available for those air contaminants, and of sufficient capacity that the worker must be protected at the measured contaminant concentration, and for the duration of the job;
(c) IDLH conditions must not be present (this includes oxygen deficient environments); and,
(d) Adequate warning properties must be present for the contaminant at concentrations below the permissible exposure limits/threshold limit values (PEL/TLV).

Given those criteria, how could the "5 ppm" level in the SOSG have been used for nearly ten years? After all, for example, for toluene, the criterion was far too conservative; for isocyantes, the criterion was far too liberal; and, for aerosols, the criterion was not relevant! The answer was three-fold:

· First, the THC monitor, especially, the photo-ionization detector (PID)-based THC version, was exceedingly easy to use. Thus, the SOSG could be applied in "real" situations by relatively untrained personnel.
· Second, the criterion in the SOSG that "IDLH conditions must not be present" seemed to supersede all other criteria. What OSC could state categorically that, during site construction or emergency response work, IDLH conditions might not occur at some time or another? What about sudden releases that had been known to occur?

Therefore, by default at any time that site construction activity took place, the IDLH criterion was usually invoked, and Level B protection was used. In those cases, Level C was only used for site walk-around activities before or after the work day, health and safety surveys, decontamination, and support activities.

· Third, OSHA rule making takes a long time.

During the 1980s, several studies were performed that showed that concentrations of air contaminants were usually very low during most hazardous waste activities [1, 27, 28]. These studies were performed using traditional NIOSH/OSHA sampling and analysis methods based on adsorbent tubes and filters with which time weighted concentration air samples were taken and sent back to the laboratory. In addition, grab samples were taken using colorimetric indicator tubes.

Unfortunately, those investigators, including the authors of this paper, and their sampling devices were invariably not present during rare but critical events. For example:

1) when acid was added to a lagoon that contained high concentrations of sulfide, which was then liberated as H_2S (Liquid Disposal Company, Utica, MI);

2) when water and concentrated H_2SO_4 were inadvertently mixed, causing massive releases of airborne H_2SO_4 (Lock Haven, PA);

3) when unknown vapors/gasses overcame guards outside the perimeter of a site during a night time period with calm winds (Chem-Dyne, Hamilton, OH);

4) when drums suddenly exploded during manipulation (Goose Farms, Trenton, NJ);

5) when workers or equipment fell into pits or trenches that were being examined or excavated, or when dramatic fires and explosions occurred (Chemical Control, Elizabeth, NJ).

The examples given above are simply a few of many such incidents.

Therefore, the IDLH conditions criterion continued to be used, and the THC monitor was frequently relegated to the role of documenting the concentration of unknown vapors during site work activities.

The SOSG has been modified by 29 CFR 1910.120. All criteria have been made consistent with the NIOSH respiratory protection criteria, and with modern practices of industrial hygiene.

However, since there are still no "universal" real-time monitors useable under routine conditions, the IDLH criterion may still be used as the "default criterion" of choice, and Level B protection may continue to be used in a majority of cases, regardless of the availability of any objective air monitoring results.

SUMMARY OF PRESENT CRITERIA FOR LEVELS OF
PROTECTION [12]

Level	Respiratory Protection	Other Protection(**)	Criteria
A	SA*, SCBA	Full Encapsulation	AIR > PEL, TLV; SKIN HAZARD/ IDLH (***)
B	SA*, SCBA	Protective Garment	AIR > PEL, TLV, ETC; IDLH (***)
C	AIR PURIFY RESPIR (****)	Protective Garment	AIR < PEL, TLV, ETC; NO IDLH (***)
D	NONE	As Needed	SUPPORT ZONE ONLY

(*)   Supplied Air (SA).
(**)   For full description of each category in table, see text and references.
(***)   IDLH conditions possible.
(****) Conditions meeting NIOSH Respiratory Protection Selection Guidelines; see references.

This is not to belittle 29 CFR 1910.120. On the contrary, most of the provisions of this regulation represent soundly-based consensus. However, the air monitoring portion will be hard to apply on a consistently useful basis.

At this point, a little-recognized, but rather significant feature of 29 CFR 1910.120 is worth noting. In "Definitions", Section a.4.D., the following is stated, "... "Published exposure level" [not to be confused with "Permissible Exposure Limits" (PELs)] means the [recommended] exposure limits (RELs) published in "NIOSH Recommendations for Occupational Health Standards" dated 1986 incorporated by reference, or if none is specified, the exposure limits published in the standards specified by the American Conference of Governmental Hygienists in their publication "Threshold Limit Values (TLVs) and Biological Exposure Indices (BEIs) for 1987-88" dated 1987 incorporated by reference."

In the body of 29 CFR 1910.120, Levels of Protection are set to "... provide protection to a level below permissible exposure levels and published exposure levels ..." (emphasis ours). Thus, after the PELs, the RELs, TLVs, and BEIs, are given the status of legally enforceable limits.

Recommendations Regarding Air Monitoring Programs

1. The EPA (and to a significant, but lesser extent, NIOSH) has active programs in research and development of field screening methods. These programs are centered at the Atmospheric Research and Environmental Assessment Laboratory (AREAL), Method Development Branch, in Research Triangle Park, N.C., the Environmental Monitoring Systems Laboratory (EMSL) in Las Vegas, Nevada, and the Environmental Response Team, in Edison, N.J., and are coordinated through the EPA Office of Emergency and Remedial Response. Annual conferences are sponsored by AREAL and EMSL on this, and related subjects. Hazardous waste professionals should keep close watch on relevant methods and technologies developed and evaluated by those groups.

2. Desirable characteristics of field screening methods have been defined by the EPA [29]: low cost, small, rugged, rapid, sensitive, specific, user-friendly, light weight, reliable, and adaptable to a broad range of samples and scenarios. Until instruments with these characteristics become available, Level B personal protective devices, centered on the use of SCBAs, may be the default choice for use at hazardous waste remedial and emergency response sites, especially when site activities are in progress.

3. All air monitoring instruments should be calibrated according to guidelines published in an international guidance document, the final version of which has been published in 1991 [30]. (For more information, see Chapter 5, Air Monitoring at Hazardous Waste Sites.)

(2)   Medical Screening and Surveillance:

In 1978, when New Jersey began one of the first medical surveillance programs (MSP) for hazardous waste workers [18], it was predicated on the belief that hazardous waste work was inherently dangerous and the workers were regularly exposed, primarily to airborne contaminants, that regularly threatened their health. It seemed reasonable to assume that hazardous waste sites exuded noxious vapors. When air monitoring failed to detect toxic levels of vapors it was sometimes presumed that the monitoring was at fault. This led to the development of elaborate medical surveillance protocols with extensive biological monitoring components, often extended to workers with little actual potential for on site exposure. During the 1980's, there was an improvement in the ability to monitor exposure [29,30] and our understanding of exposure, and of the effectiveness of protective devices. This resulted in significant modifications of medical surveillance approaches to hazardous waste workers [31,32].

Medical surveillance involves the periodic monitoring of individual workers to detect early pathophysiologic changes indicative of exposures, leading to intervention to reduce exposures and prevent disease [32]. The role of medical "surveillance" in protecting hazardous waste workers has been discussed extensively [18,31,32]. Medical "screening" involves the evaluation of a population to detect individuals with particular conditions (risk factors, exposure, disease). The terms are confused and often used interchangeably [33] with some authors trying to replace the traditional term "medical surveillance" with "medical screening" in order to avoid confusion with the term "disease surveillance", which is an entirely different epidemiologic process [34].

To complicate matters, the OSHA Hazardous Waste standard [12] includes under its medical surveillance paragraph f, procedures which have nothing to do with surveillance, e.g., determinations of fitness and respirator clearance. A recent study has shown that providers of medical services to hazardous waste contractors do a much better job at fitness determination than they do with medical surveillance [35]. Criteria for selecting medical facilities to provide such evaluation have been published [36].

Components of a medical surveillance program include: a) identification of participants (not all workers need to be in a surveillance program), b) establishment of protocol appropriate to putative or potential exposures (including appropriate tests at appropriate intervals), c) performance of the testing, d) interpretation of results and implementation of interventions (including informing the worker and record keeping), and e) evaluation of the medical surveillance in the broader context of worker protection. It is all too easy for clinically trained individuals to forget everything but c) and d). At the same time the medical surveillance examination provides the opportunity to perform fitness determination and respiratory evaluation.

WORKER SELECTION

The OSHA Standard [12] requires that the following individuals be included in a medical surveillance program: (i) "all employees who are or may be exposed to hazardous substances or health hazards at or above the permissible exposure limits" (PEL) for 30+ days per year; (ii), "all employees who wear a respirator for 30 days or more a year"; (iii) all employees who are injured due to exposure; and (iv) members of HAZMAT teams.

At first this appears to be a rather encompassing requirement. However, it allows workers who must wear a respirator or who are exposed above the PEL for up to four weeks to continue to work without medical surveillance. At the same time it requires that workers who must wear a respirator for 30+ days a year to be in a MSP, even though the only reason they must wear a respirator is that they are on sites prior to obtaining measurements.

Moreover, there are persons who must be on sites only occasionally, e.g., governmental auditors or law enforcement personnel, who may have only minimal training and who may experience intermittent exposure. These people would have no MSP, not even a baseline examination. The OSHA Standard therefore mandates a MSP for certain workers who probably have negligible exposure, while allowing those with substantial exposure (up to 30 days a year above any PEL) to work without a MSP. Fortunately, most employers in the hazardous waste industry recognize this discrepancy, and provide their basic MSP even to workers who do not meet the 30 day criterion.

ESTABLISHMENT OF PROTOCOL

A MSP must be tailored to the kinds of activities and exposures that confront a workforce. Certain basic elements such as a history and physical examination are common to all MSP examinations. However, the kinds of laboratory tests performed as well as any specific biological monitoring must be based on the kinds of exposures encountered. Workers in a single company may require different tests depending on the sites to which they are assigned. This is particularly true for companies that may assign workers to a site on a long term basis (one year or more). A careful history coupled with site specific information enables the occupational health professional to determine the necessary components for a MSP examination.

The OSHA Standard [12] requires the company to provide the examining physician with information regarding potential exposures. Ideally the workers' medical records should be linked with this air monitoring and environmental sampling data [37]. Biological monitoring (for example, measuring polychlorinated biphenyl or heavy metal levels in blood) is often expensive and seldom fruitful [38]. But there are circumstances when biomonitoring is particularly valuable [39]. Even commonly used tests such as liver function tests require careful planning. Hodgson et al. [40] discuss the values and limitations of routine biomedical evaluation of hepatotoxicity.

PERFORMANCE OF TESTS

Although the actual tests used in a MSP can be performed in many medical settings, the selection and interpretation of tests requires specialized knowledge and experience in occupational medicine and toxicology. The OSHA Standard [12] specifies that the content of the examinations shall be determined by the attending physician, but only suggests "preferably one knowledgeable in occupational medicine". (This is ironic, since a "Certified Industrial Hygienist" is a requirement, not merely "preferable", by the OSHA Standard.) A recent study [35] shows that a major weakness in MSP for hazardous waste workers is that they are being provided by people who know little about occupational health in general, much less about hazardous waste, and these physicians cannot exercise informed judgement in the selection or interpretation of tests. This also impacts on decisions regarding fitness determination and respirator clearance.

An increasing role for industrial hygiene is the selection and monitoring of the medical facilities to which ones MSP is entrusted. The industrial hygienist frequently must serve as the contract officer, assuring that the facility understands the specific features of hazardous waste work, and that it renders appropriate judgements regarding worker exposure or fitness.

INTERPRETATION OF RESULTS, INTERVENTION, AND RECORD KEEPING

One of the major criticisms of medical surveillance [41] is that results are often buried in medical records and a significant medical abnormality may not get translated into an exposure intervention. Positive findings on a MSP examination may be an individual health concern or may be related to hazardous waste exposure. In the latter case, the abnormality may reflect an accidental exposure, but often indicates that the operating procedures specified in the health and safety plan are not adequate or are not being followed. In this latter role, medical surveillance serves an important quality control capacity [32].

If workers are being exposed despite their training and use of protection, then industrial hygienists must step in to identify the source of the exposure and to modify the site plan to preclude further exposure. Some medical findings may also require that an individual worker be removed from exposure for a certain time period, or may reflect on worker fitness or vulnerability (see below).

The unique feature of medical surveillance, as opposed to medical screening or medical examinations in general, is that the results of the current test must be compared with results of previous tests or baseline tests on the same individual. All too often the examining clinician looks only at the current test results and dismisses findings that are in the normal range, regardless of how they may have changed since the previous examination.

For example, on baseline spirometry a young healthy athletic employee may have a FEV1/FVC ratio (ratio of maximal flow rate to vital capacity) of 120% of the expected value for his or her age and height. After a year of work cleaning up extremely dusty sites, the worker may have a value 100% of the expected. Failing to compare results with the baseline, the clinician may well dismiss this worker as "perfectly normal" despite the documented loss of nearly 20% of lung function.

Unfortunately the nature of hazardous waste work results in high turnover, and if a worker is in a new company this year, the facility performing this year's MSP examination is not likely to have last year's medical record [32]. Thus, many hazardous waste workers who think they are getting medical surveillance may not be receiving true surveillance at all, unless they can hand a copy of prior medical records to current examiners. This places a premium on providing all examinees with complete copies of their medical records as well as a lay language interpretation, and the instruction to bring a copy of the examination results to their next MSP examination, wherever that may be.

One of the major flaws of the OSHA Hazardous Waste Standard [12] concerns the notification of the employee and the handling of medical records. The employee, the employer and the examining physician all face serious dilemmas. In a general medical examination, results must be treated as confidential, and normally the employer is only entitled to specific work-related information regarding hazards or fitness limitations detected by the examiner. However, the OSHA Hazardous Waste Standard requires that "the employer shall obtain and furnish the employee with a copy of a written opinion from the attending physician." It does not specify that the employee shall receive a copy of the medical findings and does not require that the physician provide a copy of the medical record to the employee.

However, by reference to the OSHA Medical Records standard (29 CFR 1910.20) the employer is required to retain the medical records for a period of 30 years from the date of employee termination. The employer is not entitled to receive confidential medical records unless they have a medical department under the supervision of a trained occupational health professional capable of assuring the confidentiality of the medical records. Usually this responsibility is met by hiring or contracting with a physician or nurse to serve in this capacity. Whether an industrial hygienist fulfills this role is controversial, and some industrial hygienists we have interviewed do not feel comfortable with assuming responsibility for medical records and their contents. Site safety officers clearly are not appropriate professionals to take charge of confidential medical records.

Hazardous waste companies that do not have a medical department are understandably disturbed about their responsibility to retain the medical records that they are not entitled to possess. They are concerned that if they change medical providers or if a provider goes out of business, they may lose access to those records. Yet, the burden of having custody of those records imposes a legal liability for the content of the records, even if they do not have the professional expertise to interpret the records. Similarly, most medical providers are not aware of the responsibility they incur for retaining the medical surveillance records for 30+ years [35].

Faced by this dilemma employers have two options. They can (and should) choose to delegate the responsibility for the 30 year medical record retention to the medical facility that provides their services. Contract language should include provisions for assuring the confidentiality and the custody of records in case the medical provider ceases operations. No medical provider should be in this business if they are not capable of and prepared to assume this legal responsibility. Alternatively, on advice from their legal department, some employers are insisting that the medical provider submit a complete copy of the medical record to the company after each examination as a condition of getting paid. We argue that companies should not want to have these records unless they have a physician or nurse, because they may be liable for failure to act on information contained in the records.

This places the medical provider in a dilemma of having to breach confidentiality in order to retain a lucrative contract. In our experience, many medical providers aren't aware of the legal and ethical issues and are all too willing to submit medical records to employers without regard for confidentiality. Many employers, indeed, require as a condition of employment, that the worker sign a blanket record release. This gets the physicians off the legal hook, but places the employee in a dilemma. The result is that employees—knowing that their records may be scrutinized by people who are not health professionals—are discouraged from divulging sensitive medical information that may be of significance in their case. In virtually all cases, they simply sign the record release. Although such a release does not meet the criterion of "consent freely given" [41], it does unfortunately appear to be an increasingly common practice. (For more information, see Chapter 7, Medical Surveillance for Hazardous Waste Workers.)

PROGRAM EVALUATION

Managers are accustomed to evaluating the quality of the goods and services that they purchase, and medical providers are increasingly familiar with being evaluated like any other vendor. The evaluation of MSPs is an increasingly important role for occupational health professionals. All too often, the evaluation of an MSP has been limited to determining whether all of the papers are filled out, whether employees are seen in a timely fashion, whether there is good turnaround time on results and clearances, and whether the costs are competitive. A recent study [35] has shown that there are significant program flaws in many of the MSP services provided to hazardous waste workers. These are not necessarily fatal flaws, but they compromise the quality of the program, and place certain workers at risk. Indeed, Udasin has shown that medical providers were much better at providing fitness determination than at performing medical surveillance [35]. Common flaws identified were a) failure to document interpretation of abnormal test results; b) inadequate spirometry; c) inadequately trained personnel; and d) failure to inform employee of results. Medical program auditing will inevitably play an increasing role in monitoring the performance of MSPs in the coming years.

FITNESS DETERMINATION AND RESPIRATOR CLEARANCE

There is a substantial reliance on medical evaluations to determine that each hazardous waste worker is physically fit to perform work [42], to wear equipment, and to tolerate stress, and is not unusually vulnerable to the effects of potential toxic exposures. Specifically, the medical examiner must certify that the employee can wear and tolerate the required respiratory protective equipment. The OSHA respirator standard (29 CFR 1910.134) does not specify tests or criteria, and these are left to the discretion of the examining physicians, most of whom have not had to wear respiratory equipment more elaborate than a surgical mask. The Guidance Manual [8] provides some assistance to the examining physician, although few actually have the document, much less take the time to read and digest it. Hodous [43] provides useful background and criteria for evaluating respirator fitness. Heat stress is a special area of concern to hazardous waste workers who must use vapor barrier equipment out of doors under hot summer conditions. Medical evaluations can detect some conditions which might render individuals at risk of heat stress [44].

Respirator clearance can be provided by the examining or supervising physician at the medical facility, by an independent contractor who receives all the medical records, or by the employer's medical consultant who receives all the medical records. It is reasonable to assume that the actual examiner is the person most likely to make an informed judgement regarding a worker's ability or limitations, and the services of an experienced occupational physician would thus be particularly beneficial.

RECOMMENDATIONS REGARDING MEDICAL SURVEILLANCE PROGRAMS

1. All workers who are destined for work on hazardous waste sites should have a baseline medical examination to include: detailed health inventory questionnaire reviewed by physician or nurse practitioner, physical examination including the nervous system, spirometry, hematology, urinalysis, and blood chemistry (including liver function and renal function testing). A whole blood and a serum specimen (10 ml) should be drawn into metal-free glass containers, and archived in a freezer for future analysis. The

medical program should be under the supervision of a trained and experienced occupational physician.

2. The supervising physician and the company health and safety officer should review the individual's proposed work assignments and determine the likelihood that they will actually work on hazardous waste sites as well as the frequency. They will determine whether the employee should be examined again annually, after a longer interval (2-3 years), or not at all (until age dictates periodic screening for other reasons). In general, workers who meet the OSHA criteria will certainly be seen again after one year. Whether workers with less than 30 days of respirator use are included, depends on anticipated exposure levels and the type of sites being managed by the company. Most companies simply include all of their field personnel in their annual medical surveillance program.

3. At the time of subsequent periodic examinations, the examiner should determine that the employee is receiving mandated training (including annual updates), and that the employee is using appropriate personal protection. Any exposure incidents or changes in health status should be documented.

4. The medical record should be maintained as a confidential document by the examining facility. The employer should receive only written documentation of required clearances (or limitations). The employee should receive a complete copy of their medical record along with a lay-language interpretation and recommendations for follow-up of any identified health problems (including those not related to work).

5. Specialized testing (including biological monitoring) should be limited to those situations and employees where there is a reason to believe that a specific exposure may have occurred or may occur (i.e. because of an accident or a breakdown in work practices).

6. All occupational medical services should be periodically evaluated by a certified occupational health professional to make sure that the health of employees as well as the legal obligations of the employer are being protected.

This new edition has incorporated the experiences of the past decade from sources in academia, industry and government. The overview provided in this introduction is expanded in subsequent chapters. Maintaining the health and safety of hazardous waste workers is an ongoing challenge as the nation pursues its goals of environmental quality.

REFERENCES

1. *Protecting Personnel at Hazardous Waste Sites*, S.P. Levine and W.F. Martin, Eds. Butterworths-Ann Arbor Science, Boston, MA. (1985), page 1.
2. L.P. Andrews. *Worker Protection During Hazardous Waste Remediation*, Center for Labor Education and Research, Van Nostrand, Reinhold, New York. (1990).
3. *Hazardous Waste Site and Hazardous Substances Emergencies*, DHHS NIOSH, Cincinnati, OH, Report 83-100, December, 1982.
4. *Interim Standard Operating Safety Procedures*, U.S. EPA, Office of Emergency and Remedial Response, Hazardous Response Support Division, Environmental Response Team, Edison, NJ (Revised, June, 1982).
5. *Executive Order 12196: Occupational Safety and Health Programs for Federal Employees*, Federal Register 45 (40), Wednesday, Feb. 27, 1980, 12769-12771.
6. *Health and Safety Requirements for Employees Engaged in Field Activities*, U.S. EPA Order 1440.2. E. J. Hanley, Director, Office of Management Information and Support Services, July 12, 1981.
7. *Standard Operating Safety Guides*, U.S. EPA (OERR), OSWER Directive 9285.1-02, Washington, D.C., July 5, 1988.
8. *NIOSH/OSHA/USCG/EPA Occupational Safety and Health Guidance Manual for Hazardous Waste Site Activities*, G. Kleiner, S. Rabinovitz, D. Weitzman and G. Wiltshire, Eds., Document DHHS (NIOSH) 85-115 (1985).
9. W. F. Martin, J. M. Lippit and T. G. Prothero. *Hazardous Waste Handbook for Health and Safety*, Butterworths Publishers, Boston, MA (1987), 2nd ed. (1992).
10. *Toxic Chemicals, Health and the Environment*, L. B. Lave and A. C. Upton, Eds., Johns Hopkins Press, Baltimore, MD (1987).
11. For example: Proceedings of the National "Superfund" Conference, The Hazardous Material Control Research Institute, Washington, D.C., (Nov or Dec, 1981-present).
12. 29 CFR 1910.120, vol. 54 (42), March 6, 1989.
13. *Worker Protection Standards for Hazardous Waste Operations and Emergency Response; Final Rule*, 40 CFR 311, 54(120): 26653-26658 (July 23, 1989).
14. *Accreditation of Training Programs for Hazardous Waste Operations: Notice of Public Hearings*, Federal Register 55 (210): 45616-45618, Tuesday, October 30, 1990.

15. *Inspection Guidelines for Post-Emergency Response Operations Under 29 CFR 1910.120*, U.S. DOL (OSHA) Directorate of Compliance Programs, G. F. Scannell, CPL 2-2.51, Nov. 5, 1990.

16. P. K. Clark, Director, Directorate of Compliance, OSHA, Washington, D.C. to R. F. Boggs, Vice President, Organization Resource Counselors, Inc., Washington, D.C., Sep. 4, 1990. Personal communication distributed to the ACGIH/AIHA Hazardous Waste Committee, Dec., 1990.

17. *Hazard Ranking System; Final Rule*, Federal Register. 40 CFR 300. 55 (241): 51532-51667, Friday, December 14, 1990.

18. M. Gochfeld. *Assessment of Clinical Toxicity in Populations Exposed to Hazardous Waste,* Proc. 1st International Congress on Industrial Hazardous Waste, 1:352-365. N.J. Institute of Technology, Newark, NJ (1982).

19. Stull, J.O. *Ergonomic Criteria for the Selection of Chemical Protective Clothing*, Workplace Health Fund, Washington, D.C. 1991.

20. *Personal Protection Equipment for Hazardous Materials Incidents: A Selection Guide*, U.S. DHHS, PHS, CDC, NIOSH, (December, 1982).

21. Schwope, A.D., Costas, P.P., Jackson, J.O. and Weitzman, D.J. *Guidelines for Selection of Chemical Protective Clothing*, Third Edition, U.S. EPA, Washington, D.C., (1987), available from ACGIH, Cincinnati, OH.

22. *Focus on Protective Clothing*, Applied Industrial Hyg. 4: R1-R8 (1989).

23. *Vapor-Protective Suits for Hazardous Chemical Emergencies,* NFPA 1991, National Fire Protection Assoc., Quincy, MA (1990).

24. *Liquid Splash-Protective Suits for Hazardous Chemical Emergencies*, NFPA 1992, National Fire Protection Assoc., Quincy, MA (1990).

25. *Support Function Protective Garments for Hazardous Chemical Operations*, NFPA 1993, National Fire Protection Assoc., Quincy, MA (1990).

26. N. J. Bollinger and R. H. Schutz, *NIOSH Guide to Industrial Respiratory Protection,* U.S. DHHS (NIOSH) 87-116, NIOSH, Cincinnati, OH (1987).

27. R. J. Costello and J. Melius. Technical Assistance Determination Report: Chemical Control, Elizabeth, N.J. DHHS (NIOSH) TA 80-77. NIOSH, Cincinnati, OH (1981).

28. S. P. Levine, R. J. Costello, C. L. Geraci and K. A. Conlin, "Air Monitoring at the Drum Bulking Process of a Hazardous Waste

Remedial Action Site," *American Industrial Hygienists Journal*, 46: 192-196 (1985).

29. E. Koglin and E. Poziomek. "Advances in Field Screening Methods for Hazardous Waste Site Investigations," *Amer. Environmental Laboratory*, 18-24 (December, 1990).

30. *Guide to Portable Instruments for Assessing Airborne Pollutants Arising from Hazardous Wastes*, S. Levine, Ed., International Organization for Legal Metrology, Paris, France (1991), available from ACGIH, Cincinnati, OH.

31. Melius, J. "Medical Surveillance for Hazardous Waste Workers." *Journal Occupational Medicine*, 8:679-683 (1986).

32. M. Gochfeld and E.A. Favata. "Hazardous Waste Workers." *State-of-the-Art Reviews in Occupational Medicine*, vol. 5, Hanley & Belfus Inc, Philadelphia (1990).

33. M. Gochfeld. *Screening or Surveillance in the Workplace: Terminology and Rationales*, Environmental Research, in press.

34. W.E. Halperin, P.A. Schulte, and D.G. Greathouse (eds). "Conference on medical screening and biological monitoring for the effects of exposure in the workplace," *Journal of Occupational Medicine*, 28:547-788 (1986).

35. I. Udasin, G. Buckler and M. Gochfeld. "Quality Assurance Auditing of a Medical Surveillance Program for Hazardous Waste Workers." *Journal of Occupational Medicine*, in press.

36. "Proposed criteria for the selection of appropriate medical resources to perform medical surveillance for employees engaged in hazardous waste operations," Medical Issues Subcommittee, ACGIH/AIHA Hazardous Waste Committee, Appl. Indus. Hyg. 4: R2-R4 (1989).

37. S.P. Levine. "The role of air monitoring techniques in hazardous waste site personnel protection and surveillance strategies." *State-of-the-Art Reviews in Occupational Medicine*, 5:109-116, (1990).

38. M. Gochfeld. "Biological monitoring of hazardous waste workers: metals." *State-of-the-Art Reviews in Occupational Medicine*, 5:25-32. (1990)

39. K.H. Chase and P.G. Shields. "Medical surveillance of hazardous waste site workers exposed to polychlorinated biphenyls (PCBs)." *State-of-the-Art Reviews in Occupational Medicine*, 5:33-38. (1990)

40. M.J. Hodgson, B. Goodman-Klein and D.H. Van Thiel. "Evaluating the liver in hazardous waste workers." *State-of-the-Art Reviews in Occupational Medicine*, 5:67-78. (1990)

41. M. A. Rothstein. "Medical Screening of Workers." Bureau of National Affairs, Washington D.C. (1984)
42. B.H. Hoffman and D.W. Jones. "Evaluating physical fitness for hazardous waste work." *State-of-the-Art Reviews in Occupational Medicine*, 5:93-100. (1990)
43. T.K. Hodous. "Screening prospective workers for the ability to use respirators." *Journal of Occupational Medicine*, 28:1074-1080.
44. E.A. Favata, G. Buckler, and M. Gochfeld. "Heat stress in hazardous waste workers: evaluation and prevention." *State-of-the-Art Reviews in Occupational Medicine*, 5:79-92.

2

FEDERAL GOVERNMENT PROGRAMS AND INFORMATION GATHERING

Margo R. Dusenbury, B.S.
Kenna R. Yarbrough, B.S.
Barrett E. Benson, P.E.
William F. Martin, P.E.

The Federal government can be a valuable resource for safety and health information. A basic understanding of government programs, project-specific information needs, and sources of information will facilitate the information gathering process. The *Federal Government Programs* section of this chapter will explain the evolution of Federal government programs and hazardous waste worker safety and health laws. It also explains which Federal government programs can assist you in gathering information about personnel protection at hazardous waste sites.

Characterization is the first step in approaching a hazardous waste field investigation. The *Information Gathering* section of this chapter summarizes methods for collecting available safety information. The information gathering process is described, including suggested information needs and sources. Exhibit 2-1 at the end of the chapter lists selected databases for hazardous waste investigations.

A dominant concern during all phases of hazardous waste site characterization is safety. A comprehensive safety and health program for site investigations and subsequent remedial work at hazardous waste sites is required to protect investigators, workers, the public and the environment. Specific components of a HASP are:

- Key personnel
- Safety and health risk or hazards analysis
- Employee training assignments
- Personal protective equipment
- Medical surveillance requirements
- Employee and air monitoring
- Site control
- Decontamination
- Emergency response plan
- Confined space entry procedures

- Spill containment program
- Hazard communication plan

The appropriate level(s) of protection, emergency preparedness, potential exposures, migration pathways, and decontamination and disposal procedures must be specified in a site-specific safety plan. Each individual entering the site must read and follow the safety plan.

FEDERAL GOVERNMENT PROGRAMS

The Federal government has historically taken an active role in providing technical assistance and disseminating information. These services are provided to the general public, academia, and state and local organizations in the form of research support, supplemental funding, training programs and information programs. Provision of these services is usually mandated by legislation, and broad public access to the materials within Federal agencies is ensured by the Freedom of Information Act of 1966 [1].

The resources available on protecting worker safety and health from hazardous substances are as diverse as the many Federal programs themselves. There has been a rapid growth of available resources due to the recent emphasis in three areas: (1) research; (2) the gathering of information nationwide for identifying health risks associated with hazardous substances; and (3) the production of publications to assist state and local organizations to recognize, evaluate, and control hazardous substances. Due to modern information storage, retrieval, and database management, this vast and ever-growing body of technical information is more readily accessible to the private sector than ever before.

Even though a tremendous amount of technical data and other resources are available, much of the potential audience may never benefit from them. Some potential users will not know where they exist or how to access them, and an unfortunate few will never even know of their existence. For similar reasons, many of the users who do access Federal programs will never receive the full benefits of these programs.

This section will attempt to provide potential users with information and insights which will assist them in becoming full recipients of these services. It will, at best, serve as a starting point, since utilizing a Federal program requires skill, knowledge, and tenacity. Potential users should obtain a basic knowledge of the programs' responsibilities, purposes, and delivery mechanisms. Since this information is often provided in the legislation and public law itself, the following section, *Legislative Background*, will highlight some of the laws pertaining to hazardous substances and worker safety and health. Responsible agencies and their functions will be identified in the section, *Federal Programs Relating to Protection of Hazardous Waste Workers*. The section, *Accessing Federal Programs*, provides insight into why familiarity with the programs is necessary, and also why tenacity is essential.

Legislative Background

Historically, most of the occupational safety and health laws were enacted by states. Prior to 1960, there were relatively few Federal laws addressing worker protection, and those were only applicable to a limited number of employers or specific groups of employees [2]. During the 1960s, there was an increase of concern about worker safety and health in this nation, and the result was a proliferation of Federal legislation. Ultimately, a nationwide occupational safety and health program was designed through the Occupational Safety and Health Act of 1970 (OSHAct). The OSHAct extended safety and health coverage to most workers of business affected by interstate commerce [3].

The OSHAct established three organizations:

1. *The Occupational Safety and Health Administration.* Located within the Department of Labor, OSHA is primarily responsible for the promulgation and enforcement of standards and worker training.
2. *The Occupational Safety and Health Review Committee.* The OSHRC is an independent agency within the Executive Branch which adjudicates contested cases resulting from OSHA-initiated actions against employers.
3. *The National Institute for Occupational Safety and Health.* NIOSH is located within the Department of Health and Human Services, and is administratively under the Centers for Disease

Control. NIOSH is the principal Federal agency engaged in research, education and training, and disseminating information related to occupational safety and health.

Even though the OSHAct covers most businesses in the country, it was not specifically applied to hazardous waste handling until a 1982 amendment was made to the National Contingency Plan under Public Law 96-510, the Comprehensive Environmental Response, Compensation and Liability Act of 1980 (CERCLA or Superfund). In addition to OSHA and NIOSH, other Federal agencies have specifically defined responsibilities for assisting in protecting workers from adverse health effects from hazardous wastes.

The number of diverse Federal programs relating to hazardous waste is due to the complexities and the multidisciplinary aspect of hazardous waste management, and to the extensive amount of Federal legislation addressing hazardous materials. Much of the legislation on hazardous substances which applies to worker safety and health was developed to regulate activities other than waste site management or remedial actions. The National Contingency Plan in 40 CFR[1] Part 300 is a notable exception. Regulations and legislation applicable to worker safety and health include:

- The previously mentioned OSHAct of 1970 and the subsequent passage of regulations 29 CFR, notably Parts 1910 (Occupational Safety and Health Standards) and 1926 (Safety and Health Standards for Construction).
- The Resource Conservation and Recovery Act of 1976 (RCRA) and subsequent regulations in 40 CFR Parts 260 through 265, such as Section 265.16 (Personnel Training) and 265 Subparts C (Preparedness and Prevention) and D (Contingency Plan and Emergency Procedures).
- CERCLA of 1980 and its regulations (i.e., the National Contingency Plan) under 40 CFR 300.150 (Worker Health and Safety), stipulating which worker health and safety regulations and guidelines to follow.

---

[1] *Code of Federal Regulations*

- The Atomic Energy Act of 1954 and subsequent regulations in 10 CFR Part 20, stipulating standards for protection against radiation.
- Federal Mine Safety and Health Act (FMSHA) of 1977 and subsequent regulations in 30 CFR Part 11 (Department of the Interior, Bureau of Mines, Respiratory Protective Devices; Tests for Permissibility), providing the primary technical criteria for a permissible respirator.
- The Hazardous Materials Transportation Act of 1975 (HMTA) and regulations in 49 CFR Parts 100 to 199 which stipulate labeling, marking, packaging, placarding, manifesting and shipping papers required for handling of hazardous materials during loading, transport, and unloading.

Potential users are urged to familiarize themselves with these pieces of legislation. Other additional pieces of legislation will be of interest to the industrial hygienist working with hazardous material management; however, familiarity with those listed above will provide a good foundation for initially accessing Federal programs and resources.

Federal Programs Relating to Protection of Hazardous Waste Workers

This section identifies and highlights many of the Federal programs relating, directly and indirectly, to safety and health protection of hazardous waste workers. The informational and technical resources available through these programs will be emphasized, rather than their regulatory and policy-making functions.

Discussions of the programs will be brief, since the purpose of this section is to provide a guide for inquiry and access to services. An exception is made for the NIOSH discussion. NIOSH is engaged in research, education and training, and providing information related to occupational safety and health. NIOSH is thus a good source of information and resources on both worker safety and health and on hazardous substances found in the workplace [4, 5]. Table 2-1, located further in this chapter, provides pertinent program addresses and telephone numbers.

U.S. Department of Health and Human Services (HHS)

Centers for Disease Control and Prevention (CDC)

CDC provides assistance through its National Center for Environmental Health. Technical assistance, publications, laboratory and analytical services, and health studies are available. CDC is the focal point for HHS' responsibilities under CERCLA.

National Institute for Occupational Safety and Health (NIOSH)

NIOSH was established to ensure safe and healthful working conditions, to develop occupational safety and health standards, and to carry out research activities. Key NIOSH services include:

1. Health Hazard Evaluations (HHEs) which provide on-site evaluation of potentially hazardous chemical, physical, and biologic exposures. HHEs have both medical and industrial hygiene components. Employers or representative groups of employees may place requests by calling 1-800-35-NIOSH.
2. Providing technical information, including NIOSH criteria documents, publications, and research reports. Criteria documents contain a review of the scientific literature, required medical controls, methods of sampling and analysis and probable safe atmospheric levels. In response to inquiries, NIOSH will search two databases which relate to toxic substances and worker safety and health (RTECS® and NIOSHTIC®).
3. Technical assistance in the areas of epidemiology, engineering, industrial hygiene, and occupational medicine.
4. Training courses, provided by NIOSH and by colleges and universities through NIOSH contracts and grants. Courses are available in the fields of occupational medicine, occupational nursing, industrial hygiene, and occupational health engineering.
5. Respirator testing, called FIT testing, and certification to assure compliance with Federal requirements [see Table 2-1].
6. Because NIOSH is administratively under the CDC, inquiries to NIOSH often yield valuable environmental health information referrals to CDC's programs and specific referrals to individual professionals.

Agency for Toxic Substances and Disease Registry (ATSDR)

ATSDR was created to prevent or to mitigate adverse human health effects and diminished quality of life resulting from exposure to hazardous substances in the environment. By congressional mandate, ATSDR establishes linkages between human exposure to hazardous substances and any increased incidence of adverse health effects by applying state-of-the-art scientific methods, creating and building relevant databases, and identifying appropriate target populations for investigation.

National Institute for Environmental Health Sciences (NIEHS)

NIEHS provides toxicological data, publications, technical assistance, and research programs to study the biological effects of potentially toxic substances found in the environment. There is an emphasis on health effects from chronic low-level exposures.

U.S. Department of Labor

Occupational Safety and Health Administration (OSHA)

In addition to its enforcement responsibilities, OSHA provides technical assistance, publications, training courses, and develops and promulgates occupational safety and health standards. OSHA also provides consultation to help businesses comply with safety standards. Most of these resources can be obtained through the ten regional offices.

U.S. Environmental Protection Agency (EPA)

EPA's goal is to prevent, control and abate pollution in the areas of air, water, solid waste, pesticides, radiation and toxic substances. The EPA provides technical assistance and publications on both the management of hazardous wastes and worker safety and health at hazardous waste sites. The Office of Emergency and Remedial Response is a major resource within EPA for technical assistance, training, and environmental protection support during hazardous substance incidents. The program areas of solid waste, surface and groundwater protection, and air pollution all have extensive technical experience and current research that directly relates to hazardous waste occupational safety and health. EPA, like OSHA, has ten regional offices which can provide many of these services, or at least refer inquiries to the appropriate office within the agency.

U.S. Department of Transportation (DOT)

The DOT Office of Hazardous Materials Standards provides technical assistance and publications on the safe transport and loading of hazardous materials. DOT sponsors several hazardous materials transportation courses. They also operate the Transportation Safety Institute in Oklahoma City which provides several training courses on hazardous materials transportation.

U.S. Coast Guard

Although a branch of the uniformed services, the U.S. Coast Guard is under the jurisdiction of the DOT. The U.S. Coast Guard provides information and technical assistance in port safety. Other functions include providing a National Response Center to receive reports of oil and hazardous substance spills, investigating spills, and monitoring responsible party cleanups. In environmental emergencies, the U.S. Coast Guard may provide a strike team and public information assistance. For persons involved in oil spill response, they offer a training course which includes spill planning and response and personnel safety.

Federal Emergency Management Agency (FEMA)

FEMA participates in the development and evaluation of national, regional, and local contingency plans. It monitors responses to these plans and evaluates requests for presidential designation of disaster areas. FEMA, along with 14 additional agencies of the National Response Team 1, has developed the *Hazardous Materials Emergency Planning Guide*. FEMA also sponsors the Hazardous Materials Information Exchange (HMIX), which is a computerized bulletin board designed especially for the distribution and exchange of hazardous materials information. The HMIX provides a centralized database for sharing information pertaining to hazardous materials emergency management, training, resources, technical assistance, and regulations. To learn about accessing the system, call 1-800-PLANFOR.

U.S. Department of the Interior

U.S. Geological Survey (USGS)

The USGS provides expertise on cartography, geology, hydrology, and soil sciences. An extensive collection of topographic maps and recent and historical aerial photography is also available. These maps, photographs, and many of the USGS reports may be useful in site selection and in remedial actions. The USGS also conducts investigations of groundwater pollution and identifies sources such as waste disposal facilities. The USGS Water Resources Division's mission is to provide hydrologic information and understanding needed for the optimum utilization and management of the nation's water resources.

U.S. Department of Energy (DOE)

The DOE operates the Technical Information Center at Oak Ridge, Tennessee, which disseminates its own reports, as well as international nuclear science literature. The Office of Environmental Restoration and Waste Management provides centralized management for the Department for waste management operations, environmental restoration, and applied research and development programs and activities.

U.S. Department of Commerce

National Institute of Standards and Technology (NIST)

The NIST provides publications on its own measurement programs in physical sciences and engineering, and from its reference collection of engineering standards and specifications issued by Federal agencies, technical societies and trade associations. NIST carries out selected programs in public safety and health and environmental improvement.

National Oceanic and Atmospheric Administration (NOAA)

NOAA provides detailed state-of-the-art meteorologic data and scientific support, including expertise on living marine resources. This organization is conducting research on several topics of hazardous substances that will assist safety and health professionals.

General Services Administration (GSA) -
Federal Information Center Program

The Federal Information Center Program is a clearinghouse for information about the Federal government and can eliminate the maze of referrals that people have encountered in contacting the Federal government. People with questions about a government program or agency, and who are unsure of which office can help, may call or write the Center.

American Conference of Governmental Industrial Hygienists, Inc. (ACGIH)

ACGIH is not a Federal agency, but its membership is composed of industrial hygienists employed in government. ACGIH publishes annually a table of recommended threshold limit values for chemical substances. This can often be obtained from NIOSH or OSHA. A series of Hygienic Guides on many commonly used industrial substances with references for additional information is also available.

Accessing Federal Programs

Government publications and resources in any subject area present problems for their actual and potential audiences, due to their great number, their different distribution channels, and the number of organizations and programs producing them. In subject areas like hazardous waste, these potential problems are exacerbated by the dispersion of responsible agencies throughout the federal bureaucracy, the multidisciplinary nature of the subject, and rapid growth resulting from public concern and current legislation. Although these factors may complicate access, they are also indicators of the magnitude and diversity of the available resources. Once potential users identify these and other potential problems, strategies for accessing Federal programs can be developed. Although each user will develop his or her own unique approach, the most effective strategies will be based upon knowledge, planning and interpersonal skills.

Forethought will result in better service, less frustration, and less time expended. Planning will enable the user to obtain some familiarity with the legislation and programs related to the inquiry. It will also allow enough lead-time for proper definition of the inquiry and contacts with local resource people. Potential users are urged to consult with librarians and information specialists at public, academic, and industrial libraries. The Federal government has been modernizing in the last several years by employing information specialists to manipulate and manage their vast supply of technical information and data. These individuals are not only trained professionals, they are also "users" themselves with established methods of access. They can save both the potential and experienced user considerable time and frustration. Frequently, they can also provide sample output from automated information systems and refer users to specific individuals.

Planning should also include definition of the kind of information or services needed. Given the volume and diversity of the resources available, the user will be best served when the objective of the inquiry is clearly identified. Persistence in follow-up is as important in acquiring Federal program assistance as it is in the sales business. Program changes and staff turnover necessitate a relentless pursuing and building of communication networks. The user's skill and knowledge can be used and increased only if contact is maintained with individuals within the Federal program. It is only through these contacts and dialogues that users obtain the most comprehensive and current level of assistance available.

One characteristic shared by all Federal programs is change. All are subject to constantly changing personnel, available resources, program emphasis, and administrative organization. These can range from minor modifications of the administrative organization to major restructuring of the program emphasis. Since even minor modifications can result in personnel transfers and new telephone listings, users must monitor the program fairly frequently. A listing of Federal programs pertinent to worker safety and health, their addresses, and telephone numbers are provided as a starting point [see Table 2-1].

Keeping up to date with any specific Federal program requires obtaining pertinent information from the voluminous amount available. This is particularly true with changes in the Federal administration. The outgoing administration attempts to push through legislation and programs in its final days (e.g., EPA's Superfund) and the new administration makes changes in key staff and administrative procedures in order to institute its own agenda. During this transition, there is considerable discussion and debate creating a vast amount of information that must be sorted through to track *actual* program changes.

The task of obtaining pertinent information is even more formidable with high level public interest programs like Superfund. The Programs' potential social, economic, and environmental impact can mobilize special interest groups which further contribute to the available information. These groups can also affect rapid changes within Federal programs through their support and lobbying activities.

Due to the current level of public concern and political sensitivity, hazardous waste programs can change more quickly than other government programs. These factors and the economic implications of hazardous waste management and remedial actions will result in further Federal program modifications for some time. Even though this rapid rate of change will be a source of frustration for potential users, those tenacious enough to pursue their inquiries will be rewarded with the resources derived from changing programs.

Table 2-1 **A Partial List of Federal Programs, Addresses, and Telephone** **Numbers that can Provide Hazardous Waste Safety and Health** **Information**	

National Institute for Occupational
  Safety and Health (NIOSH)
U.S. Department of Health and
  Human Services
4676 Columbia Parkway
Cincinnati, OH 45226
(800) 356-4674
FIT Testing Information
Morgantown, WV 26505
(304) 284-5713
	Agency for Toxic Substances and Disease
	  Registry (ATSDR)
	U.S. Department of Health and
	  Human Services
	1600 Clifton Road, N.E.
	Atlanta, GA 30333
	(404) 639-0727

Centers for Disease Control and
  Prevention (CDC)
U.S. Department of Health and
  Human Services
National Center for Environmental Health
4770 Buford Highway
Chamblee, GA 30341
(404) 488-7050
	U.S. Environmental Protection Agency (EPA)
	Office of Emergency and Remedial Response
	401 M Street SW (MC5203G)
	Washington, D.C.
	(703) 603-8830

Occupational Safety and Health
  Administration (OSHA)
U.S. Department of Labor
200 Constitution Ave. NW (Rm. N3647)
Washington, D.C. 20210
(202) 219-8151
	National Institute for Environmental Health
	  Sciences (NIEHS)
	U.S. Department of Health and Human Services
	P.O. Box 12233
	Research Triangle Park, NC 27709
	(919) 541-0752 or 541-3345

U.S. Department of Transportation (DOT) Office of Hazardous Materials Standards 400 Seventh Street, SW Washington, D.C. 20590 (202) 366-4488	Federal Emergency Management Agency (FEMA) 500 C Street SW Washington, D.C. 20472 (202) 646-4600 (800) PLANFOR (HMIX bulletin board)

National Oceanic and Atmospheric
  Administration (NOAA)
U.S. Department of Commerce
Hazardous Materials Response
  and Assessment Division
7600 Sandpoint Way, NE
Seattle, WA 98115
(206) 526-6317
	U.S. Department of Energy (DOE)
	Office of Scientific and Technical Information
	P.O. Box 62
	Oak Ridge, Tennessee 37831
	(615) 576-1301
	Office of Environmental Restoration and
	  Waste Management
	(202) 586-6331

National Institute of Standards and Technology (NIST) U.S. Department of Commerce Gaithersburg, MD 20899 (301) 975-3058	U.S. Geological Survey (USGS) 12201 Sunrise Valley Dr. Reston, VA 22092 (703) 648-4460 (703) 648-5663 (NAWDEX)

Table 2-1
A Partial List of Federal Programs, Addresses, and Telephone Numbers that can Provide Hazardous Waste Safety and Health Information

EROS Data Center U.S. Geological Survey Sioux Falls, South Dakota 57102 (605) 594-6511	U.S. Coast Guard - U.S. DOT Marine Environmental Protection 2100 Second Street SW Washington, D.C. 20593 (202) 267-0518

Environmental Photographic
  Interpretation Center (EPIC)
P.O. Box 1587
Warrenton, Virginia 22186
(703) 341-7503
	Environmental Monitoring Systems
	  Laboratory (EMSL-LV)
	P.O. Box 15027
	Las Vegas, Nevada 89114
	(702) 798-2525

Earth Science Information Center (ESIC) U.S. Geological Survey Box 25046, (MS504) Denver Federal Center Denver, Colorado 80225-0046 (303) 236-5829 ESIC 507 National Center Reston, VA 22092 (703) 648-6045 ESIC 1400 Independence Road, (MS231) Rolla, MO 65401-2602 (314) 341-0851	Federal Information Center Program General Services Administration P.O. Box 600 Cumberland, MD 21502-0600 (800) 347-1997 Eastern Time Zone (800) 366-2998 Central Time Zone (800) 359-3997 Mountain Time Zone (800) 726-4995 Pacific Time Zone (800) 733-5996 Hawaii (800) 729-8003 Alaska (800) 326-2996 TDD/TTY
National Climatic Data Center U.S. Department of Commerce Federal Building Asheville, North Carolina 28801 (704) 259-0476	Soil Conservation Service U.S. Department of Agriculture P.O. Box 2890 Washington, D.C. 20013 (202) 720-1820

INFORMATION GATHERING

Information gathering is an ongoing process during all phases of a hazardous waste site investigation. As facts are discovered, leads to other previously unknown information may develop. It is essential to keep detailed records and notes of what is learned from each information source during each step of the process. All further activities, including reconnaissance and field investigations, should aid in collecting information.

The information and data gathered prior to field work can be used to determine if there is an immediate hazard present or if one will be created by remedial actions. Background and safety information should be included in a study plan for the investigation which should be distributed to all individuals participating in the investigation or remedial actions. Training, familiarity with the site safety plan, and adherence to approved technical procedures for field work are the most important aspects of protecting human health and the environment.

The first step of preparing for a site visit is to identify information needs. The information should be gathered through as many sources as possible. The information should then be evaluated to identify gaps and see if other leads develop. As much information as possible should be obtained prior to conducting a site visit. After all available information and data have been gathered, an initial evaluation of the information should be performed. The information should be used to evaluate the level of personal protective equipment to use upon site entry. If the available information is not sufficient to determine the appropriate level of protection, a conservative approach is best.

A base map depicting pertinent site information should be prepared and included in the site safety plan. Sometimes aerial photography is readily available in the right size and of sufficient quality to be used as the base map. Field notes can be written on a copy of the base map later.

The following sections, *Information Needs* and *Information Sources*, will be helpful in your final information gathering endeavors.

Information Needs

Identification of information needs begins with identification of objectives. Visualization of actually carrying out the first site visit is helpful. Answering the following questions will provide a starting point:

Who is going to the site? Have they been properly trained and informed about site activities?

What conditions and hazards will you encounter upon entry? What types of hazardous waste may be present?

Where is the site? Do you know how to get there? If so, have you informed your team?

How could planned field activities affect your team, the area and the public?

When will you go, and what weather conditions do you expect?

Why are you going? Have you adequately planned each site activity and are you prepared for unexpected difficulties?

Additional categories of information for site safety planning include 1) site surroundings, 2) hazardous waste generation process and management, 3) emergency information, 4) climate, and 5) surface and subsurface information. Each category is described below.

Site Surroundings

Before conducting a site visit, information about the surrounding area should be obtained. Sources of drinking water supplies in the area, both public and private, should be noted. It may be important to find out what kind of treatment system is used by the public water supply. Likewise, information should be gathered on the local sewer and storm drain systems to determine possible infiltration or illegal discharge points.

General land use around the site should be studied. It is important to note population densities and distances to residences, schools, commercial buildings and any other facilities in the vicinity of the waste site which may be occupied. Locations of any flammable or explosive waste, such as liquefied natural gas, stored near the site should be determined.

Hazardous Waste Generation Process and Management Information

Knowledge of raw materials and processes used onsite that may have generated hazardous wastes or other hazardous substances will assist in anticipating what level of protective clothing, equipment, or other precautions will be required. Examples of processes include manufacturing, cleaning, physical or chemical treatment, research and development, chemical analysis, petroleum refining, wood treating, electroplating, etc. Many processes have predictable chemical species associated with their operations.

Descriptions of past and present waste management activities will assist in determining logistics, work plans, hot zones, sampling locations, etc. This information will give some idea of what to expect regarding adequacy of design, conditions of tanks and containers, pollution control devices, past releases, general housekeeping, and known hazards such as unexploded ordinance, confined spaces, or exotic chemicals. A modern, operating facility will probably have abundant information available and established safety practices that must be followed, in addition to your own standard operating safety procedures. However, entering an older, poorly designed facility, or uncontrolled hazardous waste site requires more research and guesswork, and more hazard planning.

Emergency Information

At a minimum, names and telephone numbers of the local police, fire department, ambulance, and nearest hospital should appear in the site safety plan. In some cases, activities at unsecured sites may warrant keeping emergency services on standby or even onsite. Evacuation routes from the site should be determined.

Climate

Local climate and anticipated weather conditions should be factored into the safety planning. Temperature extremes, especially when combined with high humidity, can predispose workers to heat stress, cold stress and/or fatigue (for more details, see Chapter 10, Heat Stress in Industrial Protective Encapsulating Garments). When airborne contaminants may be a problem, prevailing wind patterns and velocities should be considered during preparation of the site safety plan. Such information can be obtained through the National Climatic Data Center [see Table 2-1].

Surface and Subsurface Information

Soil and overburden types and permeabilities affect the migration of contaminants from a waste management site. Highly permeable soils (i.e., 10^{-3} cm/sec) may permit rapid migration of pollutants, both vertically and horizontally, away from containment areas. Rates of attenuation of pollutants in the unsaturated zone and underlying aquifers are a function of soil chemistry and physical characteristics.

If drilling, excavation, or sampling is planned, information about subsurface contaminants and resulting potential safety hazards and/or exposures is important. Local utility companies must be notified if any excavation or drilling is anticipated, so that locations of buried pipelines and wires can be marked. Drilling in or near landfills can be very dangerous, because pockets of gas or unstable ground can be encountered.

Other pertinent information may include: depths to the water table and any underlying aquifers, characteristics of confining layers, piezometric surfaces (heads) of confined aquifers, direction(s) of flow, and types of contaminants.

Information on local bedrock types and depths may be important in understanding contaminant migration pathways, particularly where producing aquifers lie beneath the water table aquifer. Sedimentary strata (limestones, sandstones, and shales) channel groundwater flows along bedding planes and flow directions may be determined by the dip in the strata. Where limestones are present in humid climates, solution channels may develop allowing very rapid transport of pollutants over long distances with little attenuation. Igneous and metamorphic bedrock (granites, diorite, marble, quartzite, slate, gneiss, schist, etc.) may permit rapid transport of polluted groundwater along fracture zones. Sources of this information include USGS reports and files, state geological survey records, and local well driller logs.

Information Sources

As discussed in detail in earlier sections, government information sources concerning worker safety and health at hazardous waste sites are voluminous and varied. The information sources discussed in this section also include personal contacts, additional specific government sources, remote sensing data, hard copy references and databases. The list of sources is abbreviated, but will give the reader a good starting point for gathering information.

Personal Contacts

Once a site is identified for investigation or other work, the original source of information, either private citizen or government official, should be asked to provide names of any other persons who might have knowledge about the site in question. If the source is a private citizen complaint, the names of anyone who might be able to corroborate or add information to the report should be requested. If the source of information is an employee of the facility under discussion, the person is entitled to certain employee protection provisions under RCRA, Section 7001.

Additional Specific Government Sources

As mentioned earlier, the project leader should take advantage of information available through the government. Within the EPA regional offices, contacts in the Toxic Substances, Drinking Water, Solid Waste, andEnforcement programs should be consulted. Information on the site or facility may have been submitted either through the RCRA or CERCLA notification process. State and local environmental agencies may have valuable information regarding specific sites, disposal practices, and other technical data. Information on whether the site has a National Pollutant Discharge Elimination System (NPDES) permit should be sought. If the site operator has applied for this permit, the application forms may provide considerable information on waste disposal at the site and the design of the facility. Information may also be available from state inventories of surface impoundments under the Safe Drinking Water Act (SDWA) or from the *Open Dumps Inventory* conducted in the early 1980s under RCRA.

If the facility applied for a solid waste permit, a considerable amount of information may be available from state files regarding geology, hydrology, and soils. Records of site visits should be requested. State water quality agencies may have data on ambient surface water and groundwater quality.

The USGS, the Soil Conservation Service, Agricultural Extension Service Agents, state geological survey records, local well drillers, and local construction engineering companies may be able to supply soil and overburden information. Sources of subsurface hydrogeological information include the USGS, state geological surveys, local well drillers, and state and local water resources boards. A list of all state and local cooperating offices is available from the USGS Water Resources Division in Reston, Virginia. This list has also been distributed to EPA Regional Offices. Water quality data, including surface water, is available through the USGS via their automated NAWDEX system [see Table 2-1].

If limited information on wastes is available from government sources, it may be necessary to proceed with the site inspection and field investigations without benefit of background information. Sometimes it is possible to form a hypothesis on the kinds of waste present at the facility. Where a landfill contains both municipal and industrial wastes, much of the waste probably comes from local industries. If approximate dates of operation of the facility are known, local officials or the Chamber of Commerce may be able to provide information on industries operating locally during that time period. In the case of an on-site (at the generator's site) facility, it may be possible to determine the type of waste present. Information on the composition of waste streams associated with various industrial processes may be obtained from the *Kirk-Othmer Encyclopedia of Chemical Technology.*

Remote Sensing Data

Remote sensing is the science and art of obtaining information about an object, area, or phenomenon through the analysis of data acquired by a device that is not in contact with the object, area, or phenomenon under investigation [6]. Two examples of remote sensing data include aerial photography and thermal infrared imagery. Remote sensing can provide the following information:

- Location of possible hazards to inspectors
- Approximate volumes of solid and liquid waste disposal
- Illegal or unauthorized dumping
- Visible environmental effects from spills, surface runoff patterns, surface leachate flow, impoundment leakage, and damaged or stressed vegetation around disposal sites
- Geological features at ground surface such as faults or fractures on or near the site
- Container and tank storage locations
- Disposal areas not visible or accessible from the ground
- Facility configuration, boundaries, design and operation
- Historical and present land use of the site and its surroundings

Information on aerial reconnaissance and aerial data interpretation is available at these EPA offices:

- For sites located east of the Mississippi River, contact the Environmental Photographic Interpretation Center (EPIC) [see Table 2-1].
- For sites located west of the Mississippi River, contact the Environmental Monitoring Systems Laboratory (EMSL-Las Vegas) [see Table 2-1].

Each office maintains its own archive of aerial reconnaissance imagery (photography and thermal scanner data). EPIC has access to historical imagery from other government agencies.

Federal agencies have used aerial photography for many purposes for decades. Usable photographs less than five years old are usually available for a site. Frequently, however, the scale will be too small to observe details of the site without considerable magnification of the imagery. When gathering information on the locations, areal extent, and historical development of facility operations (e.g., the size and locations of old landfill cells), archival photography can be invaluable.

Usually, the requester must specify the latitude and longitude coordinates of the site when requesting photography. Archival photographs are available from the USGS Earth Science Information Center (ESIC) and EROS Data Center [see Table 2-1]. Photographs taken before 1950 are also available from the National Archives. Information on the photography available for a given site can usually be obtained through the above facilities.

Hard Copy Sources of Information

This section provides a partial list of hard copy sources of information, as follows:

Chemical Hazardous Response Information System (CHRIS). Four volume set. For sale by the Superintendent of Documents, Washington, D.C. (1986) (GPO# 0-169-147:QL 3)

Key, M., et al., Eds. *Occupational Diseases - A Guide to Their Recognition.* U.S. Department of Health, Education and Welfare, Public Health Service, Centers for Disease Control, National Institute for Occupational Safety and Health, Publication Number 77-181.

Kirk-Othmer Encyclopedia of Chemical Technology, Fourth Edition, multiple volume set, Kroschwitz, Jacqueline I., Exec. Ed., John Wiley & Sons, New York, N.Y., (1991).

The Merck Index, Eleventh Edition, Budavari, Susan, Ed., Merck & Co., Inc., Rahway, N.J., USA, (1989).

NIOSH Pocket Guide to Chemical Hazards. U.S. Department of Health and Human Services, Public Health Service, Centers for Disease Control, NIOSH, June (1990). DHHS (NIOSH) Publication Number 90-117.

NIOSH Respirator Decision Logic, U.S. Department of Health and Human Services, Public Health Service, Centers for Disease Control, NIOSH, (May 1987). DHHS (NIOSH) Publication Number 87-108.

Occupational Safety and Health Guidance Manual for Hazardous Waste Site Activities, NIOSH/OSHA/USCG/EPA, DHHS, Public Health Service, Centers for Disease Control, NIOSH, DHHS (NIOSH) Publication Number 85-115. (October 1985).

Respirator Selection Guide 1992, 3M Occupational Health & Environmental Safety Division, 3M Center Bldg. 275-6W-01, St. Paul, Minnesota 55144 (1992).

Sax, N. Irving and Richard J. Lewis, Sr.. Three volume set. *Dangerous Properties of Industrial Materials*, Seventh Edition, New York; Van Nostrand Reinhold, (1989).

Standard Operating Safety Guides, U.S. EPA, Office of Emergency and Remedial Response, (June 1992).

Student, P. J., *Emergency Handling of Hazardous Materials.* The Bureau of Explosives, American Association of Railroads, Washington, D.C., (1980).

Sweet, Doris V., Editor, *Registry of Toxic Effects of Chemical Substances*, Volumes 1 through 5, Public Health Service, Centers for Disease Control, NIOSH, Cincinnati, Ohio, (GPO# S/N 17-33-00431-5),(1985-86).

Databases

Federal databases exist in various forms: hard-copy, microfiche, compact disc, and electronic. Since Federal programs, like the rest of society, are in a transitional phase of moving from printed to electronic communication, the focus of this discussion will be on electronic systems. These are on-line, interactive computer systems maintained by various agencies. Some systems can be accessed by requests to the responsible agency or to other agencies, depending upon their information retrieval systems. All are available through one or more of the operational networks of chemical databasesequipped with computer programs that permit interactive searching and retrieval from these individual databases. Commercially operated networks include DIALOG [(800) 334-2564], BRS Search Service [(703) 442-0900], and ORBIT [(703) 442-0900]. Access is often available through public libraries and libraries within academic institutions on a fee basis. Individuals and companies may also set up their own accounts with the commercially operated networks. The following is an abbreviated list of current database systems and individual databases which are pertinent to worker safety and health. Exhibit 2-1 provides additional information on individual databases and on other databases which may be accessed by persons concerned with worker safety and health.

Chemical Information System (CIS)

The CIS is a collection of computerized data storage and retrieval modules for chemical information. The components most relevant to occupational safety and health include the Oil and Hazardous Materials/Technical Assistance Data System (OHMTADS), RTECS® (which will be described below), and Clinical Toxicology of Commercial Products (CTCP) [7]. The CIS may be accessed at (800) 247-8737.

NIOSH - Registry of Toxic Effects of Chemical Substances (RTECS®)

RTECS® is a database of toxicological information compiled, maintained, and updated quarterly by the NIOSH Division of Standards Development and Technology Transfer (DSDTT). It is a congressionally mandated activity established by the OSHAct. RTECS® is also available in hard-copy and on microfiche. Currently, there is information on over 1,000,000 compounds which is extracted from the open scientific literature. The information available on each compound includes toxicity, literature references, and specific health effects.

NIOSH - NIOSHTIC®
NIOSHTIC® is the NIOSH on-line, bibliographic database of literature in the field of occupational safety and health. The database currently contains more than 169,000 references, is updated quarterly, and is available on-line and on compact disc (CD-ROM).

NIOSH - Document Information Directory System (DIDS)
Also accessed through DSDTT, DIDS is an automated listing of all NIOSH publications, health hazard evaluations and internal NIOSH reports. Information regarding the contents and availability of DIDS can be obtained by calling (513) 533-8350.

National Technical Information Service (NTIS) - U.S. Department of Commerce
NTIS is a cross-disciplinary file of citations to federally funded research and development reports. It includes analyses prepared by Federal agencies, their contractors or grantees and nonclassified Department of Defense reports. NTIS announces 150,000 summaries of completed and ongoing U.S. and foreign government-sponsored research and development and engineering activities each year and currently has 1,500,000 records. The NTIS on-line database is available through DIALOG.

National Library of Medicine (NLM)
The NLM system contains more than five million references to journal articles and books in the health sciences published since 1965. MEDLINE® is the on-line portion of MEDLARS® which serves as a guide to worldwide medical literature. It does *not* include abstracts. It corresponds to the printed *Index Medicus*™ and currently contains 6,900,000 records.

The Toxicology Information Conversation On-Line (TOXLINE®) accesses the current literature on human and animal studies on the toxicity of substances. There are currently 1,650,000 records.

The TOXNET® system includes the Toxic Release Inventory (TRI) database. This database incorporates a national inventory of toxic chemical emissions from the majority of U.S. manufacturing facilities. There are over 300 chemicals and 20 chemical categories listed. TRI information is also available as microfiche, diskette, magnetic tape, and printed formats from the US Government Printing Office, (202) 783-3238, and the National Technical Information Service (NTIS), (703) 487-4650. The NLM can be reached at (800) 638-8480.

SUMMARY

Safety is the first and highest priority when planning field activities. Good planning minimizes wasted time and potentially dangerous mistakes. Project leaders should gather and communicate as much safety information as possible before entering or planning work activities at any site. Federal government programs offer valuable safety planning resources, given an understanding of what information is available and how to access that information. Relevant safety information can also be obtained by telephone, in hard copy literature, and by accessing databases. Preparedness gives both the project leader and team members the confidence to accomplish better, more efficient, and safer projects.

REFERENCES

1. 5 United States Code 552.
2. Bennett, G. F., et al. *Hazardous Materials Spills Handbook*, McGraw-Hill Book Co., New York, N.Y. (1982), p. 42.
3. *General Industry*, U.S. Department of Labor, Occupational Safety and Health Administration, OSHA 2206, U.S. Government Printing Office, (Revised June 1981), p.6.
4. Martin, William F., J. M. Melius, and C. A. Cottrill. *Management of Hazardous Wastes and Environmental Emergencies*, paper presented at the National Conference and Exhibition on Hazardous Wastes and Environmental Emergencies, Houston, TX: March 12-14, 1984.
5. Wallace, Lynn P., W. F. Martin, and C. A. Cottrill. *An Overview of NIOSH's Preparation of Hazardous Wastes Worker Health and Safety Guidelines*, paper presented at 4th National Conference on Management of Uncontrolled Hazardous Waste Sites, Washington, D.C., October 31-November 2, 1983.
6. Lillesand, Thomas M., and Ralph W. Kiefer. *Remote Sensing and Image Interpretation*, New York, John Wiley & Sons, Inc., (1979).
7. Heller, S.N., and G.W. Milne. *Use of the NIH-EPA Chemical Information System in Support of the Toxic Substances Control Act*, in *Monitoring Toxic Substances*, Schuetza, D., Ed., Washington, D.C., American Chemical Society (1979) pp. 255-286.

Exhibit 2-1
Selected Databases Related To Worker Safety and Health

Database Name	Subject Coverage	Coverage Dates	Update Frequency	Sponsoring Agency	Comments
Air Methods	Allows access to summarized standard methods for chemical analysis of air. Cross-indexes more than 450 air methods with 2500 compounds and their synonyms.	1990 - present	As needed	U.S. EPA (ERT) (800) 999-6990	-----
APTIC	Covers most sources for citations concerning all aspects of air pollution, its effects, prevention and control.	1966 - Oct 1978 (closed file)	-----	U.S. EPA	89,000 records
ASI	American Statistics Index covers statistical publications containing the entire spectrum of social, economic, and demographic natural resources data collected and analyzed from more than 500 U.S. and state and local agencies.	1973 - present (some material from 1960s)	Monthly	Congressional Information Service, Inc.	Over 142,000 records
BIOSIS PREVIEWS®	Covers all aspects of research in the biological and biomedical sciences, drawing upon all original published literature for citations. Corresponds to Biological Abstracts® and Biological Abstracts/RRM®.	1969 - present	Weekly	Biosis®	7,714,000 records; abstracts
CA SEARCH®	Includes citations to the literature of chemistry and its applications.	1967 - present	Biweekly	Chemical Abstracts Service	10,323,000 records
CAB ABSTRACTS	Comprehensive file of agricultural and biological information pertaining to all significant material and covering every aspect of crop and animal science.	1972 - present	Monthly	Commonwealth Agricultural Bureaux, U.K.	Over 2,878,000 records; abstracts
CANCERLIT®	Contains information on various aspects of cancer taken from over 3,500 U.S. and foreign journals as well as selected monographs, papers, reports and dissertations.	1963 - present	Monthly	U.S. National Cancer Institute	Over 823,000 abstracts of articles

Exhibit 2-1
Selected Databases Related To Worker Safety and Health

Database Name	Subject Coverage	Coverage Dates	Update Frequency	Sponsoring Agency	Comments
CHEMICAL SAFETY NEWSBASE	Provides information on the hazardous and potentially hazardous effects of chemicals and processes encountered by workers in industry and laboratories. Selected information topics include biological effects of chemicals, emergency planning, fires and explosions, occupational health and hygiene, and waste management.	1971 - present	Monthly	The Royal Society of Chemistry, U.K.	27,000 records
CHEMNAME®	Contains CAS® registry numbers, CA substance index names, molecular formulas, chemical name synonyms and periodic classification terms for chemical substances.	1967 - present	Monthly	Chemical Abstracts Service & DIALOG	Over 2,363,000 substances
CONFERENCE PAPERS INDEX	Covers approx.1,000 scientific and technical conferences worldwide and more than 100,000 papers presented. Primary subject areas covered include the life sciences, chemistry, physical sciences, geosciences, and engineering.	1973 - present	6 times yearly	Cambridge Scientific Abstracts; Bethesda, MD	1,489,000 records
DISSERTATION ABSTRACTS ONLINE	Interdisciplinary listing of almost all doctoral dissertations accepted since 1861 by accredited degree granting institutions in the U.S. plus some non-U.S. universities.	1861 - present	Monthly	University Microfilms Intl.	over 1,147,000 abstracts
ENERGY SCIENCE AND TECHNOLOGY	This energy database covers literature references on all aspects of energy and related topics. The following topics are included: nuclear, wind, fossil, geothermal energy, and the environment.	1974 - present (contains material back to late 1800s)	Biweekly	U.S. DOE	2,620,000 records

Exhibit 2-1

Selected Databases Related To Worker Safety and Health

Database Name	Subject Coverage	Coverage Dates	Update Frequency	Sponsoring Agency	Comments
ENVIRONMENTAL BIBLI-OGRAPHY	Covers the very broad field of general human ecology, atmospheric studies, energy, land resources, water resources and nutrition and health from more than 300 periodicals.	1973 - present	Bimonthly	Environmental Stud-ies Institute	Over 426,000 records; citations
Health and Safety Plan for Emergency Response (HASP)	HASP is a program that produces a site-specif-ic health and safety plan. Uses an automated decision-making process to significantly reduce data retrieval and integration time. Documents safety and health hazards, and recommended levels of protection. The plan may be edited using standard word processors.	1989 - present	As needed	U.S. EPA (ERT) (800) 999-6990	110 chemicals; 2600 chemicals avail-able
HEALTH AND SAFETY SCI-ENCE ABSTRACTS	Provides international coverage of the literature in 6 major areas: general safety, industrial and occupational safety, environmental and ecologi-cal safety, and medical safety. Available through the ORBIT system.	1982 - present	Monthly	Cambridge Scientific Abstracts	About 72,000 records
FEDERAL REGISTER	Provides the full text of the Federal Register, a daily publication of the Federal government that serves as the medium for notifying the public of official agency actions.	1988 - present	Daily	U.S. GPO	117,000 records
MEDLINE®	Bibliographic citations to worldwide bio-medi-cal literature; corresponds to Index Medicus™.	1966 - present	Weekly	National Library of Medicine (NLM)	6,857,000 records

Exhibit 2-1

Selected Databases Related To Worker Safety and Health

Database Name	Subject Coverage	Coverage Dates	Update Frequency	Sponsoring Agency	Comments
NIOSHTIC®	NIOSH's on-line, bibliographic database of literature concerned with occupational safety and health. Selected articles from about 150 current English language technical journals account for 45 percent of the 6,000 annual additions to NIOSHTIC®. Also available on compact disc.	19th century - present	Quarterly	NIOSH	165,000 records
NTIS	Complete government-sponsored research, development, and engineering reports announcement file. Contains abstracts of research reports from over 240 government agencies including EPA, DOE, HHS, etc. and some state and local government agencies.	1964 - present	Biweekly	National Technical Information Service (NTIS)	1,547,000 records
OHM-TADS	Oil and Hazardous Materials-Technical Assistance Data System contains data on materials designated as oil or hazardous materials. The system is designed to provide technical support for dealing with potential or actual dangers resulting from the discharge of oil or hazardous substances. Available through CIS system.	1978 - present	Continuous	Chemical Information System	1,400 chemicals

Exhibit 2-1
Selected Databases Related To Worker Safety and Health

Database Name	Subject Coverage	Coverage Dates	Update Frequency	Sponsoring Agency	Comments
OHS MSDS ON DISC™	Material Safety Data Sheet (MSDS) information available on a CD-ROM system. Thousands of the most frequently used chemical, plus add any additional substances you require. Is available for IBM PC/XT/AT or any of the many IBM PC compatible systems. Mainframe database is also available.	1978 - present	Daily	Occupational Health Services, Inc. (800) 445-MSDS	97,000 chemicals and chemical mixtures
OCCUPATIONAL SAFETY AND HEALTH (NIOSHTIC®)	Covers all aspects of occupational safety and health and includes such titles as biochemistry, toxicology, chemistry, education and training, safety, and hazardous wastes.	1973 - present (dating back to 1800s)	Quarterly	NIOSH	169,000 records
POLLUTION ABSTRACTS	Covers foreign and domestic reports, journals, contracts and patents, symposia, and government documents in the areas of pollution, its sources, and control. More specifically, subjects covered include: water, marine, land and thermal pollution; pesticides; sewage and waste treatments; legal developments. Corresponds in coverage to the printed abstracts publication.	1970 - present	Bimonthly	Cambridge Scientific Abstracts	175,000 records
RTECS®	Registry of Toxic Effects of Chemical Substances (RTECS®) is a comprehensive database of basic toxicity information for over 100,000 chemical substances. The toxic effects are linked to literature citations from both published and unpublished government reports and published articles from the scientific literature.	1971 - present	Quarterly	NIOSH	1,000,000+ records

Exhibit 2-1

Selected Databases Related To Worker Safety and Health

Database Name	Subject Coverage	Coverage Dates	Update Frequency	Sponsoring Agency	Comments
SCISEARCH®	Multidisciplinary index to the literature of science and technology. Based on Science Citation Index which indexes approximately 2,600 major scientific and technical journals.	1974 - present	Weekly	Institute for Scientific Information	10,707,000 records
STORET	Storage and retrieval of water quality data and a repository for water quality data that contains records of water quality parametric data by sampling site. On-line information available through NTIS.	1962 - present	Weekly	U.S. EPA	150,000,000 sampling sites at 800,000 locations
TOXLINE®	Contains data on toxicity and adverse effects of drugs, environmental pollutants and chemicals on the human food chain, laboratory animals, and biological systems.	Varies with subject file	Monthly	National Library of Medicine	1,647,000 records
WATER RESOURCES ABSTRACTS	Prepared from material collected by water research centers and academic institutes in the U.S. The file covers a wide range of water resource topics including water quality (pollution, waste treatment), ground and surface water hydrology, and water planning. Available from NTIS.	1968 - present	Monthly	U.S. Geological Survey; Water Resources	300,000 records

3

OCCUPATIONAL HEALTH AND SAFETY PROGRAMS FOR HAZARDOUS WASTE WORKERS

David L. Dahlstrom, M.S., C.I.H.

The rapid accumulation of hazardous wastes poses one of the most complex and expensive environmental control and cleanup tasks in history [1]. For this reason, numerous environmental statutes were enacted in the decades of the 1970s, 1980s and into the 1990s which have had far-reaching effects upon industry, society, and the environment [2-16]. These statutes and regulations have prescribed the means and methods to be followed to prevent significant deterioration of the overall environment in which we live, as well as to ensure the health and well-being of both the public at large and the employee within the conventional workplace. In many respects, the statutes have only begun to prescribe the means and methods necessary to properly protect the employee who must investigate, handle, dispose, and control hazardous wastes [10-16]. To carry out these tasks, health and safety professionals in the diverse industries which generate, store, transfer remediate, and/or dispose of hazardous wastes are in the process of adapting the administrative, engineering, and personal protective controls of the conventional workplace to address the varied and unique operational aspects characteristic of hazardous waste operations [39, 44, 46]. This chapter presents the current state of this technology as it is applied toward the ultimate goal of ensuring the continued good health and well-being of those who work with hazardous wastes. In particular, this chapter demonstrates the continued need for a concerted management approach which focuses program effectiveness through the coordinated integration of the multiple disciplines resources including legal, business management, industrial hygiene, industrial and construction safety, toxicology, engineering, and medicine.

56

PROGRAM DEVELOPMENT AND IMPLEMENTATION: AN OVERVIEW

Administrative Policy and Goals of a Successful Program

The development and implementation of a comprehensive Occupational Health and Safety program (OHS) for employees who work with hazardous wastes is a complex and interactive effort for which only a limited set of industry-specific codes and guidelines exist [10, 12, 33, 37, 40, 50]. As is the case for most companies, the degree of development and implementation of such a program depends upon the size of the facility (operating site), the number of employees involved, the types of operations being conducted, the variety of materials and potential hazards encountered at the work site, the type of business (consultant, waste transport, treatment, or disposal), and most importantly—management's overall philosophy towards health and safety [33, 39, 50, 52]. Irrespective of these variables, however, most successful programs have a policy on occupational safety and health which embraces certain key requirements. These requirements are listed below.

1. A policy which is explained and made available to all employees, through sufficient and frequent orientation and training sessions, in order to effect a thorough understanding of OHS program goals and individual responsibilities.
2. A clear definition of OHS program objectives and a schedule for achievement.
3. An overall commitment to support the OHS program, which acknowledges to the worker management's responsibilities to the program.
4. A mechanism which will provide for mutual representation from all functional levels within the organization in the setting of priorities and the implementation of OHS program objectives.
5. A clear definition of line and staff responsibilities and their reporting relationships. This is often best accomplished through the use of a functional organizational chart.
6. A means of periodically reviewing the progress, accomplishments, as well as the deficiencies of the OHS program [35].

Just as company OHS programs vary in their size and scope, so too do the overall goals of the program. Basically, it is imperative that for the goals set by one's company unquestionably reflect the priorities of that company with respect to employee and contractor health and safety. Developing the goals and objectives for a successfully dynamic OHS program should not be a unilateral effort. The health and safety management team should solicit the assistance and input of colleagues involved in industrial hygiene, safety, toxicology, engineering, regulatory compliance (legal) biostatistics, epidemiology, medical surveillance, environmental management, and especially from the company's overall management team [33, 34, 38, 42, 44]. Further, these goals should serve as the basis or foundation for specific company policies and operating procedures, and should provide the philosophical framework for setting more specific management objectives. It is by attaining these goals and objectives that the effectiveness of the OHS program can be evaluated over time.

The basic goals listed below, while not all inclusive, will help to ensure the continued good health and well-being of all employees who work routinely with hazardous waste materials.

1. Maintaining a safe and healthful work environment by placing all personnel in jobs according to individual physiological and psychological makeup, experience, and educational background.
2. Ensuring compliance with all legal requirements mandated by the various federal, state, and local environmental and occupational safety and health regulations.
3. Providing sufficient and periodic training to the affected employees and contractor staff (if appropriate) in the proper application of company health and safety operating procedures and the use of associated equipment. The purpose of this training is to ensure a thorough understanding of the whys and wherefores of the job [12, 13, 38, 39, 46].
4. Limiting company and personal liabilities associated with hazardous waste operations due most commonly to misinformation and negligence. This can be accomplished through the program's close adherence to the concepts and requirements of such environmental and occupational laws as the Toxic Substances Control Act (TSCA), the Resource Conservation and Recovery Act (RCRA), the Occupational Safety and Health Act (OSHA), the Comprehensive Environmental Response, Compensation and Liabilities Act (CERCLA/Superfund) and, the Superfund Amendments of 1986; "SARA"); and the ever increasing, precedent setting cases known as "Toxic Torts" [3, 8, 9, 10, 11, 12].

It is important that these goals correctly address the management priorities and current operating principles of the company. These goals must be clearly stated and communicated frequently to all of the employees. It is equally important that they are updated on a regular basis to reflect changes in related regulations or company policy and procedure.

The first major task in developing and implementing a comprehensive OHS program is providing justification for its existence. All too frequently, the problem of absorbing the related costs of the required resources has proven to be a major obstacle to the program's successful development and implementation. This is especially true in the case of smaller companies, which generally turn to its trade association or a consulting firm specializing in health and safety to provide these services on an as-needed basis [12, 13, 18]. In any case, the problem of justification can be approached from the aspects of business economics, corporate and individual liability, and the underlying responsibility of the company to its employees, its contractors and the surrounding community [20].

It is the responsibility of the OHS professional to demonstrate to the management, who is concerned with the "bottom line", that there is a need to balance the amount of resource investment and the return on that investment with the potential and actual costs associated with what we will call "negative" economics.

Here, we are referring to those costs associated with the legal liabilities pertaining to the regulatory noncompliance, toxic tort litigation, or personal damage suits. The settlement awards and court costs in these instances have continued to grow into the tens, if not hundreds of millions of dollars throughout the 1980s and into the 1990s. It has become increasingly evident that the efforts of the USEPA and OSHA are focusing on the enforcement of regulations and the assurance of corporate compliance with the respective regulations through active and aggressive inspection of facilities and remediation activities throughout the United States.

It is important to recognize further the ancillary costs associated with personal injury or regulatory compliance suits. These are the costs incurred due to the eventual increase in insurance premiums, property losses (third party or internal), and interruptions in production. There will be costs associated with labor problems which may result if the work site is perceived as being unsafe or unhealthy, and the costs associated with poor productivity due to low employee morale. Also included will be the actual and administrative costs of paying wages to injured workers who are not covered by insurance but are part of a collective bargaining agreement. Other costs that can detract from the bottom line are the costs attributable to regulatory fines and penalties; not to mention the eventual increase in OSHA/USEPA surveillance [20, 21]. Considering all these factors, it is far less costly for a company to invest in a proactive OHS program that is preventative in nature than to wait and hope an accident does not occur.

Regarding the responsibility of the company to its employees, its contractors, and the surrounding community, various environmental and occupational statutes require an employer to provide its employees and contractor personnel with a safe and healthful workplace [3, 8, 10-16]. Equally important to a company's economic health is the insurance that the surrounding environment is not adversely affected as a result of poor facility operations.

Most companies within the hazardous waste industry desire to maintain a good community image and are sincerely interested in the well-being of their employees. Most company managers readily recognize the potential impact which adverse publicity can have on the business future of a permitted hazardous waste generator, treatment, storage, or disposal facility or cleanup company; not to mention employee efficiency and productivity. To avoid negative publicity and to maintain good employee relations, management should strive to communicate to its employees and the public the *positive* actions being taken to provide acceptable levels of health and safety protection [22, 38, 51, 52]. A sound health and safety program is just such an action and can be used to demonstrate the commitment of the company to protecting the employee, public health, and the environment.

Therefore, a total commitment by management in terms of demonstrating consistent management support and the needed resources for the development and implementation of a comprehensive health and safety program is well justified. This proactive approach by management will serve not only as a preventative measure in the protection of its workers and the surrounding community, but also in the protection of the good name and assets of the company, its officers, directors, and shareholders.

Encouraging Worker Commitment to Health and Safety

Just as a total commitment by management is integral to the ultimate success of a comprehensive health and safety program, so too is the commitment of the work force. This commitment by the work force is dependent upon the manner in which policies are applied, and hence perceived, by the employee. To assist in creating a positive perception, it is essential to encourage employee involvement in achieving program goals and objectives [17, 18, 35, 38, 51, 52]. This can be done by incorporating into the OHS program the elements listed below. These elements will provide a solid foundation upon which a successful and effective OHS program can be built and maintained.

Creating a work environment that is as safe, healthful, and free from recognizable hazards as possible. Every effort must be made to provide the employee with proper and adequate training, equipment, and operating procedures with which to do his/her job safely. These efforts should be coupled with the installation of various engineering controls (e.g., positive ventilation, isolation, dust suppression) to minimize potential chemical or physical exposures. It is difficult to motivate employees to adopt safe work practices or to use protective equipment if management fails to provide an adequate work environment or fails to institute controls to protect employees from exposure to hazardous chemicals or operations.

Ensuring that there exists within the program a means for clear and open communications. The structure of the OHS Program should allow employees and management alike to communicate not only problems and recommendations, but also any modifications in programs, policies, and procedures. This can be best accomplished by including employee representatives, chosen by their co-workers, on the health and safety committee of the corporation. If suggestion boxes are used for purposes of communication, management must respond in a sincere, consistent, and meaningful fashion to reinforce the credibility of the program and management's commitment to it. Yet, it must be stressed, communications must be two way [51, 52].

Establishing both staff and line responsibilities designed to facilitate the fulfillment of the goals of the program. Line management must be given the direct responsibility of ensuring employee health and safety and preventing needless property loss. The focus of line management should be on the fulfillment of their compliance responsibilities related to the various regulatory and OHS program policies and procedures. The health and safety professional must be given the staff responsibility of assisting line management and the employee in fulfilling this goal.

The goals and objectives of the overall program should revolve around the concept of risk management. Management has the ultimate responsibility of maintaining an accurate assessment of the associated health and safety risks within each work site [3, 10-13, 16, 33, 35, 38, 42]. Management must develop the means of dealing with these defined risks in a reasonable, technical, and objective manner. This can be done through the determination of "acceptable risk." This determination entails the application of technically acceptable means of adequately evaluating and quantitating the level of chemical and physical hazards of a site; prioritizing these hazards in order of their probability to cause harm to the employees, surrounding environment, and nearby communities; and, the subsequent implementation of the appropriate administrative, engineering, and protective equipment controls in each instance to minimize the risks associated with each identified hazard [12, 19, 39, 47]. Through the application of sound industrial hygiene management techniques in monitoring both the work site environment and personnel in a consistent and conscientious manner, the proper risk evaluation can be made.

Informing the work force of the recognized risks within the work place. Federal OSHA regulations as well as many states and localities now require compliance with the requirements of established worker and community "Right-to-Know" laws [11, 12, 13, 16]. Informing employees and the appropriate community services of the risks associated with the job to be performed and demonstrating that these risks are being minimized through proper controls will encourage employee and community cooperation toward the accomplishment of the respective company's OHS program goals and objectives.

FIVE ESSENTIAL COMPONENTS OF THE HEALTH AND SAFETY PROGRAM

The specific components of a an effective OHS program are actually the bricks and mortar which solidify and structure it. They provide the means by which the employee can be assured of continued good health and a safe environment in which to work through the incorporation of administrative and engineering controls, and the use of personal protective equipment [33, 34, 44]. These controls, instituted from the aspect of prevention, serve to minimize the potential for accidents and overt exposures to occur while maximizing the professionalism and proficiency of the employees. Of course, the degree of conscientiousness in which these components are applied will determine the structural integrity (and therefore the success) of the program.

Within the hazardous waste industry, the effective implementation and management of the following program components has served to ensure the quality of the respective health and safety program:

1.   A comprehensive and dynamic employee health surveillance system;
2.   A safety program consisting of specified and consistently enforced company guidelines and standard operating procedures, whose applicability and effectiveness are evaluated by periodic compliance auditing [35], and the assignment of both company

and site-specific OHS coordinators whose responsibility it is to ensure compliance with stated OHS program requirements;

3. An industrial hygiene program which has modified conventional exposure monitoring and evaluation techniques to recognize the unique setting of each hazardous waste operation conducted [38, 44];

4. A company Health and Safety Advisory Committee whose purpose is to assist the company's management in developing, maintaining and periodically evaluating a state-of-the-art health and safety program based on current technological and regulatory advances. The Advisory Committees need to be formed at both the corporate and facility level with facility level employee participation;

5. An in-depth, hands-on training program which includes periodic refresher training on an annual basis, as a minimum [12, 33, 34, 38, 39, 42, 44].

The remainder of this chapter discusses each of these components, except for Number 5, "Training" which is discussed in greater detail in Chapter 12.

HEALTH SURVEILLANCE SYSTEM

The health surveillance system should prescribe specific fitness criteria in conjunction with periodic medical evaluations to ensure that only physically and medically sound individuals participate in field operations involving hazardous materials. The focus of this system should be the assurance that the health status of these individuals is maintained. Therefore, the objective of this system is to detect any changes in the health status of individual workers or employee groups which might be related to the nature of the job performed and the substances with which the employee comes into contact with. In consideration of the nature and variety of chemicals (and mixtures thereof) related to hazardous wastes and the frequency for potential exposure to a variety of physical and chemical hazards, it is extremely important to provide a means by which the health of personnel who work at hazardous waste sites can be periodically assessed.

To properly monitor the health status of each employee, the specific items of data needed must first be identified [38, 40-42, 45, 47-50]. Then, it must be determined how this information is to be most effectively collected, collated, analyzed, and used. It is essential that these steps be completed during the preplanning stages of surveillance system implementation so as to prevent the common mistake of collecting too much information (a scatter-gun approach); some or most of which will eventually prove to be unnecessary or inapplicable (e.g., annual heavy metal analysis or annual x-rays) [36, 40, 48, 49]. Such a mistake can be costly in terms of both money as well as time and materials spent. Only essential pieces of data that will prove most beneficial and revealing, respective of individual changes in health status, should be collected [40-42, 48-50]. Essential information to be collected is discussed below.

Complete baseline data on the health status of the individual at the time of employment in order to assure that each individual can perform their job safely [37, 38, 40, 42, 49]. This should include information on: 1) family and individual medical history; 2) prior work history, including the types of chemicals the individual has worked with; 3) any known individual abnormalities or personal habits, such as the use of alcohol, tobacco, or drugs; 4) prior surgeries, hospitalizations, and immunizations; 5) reproductive history; 6) any abnormalities found during the initial preemployment physical examination and laboratory screening; and, 7) the use of ethical and/or over-the-counter pharmaceuticals to treat existing problems.

Nature of the work to be performed. This data should include types of activities to be performed, the types of personal protective equipment to be used, the types of chemicals to be encountered, exposure data as collected through site and personal monitoring, and accident data.

Individual identification data. This should include date of employment, name and social security number, date of birth, race and sex, and current address and phone number.

Follow-up data. This will include data collected during subsequent periodic (e.g., annual) physical examination and laboratory screenings.

The orderly collection of these data on a form designed with a coding scheme will permit the information to be easily collated and analyzed on a computer, thereby easing the burden of OSHA required recordkeeping [43]. In addition, it will ensure the confidentiality of medical records and provide for rapid access to records in case of emergency.

It cannot be overemphasized that the manner in which the data is collected and analyzed be well thought out and designed so as to ensure its complete usefulness. It should also be recognized that the data collected must be complete. The same data must be collected for each member of the work force. If this is done appropriately, the relationship to work performed or exposures experienced and health status of the individual and the group can be easily and effectively correlated [43, 49].

At this point, it should be clear that the development of an employee health surveillance system requires significant preliminary work. The necessary preliminary work includes the design of data collection forms, the development of a system for coding and collating data for computer input, the development of the software necessary to generate the necessary reports, and the design of procedures to monitor data processing and report flow in order to meet defined schedules [13, 40, 42, 43]. The system also requires that a specific individual be designated as being responsible for coordinating all of these activities. This individual may either be a company employee, such as the corporate medical or health and safety director, or an occupational health consultant from outside of the company. The important factor is that a responsible person be designated to ensure the smooth operation and the quality of the system so as to provide the employee with the maximum level of protection.

Once the requirements of data collection, collation, analysis, and retention have been determined and a responsible organizational party identified, the components of the system can be easily defined. These components should include:

1. Each worker should be given an *initial medical examination* and their medical history assessed prior to the performance of hazardous waste site activities. This will establish each worker's medical baseline, overall health status, the ability to wear respirators as other protective equipment, and ensure that each individual is capable of undertaking the rigors of field operations. It will also aid in determining which job is best for that worker.

2. Each worker should undergo *subsequent medical examinations* on a periodic basis (usually annually). The examination should be geared toward the worker's job classification and the chemical and physical hazards confronted by each worker. The parameters of this examination should be consistent with those of the initial examination in order to ensure consistency.

3. An *exit examination* should be required of each individual either leaving the company or transferring to another job within the company not associated with hazardous materials. The results of this examination can serve to document the health status of the individual at that time.

4. A plan should be instituted which would require the *monthly reporting of exposures or injuries*. The system should also provide procedures which specify the design and performance

of *specific post-exposure examination protocols* based on the types of chemicals to which the employee is exposed. A *contingency plan* must include an emergency medical plan, which would include provisions for informing the attending physician with pertinent information regarding the affected individual and toxicological information specific to the chemical(s); this will facilitate proper diagnosis and treatment. There should be in-place an emergency analytical system which will quickly analyze *unknown* chemicals to which an individual has been exposed so as to provide the physician and the toxicologist with the identity of these chemicals. The plan should also specify: 1) a means for providing other job responsibilities to any women who become pregnant so as to provide for fetal protection; 2) means of evaluating male and female employees to ensure their reproductive health; and 3) the removal from work site responsibilities of any worker who shows a significant abnormality in their medical profile, at least until it has been determined that he or she has completely recovered and is in good enough health to resume work responsibilities [20-22, 33, 40-42, 45, 48-50].

5.   Specific allowances must be made to assess the applicability and appropriate implementation of procedures designed to comply with OSHA's Americans with Disabilities Act and Bloodborne Pathogen Rule [14, 15].

The implementation of such a health surveillance program is neither a trivial nor an impossible undertaking. It does require considerable attention and coordination in order to be successful, but the benefits derived from a system that has been designed to be preventative in nature are innumerable in terms of employee health, welfare, and productivity.

SAFETY PROGRAMS

The purpose of a safety program is to protect the employee from chemical, physical and health hazards during hazardous waste work. Currently, the specific guidelines and uniform code specific to the hazardous waste industry exist in the form of OSHA's Worker Protections Standard (29 CFR 1910.120), otherwise known as "HAZWOPER," for the development and implementation of a safety program [12, 13, 44, 46].

Basically, a safety program should complement and support the industrial hygiene and health surveillance systems and it must be an integral part of every aspect of site operations. Most successful safety programs, despite variations in organizational structure and technique of application, make safety a major priority with respect to company policy and action [23, 51, 52]. This attitude of management, if demonstrated in a consistent and sincere manner, lends credibility to the program, encourages employee cooperation and support, and most importantly, minimizes the frequency and severity of accidents.

The critical elements of a successful safety program are:

1. Significant employee involvement in the development and implementation of operational procedures [51, 52];
2. Openly demonstrated and consistently applied management support and leadership;
3. Assignment of responsibilities to specific persons within the corporate, divisional, and facility structures whose role it is to ensure compliance and employee understanding of company policies and procedures (e.g. OHS program director/manager);
4. Development and implementation of standard operating procedures covering all aspects of the work to be performed;
5. A personal protective equipment program which defines the decision-logic necessary to ensure that proper respiratory and dermal equipment is provided and also provides for its proper use and maintenance;
6. A safety communications system which provides for the dissemination of information to all employees regarding hazard identification, policy and procedural changes, and lessons learned [51, 52];
7. A comprehensive training program which provides for periodic classroom and hands-on training of the employee in the proper use of equipment, operational techniques, and company policy [11-13];

8. An accident record and investigation program that not only will satisfy all legal requirements, but also will prevent a similar reoccurrence;

9. An audit program to ensure consistent application of operational procedures and evaluate their effectiveness [35, 36]; and

10. The maintenance of safe working conditions.

Many of these elements are self-explanatory and require no further discussion. The remaining elements are discussed in greater detail in subsequent chapters. It should be kept in mind, however, that the role played by the safety professional in employee training often determines the effectiveness of the other elements and deserves further consideration in this chapter.

The importance of assuring that the safety program maintains a high level of visibility has already been alluded to. It therefore becomes the role of the OHS coordinator, in concert with a consistent demonstration of management's unquestioned commitment to the program, to ensure this visibility at all levels within the organizational structure. All individuals involved in safety coordination, from top management to the OHS program director of the company to the site safety officer, have the responsibility of ensuring the total compliance by each employee with all of the requirements, policies, and procedures of the OHS program. OHS coordinators must develop, implement, and evaluate the effectiveness of site-specific safety plans, operational procedures, equipment usage, and employee performance within the work setting. In cooperation with the industrial hygienist and the engineer, the OHS coordinator must ensure the application of proper site and personal monitoring techniques so as to provide the employee with pertinent information regarding site hazards and the proper selection of appropriate protective equipment [39, 44, 47]. In this way, accidents can be prevented, thereby protecting the health and welfare of the employee and the surrounding public.

In the event of an accident, the OHS coordinator must investigate its occurrence and prescribe preventative measures to preclude its reoccurrence, and should maintain records of all accidents on-site to determine accident trends. Such records are required by OSHA and, no doubt, company management. Further, the OHS coordinator must strive to instill among employees a high degree of safety consciousness through ensuring employee participation, communication, and education.

To assure that all employees are prepared to safely participate in all facets of waste site operations, a series of specific and specialized training programs must be established as an integral part of the overall health and safety program. These programs should include training the employee in a classroom setting as well as in a practical setting to allow hands-on experience. Periodic refresher courses are also important [8, 12, 16, 33, 34, 38, 39].

Prior to performing work on-site, each employee should undergo training in a classroom setting. This training should provide the new employee with information regarding: 1) company policies and procedures; 2) health and safety requirements; 3) basic toxicology and chemistry of chemicals commonly confronted on waste sites; 4) the selection, use, and limitations of the various respirators and dermal protective equipment; 5) techniques used in the decontamination of personnel and equipment; 6) sampling techniques; 7) legal requirements under "Superfund", OSHA and RCRA; 8) heavy equipment operation (if applicable); 9) the health effects of heat and cold; and 10) emergency procedures, including multimedia first aid and cardiopulmonary resuscitation [12].

Upon completion of the in-depth classroom training, each employee should be given the opportunity to gain actual hands-on experience in a field setting, where the worker learns to put classroom concepts into practice. This experience will allow each employee to gain confidence in themselves as well as the equipment and procedures upon which they ultimately must rely. Moreover, this type of training builds on the "team" concept which is so important during work on hazardous waste sites.

Refresher training should be provided annually as a minimum [12]. The purpose of this training is to keep the employee informed of new techniques, policies, and procedures as well as to improve upon skills previously learned. The frequency and setting of refresher training will vary depending upon the diversity of job settings and each employee's ability to assimilate the training provided.

The application of the elements presented earlier, in conjunction with consistent management support, will serve to maximize the employee's proficiency and professionalism in conducting work operations at hazardous waste sites.

INDUSTRIAL HYGIENE PROGRAM

During cleanup activities at hazardous waste sites, the primary objective is to minimize potential health hazards to site workers and the surrounding general public. To achieve this, a site safety plan providing specific standard operating procedures must be developed [12]. An effective site safety plan should address three key issues: *identification* of substances on-site and the hazard they represent; *evaluation* of the risk associated with those substances; and *control* of their potential impact on site personnel. Identifying substances and hazard evaluation generally involves reviewing historical and monitoring data obtained during preliminary assessment of site conditions. These data may include information obtained from manifests or facility records, as well as the results of off-site air monitoring and off-site drainage or leachate samples. Data from the identification and evaluation process provide the basis for evaluating exposure risks and determining measures to control potential impacts of exposure. These include ambient and personal monitoring, the proper selection and use of a variety of personal protective equipment, medical surveillance, safety training, and contingency planning. Proper consideration of these safety issues, including the provision for a peer review and sign-off approval by senior health and safety staff, prior to on-site activity, will result in more effective site operations [24, 38, 44, 47].

The words identification, evaluation, and control in the preceding paragraph allude to the role of the industrial hygienist who, in conjunction with the OHS coordinator and toxicologist, is responsible for assisting in protecting the worker and the general public from the hazards encountered at hazardous waste sites.

The health and safety of the worker and the public should be of primary concern in all phases of investigative and remedial activity at hazardous waste sites, from the most routine site survey involving air, water, soil, or waste sample collection to the most complex site excavation or waste treatment schemes. Therefore, the scope and sophistication of the investigation activity, plus the level of on-site effort, largely dictate the breadth of the industrial hygiene services necessary [44].

Effective implementation requires application of realistic protocols for hazard recognition, evaluation, and control, tied closely to the risks associated with the hazard potential posed by the site. These risk evaluations can vary daily or more often as a project progresses: workers will move to new locations on-site which will result in changes in their proximity in relation to contaminated zones, and/or modification of work practices. As a result, the industrial hygiene and safety monitoring performed during investigative and remedial work at a hazardous waste site differs from conventional industrial hygiene surveys in several ways, including: 1) the varied scope of safety and health concerns involved in such an effort; 2) the need for real-time as well as time-integrated analytical data; 3) the dual focus (occupational and community) of the air monitoring program; 4) the unique, multimedia, often unknown, and difficult to quantify composition of the chemical contaminants and , 5) the adaptation of traditional monitoring and sample collection instrumentation to the specific field setting [44].

It therefore becomes the role of the industrial hygienist to provide continued input during site operations to ensure operations are conducted safely. Early coordination during project planning is essential to integrate safety and industrial hygiene procedures into the operational aspects of the work plan. The industrial hygienist assists the OHS coordinator in developing a safety plan that is specifically tailored to the level of effort and the hazards associated with the work. (This occurs only after an exhaustive data review of background information and relevant toxicological data has been conducted, and the conceptual operations plan that defines the scope of work has been clarified.) The criteria used in the selection of the appropriate scope of the industrial hygiene and safety field protocols prescribed in the safety plan include toxicity-related factors and exposure potential factors [25]. Each of these factors should be defined and considered in conjunction with each of the other factors so as to best characterize the site in a comprehensive manner.

Toxicity-Related Factors	Exposure Potential Factors
absence of chemical/background data	job function
chemical agents	job function
concentrations (background, episodic)	proximity to zones of contamination
dose-response relationships	accident/major release potential
physiologic/synergistic consequences	level of site activity
TLVs, ceiling limits, STELs	physical properties of the agents
odor thresholds	frequency of exposure
percutaneous characteristics	route of exposure
carcinogenic/mutagenic/teratogenic properties	atmospheric dispersion characteristics

In addition to these risk assessment factors, the practical concerns of instrument limitations and sensitivity, sampling frequency and duration, and logistical implementation of the protocols will influence the overall focus and effectiveness of the industrial hygiene and safety program developed for each site.

As the investigation and eventual cleanup of the hazardous waste site progresses, the role of the industrial hygienist expands to address the various objectives of site operations. These objectives include: 1) the upgrading and downgrading of the levels of dermal and respiratory protection on the basis of the physical hazards and the chemical contaminants encountered and their concentrations within the worker's breathing zone; 2) documentation of ambient air and emission episodes for recordkeeping and information planning purposes; 3) on-site sample characterization using real time portable gas chromatographies, photoionization, and infrared devices for the purposes of providing a periodic survey of chemical levels and to prescreen samples so as to reduce the analytical loads or to more accurately identify constituents on a real-time basis; 4) monitoring of on-site personnel both for potential chemical exposure and the effects of heat stress or fatigue, noise, or radiation exposure; 5) the specification of engineering, administrative, or personal protective controls to mitigate any unacceptable hazards; and 6) recommending corrective actions and subsequently evaluating their effectiveness to prevent exposures to on-site or off-site locations beyond the predetermined action levels designed to protect worker or public health. Generally, separate instruments or monitoring procedures must be used to address each of these objectives because of the variable locations or time frames in which the data are needed [47].

In summary, the aspects of health surveillance, industrial hygiene, and safety must be integrated into a single program. The activities of each should serve to interrelate and support each other. Therefore, it is imperative to the success of the overall program that the roles and responsibilities of individuals in each of these areas be closely integrated.

STAFFING AND ORGANIZATION

Size and Qualifications of Health and Safety Staff

The size and organization of a health and safety staff of a company will depend upon the size of the company, the types of jobs and the variety of hazards inherent in performing these jobs, and the amount of resources available for salaries, equipment, and consultant services. Generally, the larger the company, the greater the need to develop in-house health and safety capabilities. Many companies find it more practical and cost-effective initially to hire a consulting service during the preliminary stages of its OHS program development. A consulting company may also be needed for additional support during the various stages of program implementation and for assistance with specific problems which may occur once the program becomes operational. Once the OHS program is running smoothly, however, the use of consultants is generally relegated to those situations where their services simply augment rather than substitute for in-house capabilities.

As mentioned previously, the OHS program staff is generally composed of trained and experienced individuals from the fields of medicine, industrial hygiene, toxicology, engineering, and safety. The number of individuals within an organization possessing these capabilities will depend upon the size and needs of the company. Due to the current demands for such trained and experienced individuals, their acquisition may be difficult, if not initially overwhelming. Many companies therefore attempt to train existing staff members in some of these areas through the use of short courses or through company programs for degree level studies.

At a minimum, the OHS staff should include access to a board certified occupational physician (full-time or consultant), a company OHS director, an industrial hygienist, toxicologist (full-time or consultant), and an equipment manager. The role of the occupational physician, who may either be a full-time employee in the case of a large company, or more commonly, a doctor from a nearby hospital specializing in occupational medicine, is to provide the necessary examination and emergency services as well as to assist in the continued development of a sound health surveillance program.

The OHS program director is responsible for the overall coordination and operation of the complete program. This individual generally reports directly to the company vice-president in charge of environmental affairs. He or she must understand the goals and objectives of the company and be able to develop and implement the necessary programs to achieve them. It is especially important that the director be given the authority to implement programs and procedures, to acquire the necessary funding and to make expenditures to maintain the program, and to delegate responsibilities to other personnel through their supervisors. The director must be familiar with the procedures and materials regarding all workplace operations and possess the knowledge to assess them properly based upon the principles of occupational safety and health.

The OHS director will usually be responsible for supervising a staff of industrial hygienists and safety professionals whose composition again is dependent upon the needs and the size of the company. These professionals obviously should be well trained and experienced, and must be thoroughly familiar with the types of operations being conducted on hazardous waste sites. Their roles within the company will be to fulfill the specific objectives of ensuring worker health and safety at particular waste sites and to coordinate with and support the efforts of the OHS director. Generally, larger companies will hire separate individuals to fill these positions, while small companies will commonly rely upon individuals who possess these dual capabilities.

Obviously, a certain number of support staff will be necessary to assist the health and safety staff in the day-to-day operation of the program. Primarily, clerical staff can fill this gap as well as assist in program communications and budgeting.

Budget

The OHS director is usually made responsible for the preparation of the budget for these activities, receiving assistance from the accounting and clerical staffs. In order to develop a realistic budget which is adequate to meet the needs of the program yet still within the financial bounds allowed for by management, the costs related to specific services and activities must be identified. Generally, these costs are related to the following items [26]:

Labor
- salaries - professional, clerical, and consultant
- social security payments
- unemployment and disability insurance taxes
- fringe benefits

Special Training Programs
- classroom
- hands-on refresher

Materials
- capital expenditures - industrial hygiene, laboratory and safety equipment, supplies, and uniforms
- office supplies - desks, chairs, typewriters, computers, etc.
- replacement of expendable items
- depreciation of equipment and repairs

Overhead
- rent, lights, heat, gas, water, ventilation
- telephone, postage, freight
- fire and theft insurance
- repairs, alterations, maintenance, calibration
- laboratory services
- liability insurance
- medical, toxicological, and industrial hygiene computer information services

Employee Care
- health surveillance examinations - initial, annual, post-exposure, and exit
- emergency care services
- health and safety and other employee and advisory committees

Contingency Fund
- petty cash

Miscellaneous
- travel, including transportation, lodging and meals
- professional journal and textbooks
- special educational and professional advancement training

Other factors to consider in preparing a budget may include:

- The need for new safety and health equipment to allow for better and more efficient monitoring of the employees and the workplace;
- the addition of new health maintenance programs as technology advances;
- the addition of medical and associated services as operations expand to new geographic areas; and,
- the addition of new personnel as the company expands.

Due to the differences in methods of cost accounting, it is difficult, if not impossible, to quantitate the average cost of a health and safety program for all companies within the hazardous waste industry. One company may charge the cost of certain overhead items to the health and safety department, while other companies will exclude these same items from operating costs. Therefore, how a company handles its bookkeeping items will influence the cost of the program. Generally, however, it is assumed that of the budget needed to operate a health and safety program, no more than 2.5 percent would be devoted to health and safety staff functions, while no more than 2.0 percent of the budget would be devoted to the various live organization functions, including the needed training time.

One final word: it is important to recognize that since the OHS program is generally not a revenue producing operation, it will be easy for management to slight its budget when finances get tight. However, the benefits of a preventative health and safety program will lead to:

- increased employee productivity and efficiency;
- reduced absenteeism and illness;
- reduced workmen's compensation rates;
- reduced insurance premiums;
- reduced injury, severity, and frequency rates;
- reduced legal liabilities; and
- improved employee morale and involvement.

REFERENCES

1. Magnuson, E. "The Poisoning of America," *Time Magazine*, (September 1980), pp. 58-69.
2. National Environmental Protection Act, 1969. (NEPA)
3. Occupational Safety and Health Act, 1970. (OSHA)
4. Federal Water Pollution Control Act, 1970 and Amendments, 1972 P.L. 92-500. (FWPCA)
5. Safe Drinking Water Act, 1974. (SDWA)
6. Clean Air Act, 1970 and Amended 1977, 1990. (CAA, CAAA)
7. Clean Water Act, 1977. (CWA)
8. Resource Conservation and Recovery Act and Amendments, 1976,1984. (RCRA)
9. Toxic Substances Control Act, 1976. TSCA)
10. Comprehensive Environmental Response, Compensation, and Liabilities Act, 1980. (CERCLA)
11. Superfund Amendments and Reauthorization Act of 1986. (SARA)
12. OSHA's Worker Protection Standard 29 CFR 1910.120 (HAZWOPER) 1989.
13. OSHA's Hazard Communication Standards (HAZCOMM) 29 CFR 1910.1200 and 29 CFR 1926.59.
14. OSHA - BloodBorne Pathogens Standard 29 CFR 1910.1030.(1991)
15. OSHA - Americans with Disabilities Act - 29 CFR 1910.(1992)
16. OSHA's Process Safety Management Standard 29 CFR 1910.119.(1992)
17. Dalton, J. M., and T. F. Dalton. "Personnel Safety in Hazardous Material Cleanup Operations," in *Proceedings of the 1980 National Conference on Control of Hazardous Materials Spills*, (Nashville, TN: Vanderbilt University, 1980), pp. 264-269.
18. Finch, A. C. "Small Business Needs for Occupational Safety and Health Services," in *Proceedings of Clinic Based Occupational Safety and Health Programs for Small Business*, DHEW (NIOSH) Publication Number 77-172, Cincinnati, 1977, p. 23.
19. Kerr, L. E. "Impact of National Health Insurance on Occupational Safety and Health Services for Small Businesses," in *Proceedings of Clinic Based Occupational Safety and Health Programs for Small Business*, DHEW (NIOSH) Publication Number 77-172, Cincinnati, 1977, p. 6.
20. Bridge, D. P. "Developing and Implementing an Industrial Hygiene and Safety Program in Industry," *American Industrial Hygiene Association Journal*, 40(4):255-263 (1979).

21. McRae, A. D. and K. E. Lawrence, Eds. *Occupational Safety and Health Compliance Manual*, (Germantown, MD: Aspen Systems Corp., 1978).

22. Trauth, C. A., Jr., and J. B. Sorensen. "A New Approach for Assuring Acceptable Levels of Protection from Occupational Safety and Health Hazards," Sandia National Laboratories, SAND 81-1131C, May 1981, Albuquerque, NM.

23. Edward, S. "Quality Circles are Safety Circles," *National Safety News*, 127(6):31-325 (1983).

24. Griffin, R. E. "Safety Circles are 'The New Team in Town'," *National Safety News*, 127(6):31-35 (1983).

25. Halley, P. D. "Industrial Hygiene - Responsibility and Accountability," *American Industrial Hygiene Association Journal*, 41(9):609-615 (1980).

26. Gallagher, G. A. "Health and Safety Program for Hazardous Waste Site Investigations," paper presented to the New England Section of the Association of Engineering Geologists, Boston, MA, February 7, 1981.

27. Dahlstrom, D. L. "Working in Toxic/Hazardous Environments - A question of Health Surveillance," paper presented at the 184th National Meeting of the American Chemical Society, Kansas City, MO, September 12-17, 1982.

28. Dahlstrom, D. L. "Health and Safety Programs for the Hazardous Waste Worker," paper presented at the Engineering 1982 Conference, Buffalo, NY, February 1982.

29. "The Basics of Safety," *Job Safety and Health* - Bureau of National Affairs, Inc., Washington, D.C., April 26, 1983.

30. Gartseff, G. V., and D. L. Dahlstrom. "Safety Planning for Hazardous Waste Site Activities," paper presented at the 184th National Meeting of the American Chemical Society, Kansas City, MO, September 12-17, 1982.

31. Buecker, D. Ecology and Environment, Inc., personal communication, 1982.

32. Howe, H. "Organization and Operation of an Occupational Health Program," *Journal of Occupational Medicine*, 17(6):360-400 (1975).

33. Hall, S.K. "Health Surveillance of Hazardous Materials Workers," *Pollution Engineering*, (9): 58-62 (1992).

34. Lange, J.H., P.L. Spence and P.A. Rosato. "A Medical Surveillance Program for Hazardous Waste Activities and Asbestos Abatement Operation for a Consulting Engineering Firm" *Journal of Environmental Science and Health, Part A*, 26(6) : 953-970 (1991).

35. Udasin, I.G., G. Buckler and M. Gochfeld, "Quality Assurance Audits of Medical Surveillance Programs for Hazardous Waste Workers," *Journal of Occupational Medicine*, 33(11) : 1170-1174 (1991).

36. Enright, P. and P. Scanlon, "Quality Control in Health Screening Minimizes Expensive False-Positives," *Occupational Health and Safety*, 60(4) : 38-44 (1991).

37. Burtan,R.C., "Medical Monitoring's Expanding Role," *Environmental Protection*, 2(6) :16 (1991).

38. Eisenhower, B.M., T.W. Oakes and H.M. Braunstein, "Hazardous Materials Management and Control Program at Oak Ridge National Laboratory-Environmental Protection," *American Industrial Hygiene Journal*, 45(4) : 212-221 (1984).

39. Levine, S. P., R. D. Turpin and M. Gochfeld "Protecting Personnel at Hazardous Waste Sites: Current Issues, " *Applied Occupational and Environmental Hygiene*, 6(12):1007-1014 (1991).

40. Upfel, M. and R. Butan, "Challenges in Medical Surveillance for Hazardous Waste Workers," *Applied Occupational and Environmental Hygiene*, 7(5):303-309 (1992).

41. Harber, P. and I. H. Monoeson, "Medical Surveillance: Interpreting the Results," *Handbook of Occupational Medicine*, R. J. McCunney, Editor, Little, Brown & Company, Boston, Massachusetts, pp 309-323, (1988).

42. McCunney, R. J. "Medical Surveillance: Principles of Establishing an Effective Program," *Handbook of Occupational Medicine*, R. J. McCunney, Editor, Little, Brown and Company, Boston Massachusetts, pp 297-308 (1988).

43. Stockwell, J. R., M. L. Adess, T. B. Titlow and G. R. Zabarias "Use of Sentinel Health Events (Occupational) in Computer Assisted Occupational Health Surveillance," *Aviation, Space, and Environmental Medicine*, 62(8):795-797 (1991).

44. Robinson, S. T. "Role of Industrial Hygiene in Medical Surveillance," *Occupational Medicine: State of Art Reviews*, 5(3):469-478, (1990).

45. King, E., "Occupational Hygiene Aspects of Biological Monitoring," *Annals of Occupational Hygiene*, 34(3):315-322, (1990).

46. NIOSH, "NIOSH Testimony on Hazardous Waste Operations and Emergency Response by R. A. Lemen, October 14, 1987," NIOSH, 16 pages, (1987).

47. Levine, S. P. "The Role of Air Monitoring Techniques in Hazardous Waste Site Personnel Protection and Surveillance Strategies," *Occupational Medicine*, 5(1):109-116 (1990).

48.   Gochfeld, M., "Biological Monitoring of Hazardous Waste Workers: Metals," *Occupational Medicine*, 5(1):25-31 (1990).

49.   Favata, E. A. and M. Gochfeld "Medical Surveillance of Hazardous Waste Workers: Ability of Laboratory Test to Discriminate Exposure," *American Journal of Industrial Medicine*, 15(3):255-265, (1989).

50.   Meli____, J. M., "Medical Surveillance for Hazardous Waste Workers," *Journal of Occupational Medicine*, 28(8):679-683, (1986).

51.   Delta Giustina, J. L., and D. E. Giustina, "Quality of Work Life Programs Through Employee Motivation," *Professional Safety*, 34(5):24-28, (1989).

52.   Menefee, M. L. and S. L. Owens, "Safety Circles," *Incentive*, 162(9):160-161, (1988).

4

TOXICOLOGY OVERVIEW

Virginia T. Kiefert, M.A.

Toxicology is the study of the harmful effects of substances on living organisms. Mankind has long known that there were harmful as well as beneficial consequences associated with taking materials into his body. Those materials which cause damage have been labeled poisons and are the subject matter of Toxicology.

The term "poison" is derived from a Greek word referring to the substance in which arrows were dipped. Industrial hazards or poisons have also been long identified. Clinical symptoms of lead poisoning were accurately described in 1st century A.D. literature regarding mining operations. French hatters of the 17th century discovered that mercuric nitrate aided greatly in the felting of fur. Such use led to chronic mercury poisoning so widespread among members of that trade that the expression "mad as a hatter" entered our folk language.

Our present day society is both chemically impregnated and chemically dependent. The contemporary emphasis is placed not only on man as the object being primarily threatened, but also on the environment, the biosphere. The tremendous increase in the world population, industrial development, and urbanization had a strong influence on this aspect of toxicology. The urbanization of peoples has been accompanied by a strong desire for greater quantities of foodstuffs and industrial products to satisfy the demand for an ever increasing standard of living. Production as well as consumption of energy produces mass quantities and varieties of waste products [1].

The science of Toxicology has developed three principal divisions: Environmental, Economic and Forensic. Environmental Toxicology focuses on the harmful effects to man from chemicals encountered either accidentally or by contact during occupational or recreational activities, or by ingestion as food additives. Economic Toxicology deals with the harmful effects of chemicals that are intentionally administered to achieve a desired effect (i.e., pharmaceutical drugs). Forensic Toxicology deals with the medical and legal aspects of the harmful effects of chemicals on humans [2]. The intent of this chapter is to examine the methods of Environmental Toxicology as they may impact the health and safety of workers at hazardous waste sites.

DOSE-RESPONSE RELATIONSHIP

"No substance is a poison by itself, it is the dose that makes it a poison," according to Paracelsus. Thus, the single most important factor that determines the potential harmfulness or safeness of a compound is the relationship between the concentration of the chemical and the effect that is produced upon the biological mechanism [3].

In preliminary toxicity testing, death of the animals is the response most commonly measured. Given a compound with no known toxicity data, the initial step is one of range finding. A dose is administered and, depending on the outcome, is increased or decreased until a critical range is found over which, at the upper end, all animals die and, at the lower end, all animals survive. Between these extremes is the range in which the toxicologist accumulates data that enable him to prepare a dose-response curve relating percent mortality to dose administered.

From the dose-response curve, the dose that will produce death in 50% of the animals may be calculated. This value is commonly abbreviated as LD_{50}. It is a statistically obtained value representing the best estimation that can be made from the experimental data at hand. The dose is expressed as amount per unit of body weight. The value should be accompanied by an indication of the species of experimental animal used, the route of administration of the compound, the vehicle used to dissolve or suspend the material if applicable, and the time period over which the animals were observed. For example, a publication might state "For rats, the 24hr. ip LD_{50} for 'x' in corn oil was 66 mg/kg (95% confidence limits 59-74)." This would indicate to the reader that the material was given to rats as an intraperitoneal injection of compound x dissolved or suspended in corn oil and that the investigator had limited her mortality count to 24 hours after administering the compound. If the experiment has involved inhalation as the route of exposure, the dose to the animals is expressed as parts per million, mg/m^3, or some other appropriated expression of concentration of the material in the air of the exposure chamber, and the length of exposure time is specified. In this case the term LC_{50} is used to designate the concentration in air that may be expected to kill 50% of the animals exposed for the specified length of time.

The simple determination of the LD_{50} for an unknown compound provides an initial comparative index for the location of the compound in the overall spectrum of toxic potency. Table 4-1 shows an attempt at utilizing LD_{50} and LC_{50} values to set up an approximate classification of toxic substances.

Over and above the specific LD_{50} value, the slope of the dose-response curve provides useful information. It suggests an index of the margin of safety, that is the magnitude of the range of doses involved in going from a noneffective dose to a lethal dose. It is obvious that if the dose-response curve is very steep, this margin of safety is slight. Another situation may arise in which one compound would be rated as more toxic than a second compound if the LD_{50} values alone were compared, but the reverse assessment of relative toxicity would be reached if the comparison was made of the LD_{50} values for the two compounds because the dose-response curve for the second compound had a more gradual slope. It should thus be apparent that the slope of the dose-response curve may be of considerable significance with respect to establishing relative toxicities of compounds.

Table 4-1. Toxicity Classes			
Toxicity Rating	Descriptive Term	Single Oral Dose Rates	LD_{50} wt/kg 4hr. Inhalation LC_{50} PPM Rats
1	Extremely toxic	1mg or less	10
2	Highly toxic	1-50mg	10-100
3	Moderately toxic	50-500mg	100-1000
4	Slightly toxic	0.5-5g	1000-10,000
5	Practically nontoxic	5-15g	10,000-100,000
6	Relatively harmless	15g or more	100,000

By similar experiments dose-response curves may be obtained using a criterion other than mortality as the response and an ED_{50} value is obtained. This is the dose that produced the chosen response in 50% of the treated animals. When the study of a toxic substance progresses to the point at which its action on the organism may be studied as graded response in groups of animals, dose-response curves of a slightly different sort are generally used. One might see, for example, a dose-response curve relating the degree of depression of brain choline esterase to the dose of an organic phosphorus ester or a dose-response curve relating the increase in pulmonary flow-resistance to the concentration of sulfur dioxide inhaled.

ROUTES OF EXPOSURE

Toxic chemicals can enter the body by various routes. The chemical and physical properties of each compound largely determine the route by which intentional or accidental exposure occurs. The routes of *Parenteral* (injection), *Oral, Inhalation,* and *Percutaneous* (skin) will be addressed [4].

Parenteral: Aside from the obvious use in administration of drugs, injection is considered mainly as a route of exposure of experimental animals. The injection can be into the skin (intradermal), beneath the skin (subcutaneous), in the muscle (intramuscular), into the blood of the veins (intravenous), or into the spinal fluid (intrapleural). The dose administered is known with accuracy. Intravenous (iv) injection introduces the material directly into the circulation, hence comparison of the degree of response to iv injection with the response to the dose administered by another route can provide information on the rate of uptake of the material by another route. When a material is administered by injection, the highest concentration of the toxic material in the body occurs at the time of entrance. The organism receives the initial impact at the maximal concentration without opportunity for a gradual reaction; whereas, if the concentration is built up more gradually by some other route of exposure, the organism may have time to develop some resistance or physiological adjustment that could produce a modified response. In experimental studies intraperitoneal (ip) injection of the material into the abdominal fluid is a frequently used technique. The major venous blood circulation from the abdominal contents proceeds via the portal circulation to the liver. A material administered by ip injection is subject to the special metabolic transformation mechanisms of the liver, as well as the possibility of excretion via the bile before it reaches general circulation. If the LD_{50} of a compound given by ip injection was much higher (i.e., the toxicity is lower) than the LD_{50} by iv injection, this fact would suggest that the material was being detoxified by the liver or that the bile was a major route of excretion of the material. If the values for LD_{50} were very similar for ip and iv injection, it would suggest that neither of these factors played a major role in the handling of that particular compound by that particular species of animal.

Oral: Ingestion occurs as a route of exposure of workers through eating or smoking with contaminated hands or in contaminated work areas. Ingestion of inhaled materials also occurs. One mechanism for the clearance of particles from the respiratory tract is the carrying up of the particles by the action of the ciliated lining of the respiratory tract. These particles are then swallowed and absorption of the material may occur from the gastrointestinal tract. This situation is most likely to occur with larger size particles although smaller particles deposited in the alveoli may be carried by phagocytes to the upward moving mucous carpet and eventually to be swallowed. The toxicity of orally administered chemicals may vary with the frequency with which they are given, and with the conditions under which they are given; that is, whether they are mixed with food or given on an empty stomach.

In experimental work, compounds may be administered orally as either a single or multiple dose given by stomach tube or the material may be incorporated in the diet or drinking water for periods varying from several weeks or months up to several years or the lifetime of the animals. In either case, the dose the animals actually receive may be ascertained with considerable accuracy. Except in the case of a substance that has a corrosive action or in some way damages the lining of the gastrointestinal tract, the response to a substance administered orally will depend on how readily it is absorbed from the gut. Uranium, for example, is capable of producing kidney damage, but is poorly absorbed from the gut and so oral administration produces only low concentrations at the site of action. On the other hand, ethyl alcohol, which has as a target organ the central nervous system, is very rapidly absorbed and within an hour 90% of an ingested dose has been absorbed.

The epithelium of the gastrointestinal tract is poorly permeable to the ionized form of organic compounds. Absorption of such materials generally occurs by diffusion of the lipid-soluble non-ionized form. Weak acids that are predominately nonionized in the high acidity (pH 1.4) of gastric juice are absorbed from the stomach. The surface of the intestinal mucosa has a pH of 5.3. At this higher pH weak bases are less ionized and more readily absorbed. The pH of a compound thus becomes an important factor in predicting absorption from the gastrointestinal tract.

Inhalation: Inhalation exposures are of prime importance to the industrial toxicologist. Exposure to chemicals in the atmosphere is accomplished by unavoidable inhalation of such agents unless devices are used to remove the atmospheric contaminants before they enter the respiratory tract. In experimental work, the dose actually received and retained by the animals is not known with the same accuracy as when a compound is given by the routes previously discussed. This route depends on the ventilation rate of the individual. In the case of a gas, it is influenced by *solubility* and in the case of an aerosol by *particle size*. The concentration and time of exposure can be measured and this gives a working estimate of the exposure. Two techniques are sometimes utilized in an attempt to determine the dose with precision and still administer the compound via the lung. One is intratracheal injection, which may be used in some experiments in which it is desirable to deliver a known amount of particulate material into the lung. The other is so-called precision gassing. In this technique the animal or experimental subject breathes through a valve system and the volume of exhaled air and the concentration of toxic material in it are determined. A comparison of these data with the concentration in the atmosphere of the exposure chamber gives an indication of the dose retained.

Percutaneous: Cutaneous exposure ranks first in the production of occupational disease, but not necessarily first in severity. In order to pass into the skin, the chemical must either traverse the epidural cells or enter through the follicles. Although the transfollicular pathway provides access to the deeper layers of the skin via relatively permeable cells of sebaceous glands and the follicular walls, the pathway through the epidermal cells is probably the main avenue of penetration because this tissue constitutes the majority of the surface area.

The skin and its associated film of lipids and sweat may act as an effective barrier. The chemical may react with the skin surface and cause primary irritation. The agent may penetrate the skin and cause sensitization to repeated exposure. The material may penetrate the skin in an amount sufficient to cause systemic poisoning. In assessing the toxicity of a compound by skin application, a known amount of the material to be studied is placed on the clipped skin of the animal and held in place with a rubber cuff. Some materials such as acids, alkalis, and many organic solvents are primary skin irritants and produce skin damage on initial contact. Other materials are sensitizing agents. The initial contact produces no irritant response, but may render the individual sensitive and dermatitis may result from future contact. Ethyleneamines and the catechols in the well-known members of the Rhus family (poison ivy and poison oak) are examples of such agents. The physicochemical properties of a material are the main determinant of whether or not a material will be absorbed through the skin. Among the important factors are pH, extent of ionization, water and lipid solubility, and molecular size. Some compounds, such as phenol and phenolic derivatives, can readily penetrate the skin in amounts sufficient to produce systemic intoxication. If the skin is damaged, the normal protective barrier to absorption of chemicals is lessened and penetration may occur. An example of this is a description of cases of mild lead intoxication that occurred in an operation that involved an inorganic lead salt and also a cutting oil. Inorganic lead salts would not be absorbed through intact skin, but the dermatitis produced by the cutting oil permitted increased absorption.

CRITERIA OF RESPONSE

After the toxic material has been administered by one of the routes of exposure discussed above, there are various criteria to evaluate the response. These criteria are oriented whenever possible towards elucidating the mechanisms of action of the material.

Mortality: As has been indicated, the LD_{50} of a substance serves as an initial test to place the compound appropriately in the spectrum of toxic agents. Mortality is also a criterion of response in long-term chronic studies. In such studies, the investigator must be certain that the mortality observed was due to the chronic low level of the material she is studying; hence, an adequate control group of untreated animals subject to otherwise identical conditions is maintained for the duration of the experiment.

Pathology: Organ toxicity covers a wide range of organ systems and toxic effects. In addition to the heart, lungs, kidneys, and liver, toxic effects can also decrease functioning of the pancreas, spleen, thymus, and even nondiscrete organs, such as the skin. In many cases, the effects on one organ system may be manifested throughout the body. For example, depression of thymus function may reduce the efficacy of the immune system and so make the organism susceptible to infectious diseases. Effects may be less general in other cases such as skin lesions, e.g., chloracne. The liver and the kidneys are organs particularly sensitive to the action of a variety of toxic agents. In some instances the pathological lesion is typical of the specific toxic agents; for example, the silicotic nodules in the lungs produced by inhalation of free silica or the pattern of liver damage resulting from exposure to carbon tetrachloride and some other hepatotoxins. In other cases the damage may be more diffuse and less specific in nature.

Growth: In chronic studies the effect of the toxic agent on the growth rate of the animals is another criterion of response. Levels of the compound that do not produce death or overt pathology may result in a diminished rate of growth. A record is also made of the food intake. This will indicate whether diminished growth results from lessened food intake or from less efficient use of food ingested. It sometimes happens that when an agent is administered by incorporation into the diet, especially at high levels, the food is unpalatable to the animals and they simply refuse to eat it.

Organ weight: The weight of various organs, or more specifically the ratio of organ weight to body weight, may be used as a criterion of response. In some instances such alterations are specific and explicable, as for example, the increase of lung weight to body weight ratio as a measure of the edema produced by irritants such as ozone or oxides of nitrogen. In other instances the increase is a less specific general hypertrophy of the organ, especially of the liver and kidney.

Physiological Function Tests: Physiological function tests are useful criteria of response both in experimental studies and in assessing the response of exposed workers. (For more information, see Chapter 7, Medical Surveillance for Hazardous Waste Workers.) They can be especially useful in chronic studies in that they do not necessitate the killing of the animal and can, if desired, be done at regular intervals throughout the period of study. Tests in common clinical use such as bromsulphalein retention, thymol turbidity, or serum alkaline phosphatase may be used to assess the effect of an agent on liver function. The examination of the renal clearance of various substances helps give an indication of localization of kidney damage. The ability of the kidney (especially in the rat) to produce a concentrated urine may be measured by the *osmolality* of the urine produced. This has been suggested for the evaluation of alterations in kidney function. Alterations may be detected following inhalation of materials such a chlorotrifluoroethylene at levels of reversible response. In some instances measurement of blood pressure has proved a sensitive means of evaluating response. Various tests include relatively simple tests that are suitable for use in field surveys as well as more complex methods possible only under laboratory conditions. Simple tests include such measurements as peak expiratory flow rate (PEFR), forced vital capacity (FVC), and 1 second forced expiratory volume (FEV), More complex procedures include the measurement of pulmonary mechanics (flow-resistance and compliance).

Biochemical Studies: The study of biochemical response to toxic agents leads in many instances to an understanding of the mechanism of action. Tests of toxicity developed in animals should be oriented to determination of early response from exposures that are applicable to the industrial scene. Many toxic agents act by inhibiting the action of specific enzymes. This action may be studied *in vitro* and *in vivo*. In the first case, the toxic agent is added to tissue slices or tissue homogenate from normal animals and the degree of inhibition of enzymatic activity is measured by an appropriate technique. In the second case, the toxic agent is administered to the animals; after the desired interval the animals are killed and the degree of enzyme inhibition is measured in the appropriate tissues. A judicious combination of in vivo and in vitro studies is especially useful when biotransformation to a toxic compound is involved. The classic example of this is the toxicity of fluoroacetate. This material, which was extremely toxic when administered to animals of various species, did not inhibit any known enzymes in vitro. Fluoroacetate entered the carboxylic acid cycle of metabolism as if it were acetic acid. The product formed was fluorocitrate, which was a potent inhibitor of the enzyme aconitase. Biological conversion in the living animal had resulted in the formation of a highly toxic compound. The term lethal synthesis describes such a transformation.

DETOXICATION MECHANISMS

Because of the proliferation of chemicals in working environments and the resulting exposure of workers to potentially toxic substances, it has become necessary to establish some standards regarding the limits of contamination of the atmosphere which could be considered safe.

Threshold Limit Values: (TLVs) have been compiled by the American Conference of Governmental Industrial Hygienists for approximately 400 substances. TLVs refer to airborne concentrations of substances and represent conditions under which it is believed that nearly all humans may be repeatedly exposed day after day without adverse effects. TLVs for air contaminants that exist as gases or fumes are expressed as ppm (parts per million parts of air by volume at 25° C and 760mm Hg pressure). TLVs for respirable dusts, which are suspended in the air are in terms of mppcf (millions of particles per cubic foot of air).

The use of biologic threshold limit values provides a valuable adjunct to TLVs, which are based on air analysis. The analysis of blood, urine, hair, or exhaled air for a toxic material per se (e.g., Pb, As) or for a metabolite of the toxic agent (e.g., thiocyanate, phenal) gives an indication of the exposure of an individual worker. These tests represent a very practical application of data from experimental toxicology. Research in industrial toxicology is often oriented toward the search for a test suitable for use as a biologic threshold that will indicate exposure at a level below which damage occurs. Biological monitoring determines both the occurrence of exposure and the uptake (or presence) of a particular substance or its metabolites in body fluids or organs; it can be used to estimate the dose to effector organs and possibly the concentration at binding sites (receptor compartment) in the critical organs. It may complement both medical surveillance and environmental monitoring [5]. (For more information, see Chapter 7, Medical Surveillance for Hazardous Waste Workers.)

HEALTH & SAFETY STANDARDS AND THEIR DEVELOPMENT

Historically, there has been very little concern for protecting the health of the worker prior to 1900. The English Factory Acts of 1833 were the first example of government's interest in the health of the working man. This interest was more toward providing compensation for accidents than in the area of prevention. In 1908, the U.S. Government passed a compensation act for certain civil employees and by 1948 all states had passed such legislation. This focus on compensation led to the development of industrial health and safety as it became more profitable to control the environment than to pay for its negative health effects [6].

In 1912, the U.S. Public Health Service was given the authority to investigate conditions relating to worker health and safety in many industries and to make recommendations for concrete, workable solutions. NIOSH, a division of the U.S. Public Health service has formalized a system for developing criteria on which to base standards for ensuring the health and safety of workers exposed to hazardous chemicals and physical agents. The resulting criteria and recommended standards are intended to help management and labor develop better engineering controls and more healthful work practices. The established criteria and the published recommendations (criteria documents) of NIOSH are the scientific bases for the standards setting and enforcement work of OSHA [7].

TYPES OF TOXIC EFFECTS

There are two generally recognized kinds of adverse health effects induced by chemical exposures at work. *Acute* health effects result in undesirable and irreversible health changes in short periods of time (in the order of magnitude of a few seconds or minutes). *Chronic* effects reflect the cumulative bodily damage resulting from repetitive exposures that do not produce immediately irreversible consequences. The techniques for measuring the lower levels of exposure that typically produce chronic health effects frequently differ from those used to measure exposures which may result in acute effects. Because immediate decisions concerning protection are usually required, direct-reading instruments are ordinarily used to evaluate exposures likely to result in acute effects [5]. (For more information, see Chapter 5, Air Monitoring at Hazardous Waste Sites.)

Although toxic effects are divided into acute, subacute, and chronic on the basis of time course, it is not possible to categorize each type of toxicity or the effects of individual chemicals into one of these three classifications. For example, lung toxicity may be an acute, subacute, or chronic effect. Similarly, a particular chemical may produce an acute effect at one exposure level and a subacute or chronic effect at another. Despite these classification difficulties, it has been common practice to identify the different types of toxicity with one of the three time-course categories. Thus organ damage has been classified as an acute or subacute effect, and most other types of toxicity have been assigned to the chronic classification. The effects generally included in the chronic category are carcinogenesis, teratogenesis, reproductive toxicity, and mutagenesis [6].

Lung Toxicity: The lung can be acutely affected in various ways by toxic substances. Direct damage to lung cells and thereby lung function can be caused by inhalation of oxidizing gases such as oxygen, ozone or nitrogen dioxide. Indirect lung damage can result from the ingestion of chemicals or via cutaneous absorption. An example of this indirect process of lung damage is seen in the results of exposure to paraquat (agricultural insecticide). This chemical causes lung cell damage following absorption through the skin or gastrointestinal tract.

In contrast, chronic lung damage can result from long term exposure to a toxicant. Two examples that are well documented are emphysema from smoking and asbestosis from prolonged exposure to asbestos.

Respiratory illness in workers of an indoor Shitake mushroom farm was investigated by Lenhart and Cole [9]. Predominant symptoms were dry cough, nasal discharge, sneezing, productive couch and dyspnea. Shitake mushrooms are grown on logs, usually outdoors, but more recently indoors as well and are harvested in the mature state when there is active sporulatim. Upon reviewing the results of an acute symptoms questionnaire and learning that allergenic mold and mushroom spores were available for inhalation in high concentrations during harvesting work, the management decided to implement a respiratory protection program which included half mask air-purifying respirators, disposable uniforms, a medical surveillance program and pulmonary function tests.

Kidney Toxicity: Toxicants that interfere with kidney function can produce severe adverse effects. The most common and well studied example is lead. The presence of lead inhibits the blood filtering capacities of the kidney and allows increasing concentrations of damaging chemicals in tissues and organs throughout the body. Thus while the kidney is the original site of toxicity, the damage is more universal.

Carcinogenesis: Cancer is the chronic toxic effect that is of most concern to the general population and is the most well studied. Carcinogenesis results from uncontrollable cell proliferation and may result from toxic alterations of only a single cell. The study of the carcinogenic effects of a toxic chemical is a complex experimental problem. Such testing involves the use of sizable groups of animals observed over a period of two years in rats or four to five years in dogs because of the long latent period required for the development of cancer. Efforts to shorten the time lag have led to the use of aging animals. This may reduce the lag period one third to one fourth. Various strains of inbred mice or hamsters are frequently used in such experiments. Quite frequently materials are screened by painting on the skin of experimental animals, especially mice. Industrial experience down through the years has made plain the hazard of cancer from exposure to various chemicals. Among these are many of the polynuclear hydrocarbons, beta-naphylamine, which produces bladder cancer, chromates, and nickel carbonyl, which produce lung cancer.

A common industrial hazard is the process of welding [10]. Metal fume fever is an acute respiratory disease that is usually of short duration [11]. Studies have taken in effect the smoking habits of welders [12]. As expected, welders and controls that smoked reported a higher frequency of respiratory symptoms than corresponding non-smokers.

Teratogenesis: Teratogenesis is the formation of birth defects in offspring, often as a result of maternal or paternal exposure to a toxicant. It is usually classified as a chronic effect, even though the toxicity appears within a relatively short period of time (the term of the pregnancy). Since some birth defects caused by toxicity are inheritable, the time course is much longer. Chemicals administered to the pregnant animal may, under certain conditions, produce malformations of the fetus without inducing damage to the mother or killing the fetus. The experience with the birth of many infants with limb anomalies resulting from the use of thalidomide by the mothers during pregnancy alerted the toxicologists to the need for more rigid testing in this difficult area. Recent studies have reported the occurrence of hypospadias (malformation of the sexual organs) at birth in two boys whose mother had been occupationally exposed to EGMEA (ethylene glycol monomethyl ether acetate) during her pregnancies [13]. She had worked in an industrial laboratory that produced lacquers and enameled wire [14].

Another example of human experience in recent times was the teratogenic effect of methyl mercury as demonstrated in the incidents of poisoning in Minamata Bay, Japan. The study of the teratogenic potential poses a very complex toxicological problem. The susceptibility of various species of animals varies greatly in the area of teratogenic effects. The timing of the dose is very critical as a chemical may produce severe malformations of one sort if it reaches the embryo at one period of development and either no malformations or malformations of a completely different character if it is administered at a later or earlier period of embryogenesis.

Reproductive Toxicity: Reproductive Toxicity is a broad category that includes a variety of effects on the reproductive capacity of living systems. These effects can involve decreases in fertility, decreases in percent of conceptions leading to live birth, or fetal or embryonic toxicity. This last category may be distinguished from teratogennicity in that the toxicity does not lead to birth defects, but instead, may lead to reduced birth weight or size. Two common toxicants that can lead to such phytotoxicity are alcohol and tobacco [7].

The effects of combined EGME (ethylene glycol monomethyl ether) and EGEE (ethylene glycol monomethyl ether) exposure on the reproductive potential of men working in a large ship building facility was recently studied [15]. The authors concluded that exposure to EBME and EGEE caused functional impairment by lowering sperm counts, in addition, when the results were controlled for the effects of smoking, there was an increased odds ratio for a lower sperm count per ejaculate.

It is possible that a level of a toxic material can have an effect on either male or female animals that will result in decreased fertility. In fertility studies the chemical is given to males and females in daily doses for the full cycle of oogenesis and spermatogenesis prior to mating. If gestation is established, the fetuses are removed by caesarean section one day prior to delivery. The litter size and viability are compared with untreated groups. The young are then studied to determine possible effects on survival, growth rate, and maturation. The tests may be repeated through a second and third litter of the treated animals. If it is considered necessary the test may be extended through the second and third generation.

FACTORS INFLUENCING INTENSITY OF TOXIC ACTION

One of the factors influencing the intensity of the toxic action has already been mentioned; i.e., the route of exposure. For example, when a substance is administered as an iv injection, the material has maximum opportunity to be carried by the blood stream throughout the body, whereas other routes of exposure interpose a barrier to distribution of the material. The effectiveness of this barrier will govern the intensity of toxic action of a given amount of toxic agent administered by various routes. Lead, for example, is toxic both by ingestion and by inhalation. An equivalent dose, however, is more readily absorbed from the respiratory tract than from the gastrointestinal tract, and hence produces a greater response.

There is frequently a difference in intensity of response and sometimes a difference even in the nature of the response between the acute and chronic toxicity of a material. If a material is taken into the body at a rate sufficiently slow that the rate of excretion and/or detoxification keeps pace with the intake, it is possible that no toxic response will result even though the same total amount of material taken in at a faster rate would result in a concentration of the agent at the site of action sufficient to produce a toxic response. Information of this sort enters into the concept of a threshold limit for safe exposure. Hydrogen sulfide is a good example of a substance that is rapidly lethal at high concentrations as evidenced by the many accidental deaths it has caused. It has an acute action on the nervous system with rapid production of respiratory paralysis unless the victim is promptly removed to fresh air and revived with appropriate artificial respiration. On the other hand, hydrogen sulfide is rapidly oxidized in the plasma to nontoxic substances, and many times the lethal dose produces relatively little effect if administered slowly. Benzene is a good example of a material that differs in the nature of response depending on whether the exposure is an acute one to a high concentration or a chronic exposure to a lower level. If one used as criteria the 4 hr LC_{50} for rats of 16,000 ppm, which has been reported for benzene, one would conclude that this material would be "practically nontoxic" which, of course, is contrary to fact. The mechanism of acute death is narcosis. Chronic exposure to low levels of benzene on the other hand produces damage to the blood-forming tissue of the bone marrow, and chronic benzene intoxication may appear even many years after the actual exposure to benzene has ceased.

Other factors that directly influence the intensity of a toxic effect are the *age*, *state of health*, and *previous exposure history* of the worker. Some work environments also introduce environmental variables that have bearing on toxic intensity. (For more information, see Chapter 7, Medical Surveillance for Hazardous Waste Workers.)

Age: It is well known that, in general, infants and the newborn are more sensitive to many toxic agents than are adults of the same species, but this has relatively little bearing on a discussion of industrial toxicology. Older persons or older animals are also often more sensitive to toxic action than are younger adults. With aging comes a diminished reserve capacity in the face of toxic stress. This reserve capacity may be either functional or anatomical. The excess mortality in the older age groups during and immediately following the well-known acute air pollution incidents is a case in point. There is experimental evidence from electron microscope studies that younger animals exposed to pollutants have a capacity to repair lung damage that was lost in older animals.

State of Health: Pre-existing disease can result in greater sensitivity to toxic agents. In the case of specific diseases that would contraindicate exposure to specific toxic agents, pre-placement medical examination can prevent possible hazardous exposure. For example, an individual with some degree of pre-existing methemoglobinemia would not be placed in a work situation involving exposure to nitrobenzene. Since it is known that the uptake of manganese parallels the uptake of iron, it would be unwise to employ a person with known iron deficiency anemia as a manganese miner. It has been shown that viral agents will increase the sensitivity of animals to exposure to oxidizing type air pollutants. Nutritional status also affects response to toxic agents.

Previous Exposure: Previous exposure to a toxic agent can lead to either tolerance, increased sensitivity, or make no difference in the degree of response. Some toxic agents function by sensitization and the initial exposures produce no observable response, but subsequent exposures will do so. In these cases the individuals who are thus sensitized must be removed from exposure. In other instances, if an individual is re-exposed to a substance before complete reversal of the change produced by a previous exposure, the effect may be more dangerous. A case in point would be an exposure to an organophosphorus insecticide that would lower the level of acetylcholine esterase. Given time, the level will be restored to normal. If another exposure occurs prior to this, the enzyme activity may be further reduced to dangerous levels. Previous exposure to low levels of a substance may in some cases protect against subsequent exposure to levels of a toxic agent that would be damaging if given initially. This may come about through the induction of enzymes that detoxify the compound or by other mechanisms often not completely understood. It has been shown, for example, that exposure of mice to low levels of ozone will prevent death from pulmonary edema in subsequent high exposures. There is also a considerable cross tolerance among the oxidizing irritants such as ozone and hydrogen peroxide, an exposure to low levels of the one protecting against high levels of the other.

Environmental Factors: Physical factors can also affect the response to toxic agents. In industries such as smelting or steel making, high temperatures are encountered. Pressures different than normal ambient atmospheric pressure can be encountered in caissons or tunnel construction.

CLASSIFICATION OF TOXIC MATERIALS

Toxic agents may be classified in several ways. No one of these is of itself completely satisfactory. A toxic agent may have its action on the organ with which it comes into first contact. Let us assume for the moment that the agent is inhaled. Materials such as irritant gases or acid mists produce a more or less rapid response from the respiratory tract when present in sufficient concentration. Other agents, such as silica or asbestos, also damage the lungs but the response is seen only after lengthy exposure. Other toxic agents may have no effect on the organ through which they enter the body, but exert what is called systemic toxic action when they have been absorbed and translocated to the site of biological action. Examples of such agents would be mercury vapor, manganese, lead, chlorinated hydrocarbons, and many others that are readily absorbed through the lungs, but produce typical toxic symptoms only in other organ systems.

Physical Classifications: This type of classification is an attempt to base the discussion of toxic agents on the form in which they are present in the air. These are discussed as *gases* and *vapors* or as *aerosols*.

1. *Gases and Vapors*: In common industrial hygiene usage the term *gas* is usually applied to a substance that is in the gaseous state at room temperature and pressure and the term *vapor* is applied to the gaseous phase of a material that is ordinarily a solid or a liquid at room temperature and pressure. In considering the toxicity of a gas or vapor, the solubility of the material is of the utmost importance. If the material is an irritant gas, solubility in aqueous media will determine the amount of material that reaches the lung and hence its site of action. A highly soluble gas, such as ammonia, is taken up readily by the mucous membranes of the nose and upper respiratory tract. Sensory response to irritation in these areas provides the individual with warning of the presence of an irritant gas. On the other hand, a relatively insoluble gas such as nitrogen dioxide is not scrubbed out by the upper respiratory tract, but penetrates readily to the lung. Amounts sufficient to lead to pulmonary edema and death may be inhaled by an individual who is not at the time aware of the hazard. The solubility coefficient of a gas or vapor in blood is one of the factors determining rate of uptake and saturation of the body. With a very soluble gas, saturation of the body is slow, is largely dependent on ventilation of the lungs, and is only slightly influenced by changes in circulation. In the case of a slightly

soluble gas, saturation is rapid, depends chiefly on the rate of circulation, and is little influenced by the rate of breathing. If the vapor has a high fat solubility, it tends to accumulate in the fatty tissues that it reaches carried in the blood. Since fatty tissue often has a meager blood supply, complete saturation of the fatty tissue may take a longer period. It is also of importance whether the vapor or gas is one that is readily metabolized. Conversion to a metabolite would tend to lower the concentration in the blood and shift the equilibrium toward increased uptake. It is also of importance whether such metabolic products are toxic.

2. *Aerosols*: An aerosol is composed of solid or liquid particles of microscopic size dispersed in a gaseous medium (for our purposes, air). Special terms are used for indicating certain types of particles. Some of these are; *dust*, a dispersion of solid particles usually resulting from the fracture of larger masses of material such as in drilling, crushing, or grinding operations; *mist*, a dispersion of liquid particles, many of which are visible; *fog*, visible aerosols of a liquid formed by condensation; *fume*, an aerosol of solid particles formed by condensation of vaporized materials; *smoke*, aerosols resulting from incomplete combustion that consists mainly of carbon and other combustible materials. The toxic response to an aerosol depends obviously on the nature of the material, which may have as a target organ the respiratory system or may be a systemic toxic agent acting elsewhere in the body. In either case, the toxic potential of a given material dispersed as an aerosol is only partially described by a statement of the concentration of the material in terms of weight per unit volume or number of particles per unit volume. For a proper assessment of the toxic hazard, it is necessary to have information also on the particle size and distribution of the material. Understanding of this fact has led to the development of instruments that sample only particles in the respirable size range. (See Chapter 5, Air Monitoring at Hazardous Waste Sites.)

The particle size of an aerosol is the key factor in determining its site of deposition in the respiratory tract and as a sequel to this, the clearance mechanisms that will be available for its subsequent removal. The deposition of an aerosol in the respiratory tract depends on the physical forces of impaction, settling, and diffusion or Brownian movement that apply to the removal of any aerosol from the atmosphere, as well as on anatomical and physiological factors such as the geometry of the lungs and the air-flow rates and patterns occurring during the respiratory cycle.

In the limited space available only one point will be emphasized here, namely, the toxicological importance of particles below 1 m in size. Aerosols in the range of 0.2-0.4 μm tend to be fairly stable in the atmosphere. This comes about because they are too small to be effectively removed by forces of settling or impaction and too big to be effectively removed by diffusion. Since these are the forces that lead to deposition in the respiratory tract, it has been predicted theoretically and confirmed experimentally that a lesser percentage of these particles is deposited in the respiratory tract. On the other hand, since they are stable in the atmosphere, there are large numbers of them present to be inhaled, and to dismiss this size range as of minimal importance is an error in toxicological thinking that should be corrected whenever it is encountered. Aerosols in the size range below 1.0 μm are also of major toxicological importance. The percentage deposition of these extremely small particles is as great as for 1 μm particles and this deposition is alveolar. Particles in the submicron range also appear to have greater potential for interaction with irritant gases, a fact that is of importance in air pollution toxicology.

Chemical Classification: Toxic compounds may be classified according to their chemical nature. The most recent volume of the Merck Index is an excellent reference [18]. Knowledge of the chemical nature of a compound, i.e., oxidizers, reducers, corrosives, etc. is required by the user. Another approach more accessible to the health and safety personnel is the NIOSH Pocket Guide to Chemical Hazards®.

Physiological Classification: Such classification attempts to frame the discussion of toxic materials according to their biological action.

Irritants: The basis of classifying these materials is their ability to cause inflammation of mucous membranes with which they come in contact. While many irritants are strong acids or alkalis familiar as corrosive to nonliving things such as lab coats or bench tops, bear in mind that inflammation is the reaction of a living tissue and is distinct from chemical corrosion. The inflammation of tissue results from concentrations far below those needed to produce corrosion. As was indicated earlier in discussing gases and vapors, solubility is an important factor in determining the site of irritant action in the respiratory tract. Highly soluble materials such as ammonia, alkaline dust and mists, hydrogen chlorides and hydrogen fluoride affect mainly the upper respiratory tract. Other materials of intermediate solubility such as the halogens, ozone, diethyl or dimethyl sulfate, and phosphorus chlorides affect both the upper respiratory tract and the pulmonary tissue. Insoluble materials, such as nitrogen dioxide, arsenic trichlorides, or phosgene, affect primarily the lung. There are exceptions to the statement that solubility serves to indicate site of action. One such is ethyl ether and other insoluble compounds that are readily absorbed unaltered from the alveoli and hence do not accumulate in that area. In the upper respiratory passages and bronchi where the material is more readily absorbed, it can accumulate in concentrations sufficient to produce irritation. Another exception is in materials such as bromobenzyl cyanide that is a vapor from a liquid boiling well above room temperature. It is taken up by the eyes and skin as a mist. In initial action, then, it is a powerful lachrymator and upper respiratory irritant, rather than producing a primarily alveolar reaction as would be predicted from its low solubility.

Irritants can also cause changes in the mechanics of respiration such as increased pulmonary flow-resistance or decreased compliance (a measure of elastic behavior of the lungs). One group of irritants, among which are sulfur dioxide, acetic acid, formaldehyde, formic acid, sulfuric acid, acrolein, and iodine, produce a pattern in which the flow-resistance is increased, the compliance is decreased only slightly and at higher concentrations the frequency of breathing is decreased. Another group, among which are ozone, and oxides of nitrogen, has little effect on resistance, produces a decrease in compliance and an increase in respiratory rate. There is evidence that in the case an irritant aerosol, the irritant potency of a given material tends to increase with decreasing particle size as assessed by the increase in flow-resistance. Following respiratory mechanics measurements in cases exposed to irritant aerosols, the histologic sections prepared after rapid freezing of the lungs showed the anatomical sites of constriction. Long-term chronic lung impairment may be caused by irritants either as sequelae to a single very severe exposure or as the result of chronic exposure to low concentrations of the irritant. There is evidence in experimental animals that long-term exposure to respiratory irritants can lead to increased mucous secretion and a condition resembling the pathology of human chronic bronchitis without the intermediary of infection. The epidemiological assessment of this factor in the health of residents of polluted urban atmospheres is currently a vital area of research.

Irritants are usually further subdivided into primary and secondary irritants. A primary irritant is a material that for all practical purposes exerts no systemic toxic action either because the products formed on the tissues of the respiratory tract are nontoxic or because the irritant action is far in excess of any systemic toxic action. Examples of the first type would be hydrochloric acid or sulfuric acid. Examples of the second type would be materials such as Lewisite or mustard gas, which would be quite toxic on absorption but death from the irritation would result before sufficient amounts to produce systemic poisoning would be absorbed. Secondary irritants are materials that do produce irritant action on mucous membranes, but this effect is overshadowed by systemic effects resulting from absorption. Examples of materials in this category are hydrogen sulfide and many of the aromatic hydrocarbons and other organic compounds. The direct contact of liquid aromatic hydrocarbons with the lung can cause chemical pneumonitis with pulmonary edema, hemorrhage, and tissue necrosis. It is for this reason that in the case of accidental ingestion of these materials the induction of vomiting is contraindicated because of possible aspiration of the hydrocarbon into the lungs.

Asphyxiants: The basis of classifying these materials is their ability to deprive the tissue of oxygen. In the case of severe pulmonary edema caused by an irritant such as nitrogen dioxide or laryngeal spasm caused by a sudden severe exposure to sulfuric acid mist, the death is from asphyxia, but this results from the primary irritant action. The materials we classify here as asphyxiants do not damage the lungs. Simple asphyxiants are physiologically inert gases that act when they are present in the atmosphere in sufficient quantity to exclude an adequate oxygen supply. Among these are such substances as nitrogen, nitrous oxide, carbon dioxide, hydrogen, helium, and the aliphatic hydrocarbons such as methane and ethanol. All of these gases are not chemically unreactive and among them are many materials that pose a major hazard of fire and explosion. Chemical asphyxiants are materials that have as their specific toxic action the ability to render the body incapable of utilizing an adequate oxygen supply. They are thus active in concentrations far below the level needed for damage from the simple asphyxiants. The two classic examples of chemical asphyxiants are carbon monoxide and cyanides. Carbon monoxide interferes with the transport of oxygen to the tissues by its affinity for hemoglobin. The carboxyl-hemoglobin thus formed is unavailable for the transport of oxygen. Over and above the familiar lethal effects, there is concern about how low level exposures will affect performance of such tasks as automobile driving and so on.

In the case of cyanide, there is no interference with the transport of oxygen to the tissues. Cyanide transported to the tissues forms a stable complex with the ferric iron of ferric cytochrome oxidase resulting in inhibition of enzyme action. Since aerobic metabolism is dependent on this enzyme system, the tissues are unable to utilize the supply of oxygen, and tissue hypoxia results. Therapy is directed toward the formation of an inactive complex before the cyanide has a chance to react with the cytochrome. Cyanide will complex with methemoglobin so nitrite is infected to promote the formation of methemoglobin. Thiosulfate is also given as this provides the sulfate needed to promote the enzymatic conversion of cyanide to the less toxic thiocyanate.

Primary Anesthetics: The main toxic action of these materials is their depressant effect on the central nervous system, particularly the brain. The degree of anesthetic effect depends on the effective concentration in the brain as well as on the specific pharmacologic action. Thus, the effectiveness is a balance between solubility (which decreases) and pharmacological potency (which increases) as one moves up a homologous series of compounds of increasing chain length. The anesthetic potency of the simple alcohols also rises with increasing number of carbon atoms through amyl alcohol, which is the most powerful of the series. The presence of multiple hydroxyl groups diminishes potency. The presence of carboxyl groups tends to prevent anesthetic activity, which is slightly restored in the case of an ester. Thus acetic acid is not anesthetic, but ethyl acetate is mildly so. The substitution of a halogen for a hydrogen of the fatty hydrocarbons greatly increases the anesthetic action, but confers toxicity to other organ systems, which out-weighs the anesthetic action.

Occupational Exposure Limits (OEL) are set using a variety of criteria, but human experience, animal testing and analogy with similar materials are three primary sources of information. One study recently published in AOEH suggests that in the production of oil and gas with its workers' exposure to high levels of hydrocarbon gas, first alarm levels should be set at 10% of the LEL based on knowledge of narcosis onset. This criteria is drawn from studies of anesthetic gases and the literature from diving [20, 21].

Ethanol is the only alcohol that has wide spread intentional human use. Ethanol is one of the oldest drugs recognized by man and is the primary alcohol present in beers, wines, and distilled spirits. Ethanol is a clear, colorless liquid that imparts a burning sensation to the mouth and throat when swallowed. Pure ethanol has a very slight, pleasant odor. It is freely soluble in water. Contrary to popular belief, ethanol is a powerful central nervious system (CNS) depressant that works primarily on the reticular activation system. In fact, its actions are qualitatively similar to those of the general anesthetics. It has a relatively low order of toxicity compared to methanol or isopropanol.

The exact mechanism by which ethanol produces its actions is not entirely understood. The CNS is selectively affected. Ethanol is thought to act directly on neuronal membranes and not at the synapses. At the membrane, it may interfere with ion transport. In vitro studies indicate that Na, K ATPase is inhibited by ethanol. Concentrations of 5 to 10% block the neuron's ability to produce electrical impulses. These concentrations are far greater than the concentrations of ethanol in the CNS in vivo.

The effect of ethanol on the CNS is directly proportional to the blood concentration. The first region of the brain affected is the reticular activating system. This causes disruption of the motor and thought processes. In addition, suppressing the cerebral cortex with ethanol will cause behavioral changes. Which specific types of behavior will be suppressed and which will be released from inhibition depends on the individual. In general, complex, abstract, and poorly learned behaviors are disrupted at low alcohol concentrations [22].

Ethanol depresses the CNS irregularly in a descending order from the cortex to the medulla. Table 4-2 illustrates the correlation between blood alcohol concentration and the area of the brain which is affected. Also, subjective feelings are noted based on blood alcohol concentration and the area of the brain where ethanol produces its effect.

Table 4-2. Range of Toxicity of Ethanol		
Clinical Description/Symptoms	**Blood Alcohol Concentration**	**Brain**

Mild
  Decreased inhibitions
  Slight visual impairment
  Slowing of reaction time
  Increased confidence
	0.05 - 0.010%	Frontal lobe

Moderate
  Ataxia
  Slurred speech
  Decreased motor skills
  Decreased attention
  Diplopia
  Altered perception
  Altered equilibrium
	0.15 - 0.30%	Parietal lobe
		
		Occipital lobe
		
		Cerebellum

Severe
  Vision impairment
  Equilibrium
  Stupor
	0.30 - 0.5%	Occipital lobe
		Cerebellum
		Diencephalon

Coma Respiratory failure	0.5%	Medulla

Figure 4-1 demonstrates a good relationship between hydrocarbon gases in the atmosphere and the development of nitrogen narcosis.

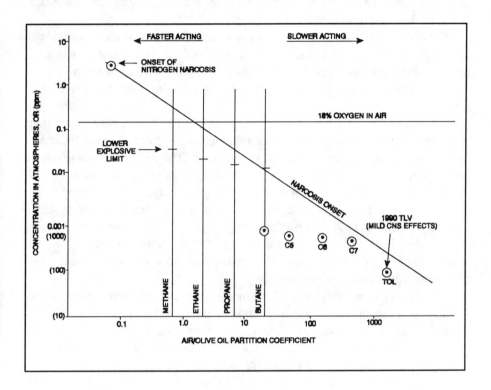

Figure 4-1 [20]. *The prediction of the concentration in air to induce narcosis from olive oil solubility. The graph allows ready comparison between the ability of a material to form an atmosphere which might be narcosis inducing, explosive or oxygen deficient. For example, propane has an oil solubility of 5.9, a lower explosive limit of 21,000 ppm, it is predicted to cause overt narcotic effects at 47,000 ppm, and at 140,000 ppm has displaced oxygen to 18 percent.*

courtesy of APPL. OCCUP. ENVIRON. HYG. 8(2)

Hepatoxic Agents: These are materials that have as their main toxic action the production of liver damage. Carbon tetrachloride produces severe diffuse central necrosis of the liver. Tetrachloroethane is probably the most toxic of the chlorinated hydrocarbons and produces acute yellow atrophy of the liver. Nitrosamines are capable of producing severe liver damage. There are many compounds of plant origin such as some of the toxic components of the mushroom Amanita phalloides, alkaloids from Senecio, and aflatoxins that are capable of producing severe liver damage and in some instances are powerful hepatocarcinogens.

Nephrotoxic Agents: These are materials that have as their main toxic action the production of kidney damage. Some of the halogenated hydrocarbons produce damage to the kidney as well as to the liver. Uranium produces kidney damage, mostly limited to the distal third of the proximal convoluted tubule.

Neurotoxic Agents: These are materials that in one way or another produce their main toxic symptoms on the nervous system. Among them are metals such as manganese, mercury, and thallium. The central nervous system seems particularly sensitive to organometallic compounds, and neurological damage results from such materials as methylmercury, and tetraethyl lead. Trialkyl tin compounds may cause edema of the central nervous system. Carbon disulfide acts mainly on the nervous system. The organic phosphorus insecticides lead to an accumulation of acetyl choline because of the inhibition of the enzyme that would normally remove it and hence cause their main symptoms in the nervous system.

Agents That Act on the Blood or Hematopoietic System: Some toxic agents such as nitrates, aniline, and toluidine convey hemoglobin to methemoglobin. Nitrobenzene forms methemoglobin and also lowers the blood pressure. Arsine produces hemolysis of the red blood cells. Benzene damages the hematopoietic cells of the bone marrow.

Agents That Damage the Lung: In this category are materials that produce damage of the pulmonary tissue but not by immediate irritant action. Fibrotic changes are produced by materials such as free silica, which produces the typical silicotic nodule. Asbestos also produces a typical damage to lung tissue and there is newly aroused interest in this subject from the point of view of possible effects of low level exposure of individuals who are not asbestos workers. Other dust, such as coal dust, can produce pneumoconiosis that, with or without tuberculosis superimposed, has been of long concern in mining. Many dusts of organic origin such as those arising in the processing of cotton or wood can cause pathology of the lungs and/or alterations in lung function. The proteolytic enzymes added to laundry products are an occupational hazard of current interest. Toluenediisocyanate (TDI) is another material which can cause impaired lung function at very low concentrations and there is evidence of chronic as well as acute effects.

SUMMARY

This toxicology overview is intended to acquaint the reader with some of the terminology that health scientists use to communicate toxicological information to public health, industrial hygienists and environmental health workers. The reader should be aware throughout this overview of the complexity of the issue and the difficulty of establishing specific, definitive exposure limits to hazardous substances. The range of responses from individuals to the same toxic substance plus the imprecise process of extrapolating animal exposure to human tolerance must be appreciated by the hazardous waste worker. Great care should be taken to prevent and/or limit hazardous waste worker exposure to the lowest practical level.

Any program to protect the health and safety of hazardous waste workers will be made more effective by a basic understanding of the science of toxicology. The detection of potentially toxic substances before damaging concentrations are reached is important for the prevention of worker injury. The ability to recognize the workers' symptomatic responses to toxic exposures is fundamental for timely intervention. The perspective that toxicology provides to site supervisors, project managers and others involved in worker health and safety is an essential part of any successful health and safety program.

REFERENCES

1.   Ariens, E., *Introduction to General Toxicology*, Academic Press, NY, NY, 1976, pg. 3.
2.   Loomis, Ted, PhD, MD, *Essentials of Toxicology*, Lea & Febiger, Philidelphia, PA, 1968, pg. 5.
3.   Loomis, pg. 13.
4.   Amdur, Mary O. PhD, *The Industrial Environment, Its Evaluation & Control*, US Dept. of Health, Education & Welfare, Public Health Service, 1973. pg. 61.
5.   Costello, Richard J.,PE, CIH, *Protecting Personnel at Hazardous Waste Sites*, Chapter 5, 1st Edition, Butterworth Publishers, Stoneham, MA, pg. 99.
6.   Kamin, Michael A., *Toxicology; a Primer on Toxicology Principles & Applications*, Lewis Publishers, Inc., Chelsea, Michigan, 1988, pg. 33.
7.   Kamin, pg. 39.
8.   Clayton, George, *The Industrial Environments. Its Evaluation and Control*, U.S. Dept. of Health, Education and Welfare, Public Health Service. 1973, pg. 2.
9.   Occupational Exposure to Ethylene Glycol Monobutyl Ether and Ethylene Glycol Monobutyl Ether Acetate, NIOSH, 90-118, Sept. 1990, pg. 17.
10.   Costello, pg. 100.
11.   Lenhart, Steven W. and Eugene C. Cole, "Respiratory Illness in Workers of an Indoor Shitake Mushroom Farm," ACEH, Vol. 6, No. 2, Feb. 1993, pg. 112.
12.   Welding, Brazing and Thermal Cutting, NIOSH, 88-110, April 1988, pg. 116.
13.   Johnson, J.S., Kilburn K.H., 1983, "Cadmium Induced Metal Fume Fever, Results of Inhalation Challenge." Am. J. Ind. Med. 4(4), 533-540.
14.   Sjogren B. Ulfvarson U, 1985, "Respiratory Symptoms and Pulmonary Function Among Welders Working With Aluminum, Stainless Steel, and Railroad Tracks." Scand. J. Work Environ. Health 11: 27-32.
15.   Bolt, H.M., Golka K, 1990, "Material Exposure to EGMEA and Hypospadia in Offspring: a case report," Br. J. Ind. Med. 47: 352-353.

16. "Occupational Exposure to Ethylene Glycol Monomethyl Ether and Ethylene Glycol Monoethyl Ether and Their Acetates," DHHS (NIOSH) 91-119, 1991, pg. 29-35.
17. Welch, L.S. et al, "Effects of Exposure to Ethylene Glycol Ethers on Shipyard Painters," Am. J. Ind. Med. 1988, 14: 509-526.
18. The Merck Index 11th ed., Rathway, N.J., Merck & Co., 1989.
19. "NIOSH Pocket Guide to Chemical Hazards," DHHS (NIOSH) 90-117, latest ed.
20. Drummond, San, "Highest Hydrocarbon Gases: A Narcotic, Asphyxiant, or Flammable Hazard?" AOEH, Vol. 8, 2 1993, pg. 120-125.
21. Graves, D., Wohlers R: "PAD1 Advanced Diving Manual," pp180-181, Santa Anna, CA, (1984).
22. Gossel, Thomas, "Principles of Clinical Toxicology," Raven Press., NY, NY. 1984, pg. 23.

5

AIR MONITORING AT HAZARDOUS WASTE SITES

Edward C. Bishop, Ph.D., C.I.H.

INTRODUCTION

This chapter discusses strategies for assessing inhalation exposure to chemicals at hazardous waste sites; monitoring strategies; PPE upgrade level selection; commonly used methods for measuring exposures; operating principles and limitations of common direct reading instruments; instrument selection considerations; and hazardous atmosphere classification.

Reliable measurements of airborne contaminants are necessary:

1) to select appropriate protective equipment based on the potential health effects of the exposure;
2) to differentiate between areas where protection is needed and areas where it is not needed;
3) to determine when operations must be halted for safety or health reasons (e.g., well drilling in potentially explosive atmospheres); and
4) to determine medical surveillance requirements.

Industrial hygiene measurements at hazardous waste sites are similar to other workplaces. However, development of sampling protocols and interpretation of the measurements made at hazardous waste sites are more difficult because many complicating factors are present. The factors peculiar to hazardous waste sites include:

1) Workers may receive multiple exposures due to the large number of (often unidentified) bulk chemicals present and the complexity of the mixtures. Compared to hazardous wastes, the composition of industrial chemicals is well known based upon material safety data sheet information. Wastes are at best unknown mixtures of known constituents and more likely mixtures of unknown constituents. Since most hazardous waste site work involves pre Resource Conservation and Recovery Act (RCRA) wastes, drums, etc., are rarely labeled.

2) The variability of exposure with location without a corresponding change of process or unit operation. Traditionally, industrial hygienists have categorized exposures in terms of their location in the production of a product. For example, production line station #1 is associated with particulate heavy metal exposures, while station #2 is associated with acutely toxic vapors. Workers from station #1 would not ordinarily be assigned to station #2, and so the exposure populations are mutually exclusive. At waste sites, the composition and concentration of chemical substances in a worker's breathing zone varies substantially from point to point on the site. This is due to the different processes or types of operation at various site locations and to the variable composition of the waste from point to point. Differences in exposure with site location have been demonstrated for individuals who work full shifts in and around trenches in contaminated soils and workers who handle contaminated materials directly [1, 2].

3) Hazardous waste cleanup usually occurs in an outdoor environment. In-plant exposures are ordinarily confined to the immediate vicinity of their source. Given a localized source, contaminants are not usually transported from one part of the plant to another. In outdoor environments, airborne contaminants are readily transported from one part of the site to another. Workers are not only exposed to the materials which they handle directly, they are also exposed to materials handled elsewhere on the site.

4) The quality of the waste containers is poor. Commercial products are packaged in containers that do not leak under ordinary circumstances. However, deteriorated containers at waste sites routinely rupture and release their contents.

5) The lack of containment vessel integrity and the incomplete identification of contaminants increase the possibility that waste mixing will occur, resulting in dangerous reaction products.

6) Dusts, including both finely divided hazardous solids and other hazardous materials coated onto soil particles, are highly sensitive to a number of factors that can vary significantly with location and time, especially soil moisture content. Vapor emissions can be produced by mechanical displacement of saturated vapors, which can produce relatively high short-term concentrations;

direct evaporations, which can produce moderate short-term concentrations; or diffusion mechanisms, which can produce relatively low short-term concentrations. Direct evaporation and diffusion can also be important long-term phenomena since they may continue for long periods of time and involve large areas.

7) Weather is an important factor. Seasonal temperature changes may greatly influence conditions. An increase in soil temperature will markedly increase the vapor pressure of volatile materials. Rain or other moisture can cap or plug vapor emission routes and greatly reduce airborne emissions.

MONITORING TECHNIQUES

Industrial hygiene has three primary methods for quantification of airborne contaminants at hazardous waste sites: direct reading instruments, chemical detector tubes, and traditional personal/area sampling methods.

Direct Reading Instruments

Direct reading instruments provide instantaneous indications of the level of contaminants in the work area. These instruments are commonly used to monitor the work site to indicate if the personal protective equipment should be upgraded. The site specific health and safety plan (HASP) required by 29 CFR 1910.120 [3] should specify predetermined trigger levels for upgrading PPE or leaving the area depending upon the contaminants likely to be found and readily measured. The HASP often specifies entry level PPE based upon the direct reading instrument.

Generally these instruments detect properties common to a class or classes of chemicals. As such, these instruments are often non-specific and may be subject to interferences. That is, they usually indicate total concentrations of components with similar measurement properties. For example, a typical photoionization detector (PID) will provide a readout of the concentration of benzene, toluene, ethyl benzene, and xylenes (BTEX) and other hydrocarbons in the area. While this is useful information, the instrument is unable to distinguish and isolate the more toxic benzene from other the other contaminants. Without additional sampling, a higher level of PPE is required based upon the higher PPE levels required to protect against benzene exposure.

Chemical Detector Tubes

Chemical detector tubes are more generally more specific than direct reading instruments. While these chemical detector tubes may also be subject to interferences, the interferent's direction (positive or negative) of interference is usually documented. For example, in the situation above, a benzene chemical detector tube could be used to verify the level of benzene present. Documentation from one manufacturer as an example, indicates toluene, xylene, and ethyl benzene are positive interferents. In addition, the degree of interference may also be reported.

Personal/Area Sampling

Personal/area sampling uses personal dosimeters or sample pumps and adsorption media tubes or filters with subsequent analysis by a full scale analytical laboratory. As such, results require additional time for analysis, often several days, if not several weeks. While this is of little use for determining PPE levels, personal sampling should be used to supplement direct reading instruments. These samples can be used to verify direct reading instrumentation and the selection of PPE after the fact. This monitoring is also essential for medical surveillance purposes.

HEALTH AND SAFETY PLAN

Hazardous Waste Operations and Emergency Response, 29 CFR 1910.120 [3], requires a written health and safety plan (HASP) for all hazardous waste operations. From an air monitoring standpoint, the key requirements of the HASP are the scope of work to be accomplished, identification of potential chemical hazards, and personal protection equipment (PPE) trigger levels. The air monitoring program will vary depending on the length of the operation, the suspected or known hazards, and the potential concentrations.

Scope of Operations

The scope of hazardous waste operations varies from preliminary assessment/site investigation, through remedial investigation/feasibility study, interim removal action, remedial design and remedial action and emergency response. The primary air monitoring considerations for different scopes of operations are the duration of the operation and the number of workers potentially exposed. For example, remedial investigation activities such as well installation, hydropunching, or soil gas surveys, are generally characterized by short durations, few workers (2-3), small and localized exposure sources (e.g., well bore hole), and relatively large geographical separations. In contrast, a remedial action or interim removal action at a drum disposal location could involve many workers and the potential for large releases of hazardous materials.

Initial Entry and Emergency Response

Initial entry should only be made by properly protected personnel with appropriate direct reading instrumentation to determine contaminant levels. In the case of an emergency response to a spill, Level A PPE is probably required. At undefined hazardous waste sites, Level B PPE is the minimum recommended for initial entry. If contaminants are known and are low hazards, a lower PPE level can be used. The initial entry team should make an sweep using a broad spectrum of instrumentation. This should include an oxygen meter, combustible gas indicator, detector tubes for contaminants known to be present, and a radiation survey meter if applicable. Once contaminant levels are identified, the exclusion zone or hot area is defined, appropriate PPE levels are determined, and other teams can enter the area.

Immediately Dangerous to Life and Health (IDLH) Locations

All confined spaces are potential IDLH locations. These include sumps, silos, cargo holds, storage tanks, and mine shafts. Bermed areas around storage tanks may also be considered confined spaces. IDLH conditions are less likely in open areas because toxic materials emitted into the atmosphere tend to be transported away from the source and simultaneously diluted. Unless there is a very large (and hence readily identifiable) source, such as an overturned tankcar, IDLH conditions in the open atmosphere are likely to be localized and last for only brief periods. An example is the immediate vicinity of a leaking gas cylinder. The initial entry team must identify all potential IDLH locations. This information must be briefed to other personnel working on the site and should be included in the HASP.

Routine Hazardous Waste Site Operations

Since direct reading instrumentation is the primary air monitoring process, the site HASP should identify direct reading instrument trigger levels for all known or suspected contaminants. Since direct reading instruments generally respond to a range of components, chemical detector tubes can be used to further define the atmosphere. In addition, personal sampling may also be used to support the direct reading results. Charcoal tube or charcoal passive dosimeter samples submitted for off-site analysis will verify the presence of benzene or other contaminants. This can be used to refine the HASP based upon the more detailed information. For the long duration remedial action, more elaborate air monitoring programs may be required. These could include scheduled personal sampling for different contaminants of concern, real-time and adsorption media fenceline sampling, etc.

Potential Contaminants

Whether the site is an emergency response to a spill, the first visit to a known hazardous waste site, or a long term remedial action, accurate identification of the potential contaminants is essential. Similar to workplace evaluations, a presurvey is required to identify potential contaminants to determine the proper sampling method.

At emergency response sites, identification of potential contaminants should be determined from tank/vessel placards or bill of laden prior to initial site entry whenever possible. At hazardous waste sites, identification is complicated by complex mixtures of contaminants, the potential for unknown contaminants, and reactions of wastes resulting in other contaminants. There can be a large number of potential airborne contaminants coexisting in the workplace atmosphere even at small sites (see Tables 5-1 and 5-2). However, a thorough document review, record search, and personal interviews should narrow the list of potential hazardous materials.

Potential Hazardous Effects

The HASP and air monitoring plan at hazardous waste sites must address acute and chronic health effect levels and the explosive ranges for flammable materials.

Acute Effects. Acute effects are adverse health changes which occur after a short period of time (in the order of magnitude of a few seconds or minutes) following exposure. In hazardous waste operations, an important consideration is the immediately dangerous to life or health concentration level. This is the maximum concentration from which, in the event of respirator failure, one could escape within 30 minutes without a respirator and without experiencing any escape-impairing (e.g., severe eye irritation or irreversible health effects [4]. Because immediate decisions concerning protection are usually required, direct reading instruments are ordinarily used to evaluate exposures likely to result in acute effects.

The short term exposure level, or STEL, and ceiling levels are other considerations. The STEL is the level at which the average worker can be exposed for 15 minutes without adverse effect [5]. Ceiling levels are concentrations which should not be exceeded. The potential harmful effects of short duration exposures above the STEL or ceiling value dictate the use of direct reading instruments or chemical detector tubes.

Chronic Effects. Chronic effects reflect the cumulative bodily damage resulting from repetitive exposures that do not produce immediately irreversible consequences. The exposures occur again and again during long periods of time (on the order of magnitude of years). The applicable standards at hazardous waste sites include the OSHA permissible exposure levels (PELs), NIOSH recommended exposure levels (RELs), and ACGIH Threshold Limit Values (TLVs). Unlike typical industrial workplaces, the latter guidelines are given legally enforceable status for hazardous waste operations per 29 CFR 1910.120 [6].

The techniques for measuring the lower levels of exposure that typically produce chronic health effects frequently differ from those used to measure exposures which may result in acute effects. Full-shift personal air samples, analyzed in an off-site laboratory, are ordinarily used to assess these exposures.

Explosive Limits. Flash fires may occur in the explosive range defined as the concentration range between the lower explosive limit (LEL) and the upper explosive limit (UEL). These levels are typically in the percent by volume range for common flammable materials. The NIOSH Pocket Guide to Chemical Hazards [4] provides the LEL for chemicals likely to be encountered in hazardous waste operations. In industrial operations, health based concentration standards are normally the limiting concentrations. However, hazardous waste operations present unique situations. For example, since properly selected Level A protection should be suitable for all concentrations, there may be a tendency to not perform air monitoring since the highest level of protection is already used. Workers could be in a potentially explosive atmosphere without instrumentation warning of the dangers. Note also the OSHA Confined Space Entry Regulation, 29 CFR 1910.146 [7] defines hazardous atmospheres as greater than 10% of the LEL. Direct reading combustible gas indicators which read in percent LEL are the instruments of choice. However, other instrumentation may be used if the LEL is presented in ppm is the range of the instrument.

Personal Protection Equipment Trigger Levels

Selecting the proper level of PPE for each task is a critical part of the HASP and requires detailed knowledge of the likely contaminants and the work to be performed. Selection of proper PPE is crucial to safe and healthful hazardous waste operations. Too low a level and workers are unnecessarily exposed. However, over protection increases the risk of heat stress, may introduce additional safety hazards from air lines and reduce visibility, reduces productivity, and is more costly in terms of equipment and training [6]. In the absence of knowledge of the components, Level B is the minimum protection that can be used [3].

PPE trigger levels to downgrade or upgrade PPE levels must be based upon the most components known or suspected to be present in sufficient quantity to present a hazard. This can produce a dilemma when more hazardous components have similar analytical properties as other less hazardous and potentially more prevalent components. A common example is benzene present with other hydrocarbons such as might occur at a leaking underground storage tank site. The upgrade from Level D to Level C occurs when the benzene concentration exceeds the 1.0 ppm benzene PEL or gasoline vapors exceed the 300 ppm gasoline TLV. Since a PID or FID responds to most if not all gasoline components (i.e., it cannot distinguish benzene from the other gasoline components), the upgrade may be ordered unnecessarily.

This situation is further confused when the instrument is calibrated to benzene. Inexperienced users may assume the instrument is reading benzene because it is calibrated to benzene. In the absence of other contaminants, the instrument will correctly respond to benzene. However, when other contaminants are present, it will respond to those contaminants also, although not in a predictable manner. To prove this, calibrate an instrument to benzene (or hexane, etc.) and expose the instrument to a permanent marker (alcohol based) or nail polish remover (acetone based) and note the effect.

Calculations of maximum concentrations are valuable in predicting which contaminants may result in greatest potential hazard. Contaminants which cannot be present in potentially hazardous concentrations can be eliminated from consideration.

There are two common equations for estimating the partial pressure of a particular contaminant. These are Raoult's Law and Henry's Law.

Raoult's Law: $p_i = x_i P_i^{sat}$

where: p_i = the partial pressure of the ith component
x_i = the mole fraction of the ith component
P_i^{sat} = the saturated vapor pressure of the ith component

Henry's Law for dilute aqueous solutions: $p_i = k_i m_i$

where: p_i =   the partial pressure of the ith component
k_i =   Henry's Law constant of the ith component
m_i =   molality of the ith component = moles per 1000 grams solvent (approximately moles/L for water)

Raoult's Law is exact as the mole fraction approaches one and Henry's Law is exact as the mole fraction approaches zero [8].

Raoult's Law will provide sufficiently reliable estimates of vapor pressures of components in drums or similar high concentration mixtures, especially if the components are from the same chemical family (e.g., alkanes) and not mixtures of families. Henry's Law will provide reliable estimates of equilibrium vapor pressures for dilute sources such as contaminated groundwater sources such as might occur during well drilling, aquifer pump tests, etc. Henry's Law constants are specific for the component. A good source of these constants is Tomes [9].

Two cautions should be exercised when using these equations. First, ensure the units are compatible. Unit conversions may be necessary to convert the Henry's Law constant to yield the partial pressure in units of mm Hg. Second, these equations predict equilibrium vapor pressures—the saturated vapor pressure at the liquid surface (e.g., the concentrated liquid [Raoult's Law] or water [Henry's Law]). Additional dilution will occur and should be estimated. Outdoors, a conservative estimate is a three fold dilution based upon the general dilution equation for liquids evaporating into an enclosed room and assuming maximum mixing [10] - a valid assumption outdoors without major wind obstructions.

To convert to parts per million:

$$(p_i \text{ [in mm Hg]}/760) \times 10^6 = \text{ppm}$$

The PPE upgrade occurs whenever a trigger level is exceed. As examples:

Raoult's Law

Conservatively, gasoline contains 5% benzene by volume. Table 5-1 shows the results of the mole fraction calculations assuming gasoline can be described as a mixture of benzene, hexane, and octane.

Table 5-1 Calculation of Mole Fraction of Benzene in Gasoline						
	MW, gm/mole	Density, gm/cm³	Mole Fraction, Liquid [1]	P_i^{sat}, mm Hg	p_o mm Hg	Mole Fraction, Vapor
Benzene, 5 cm³	78.1	0.88	0.08	80.1	6.4	0.07
Hexane, 50 cm³	86.2	0.66	0.54	68.7	37.1	0.41
Octane, 45 cm³	114.2	0.70	0.38	125.6	47.7	0.52

[1] (Vol, cm³)(Density, gm/cm³)/(MW, gm/mole) = Moles

At this composition, what concentration of gasoline vapors contains 1 ppm benzene?

$$1 \text{ ppm benzene} = 0.07(\text{gasoline vapor concentration})$$

At 14 ppm total gasoline vapor, the estimated benzene concentration is 1 ppm. Therefore, the HASP should specify upgrade to PPE Level C when the PID or FID exceeds 14 ppm. To refine the trigger procedures, the HASP could specify using a benzene specific chemical detector tube at the same trigger point to verify the presence of benzene. Air monitoring continues and PPE is upgraded to Level C whenever the benzene concentration exceed 1 ppm by chemical detector tube or gasoline vapors exceed 300 by PID or FID.

Henry's Law

Well drilling and well sampling operations may also present hazards to workers. Many contaminants may be present in the water at the part per billion range. Again, different trigger levels are common for components having similar analytical properties. Use of Henry's Law predicts the maximum concentration of dilute contaminants at the air-water interface. This is demonstrated as follows for 1,2,3 trichloropropane in water at 5mg/L:

$$k = 3.44 \times 10^{-4} \text{ atm m}^3/\text{mole in water}$$
$$MW = 147.5 \text{ gm/mole}$$

$$p = (3.44 \times 10^{-4} \text{ atm m}^3/\text{mole})(5 \text{ mg}/10^{-3} \text{ m}^3)/(147.5 \text{ gm/mole})$$

$$p = (1.2 \times 10^{-5} \text{ atm})$$

$$(1.2 \times 10^{-5} \text{ atm})(10^6 \text{ ppm/atm}) = 12 \text{ ppm}$$

A threefold dilution yields a maximum estimated concentration of 4 ppm which is safely below the PEL of 10 ppm. An appropriate trigger level is based upon the next most restrictive component which could be present in greater concentration.

Summary

Development of appropriate trigger levels requires knowledge of the contaminants and their toxicological and physical properties, and knowledge of the available instrumentation and its strengths and weaknesses. Continual or frequent direct reading air monitoring is performed during the entire operation. PPE is upgraded whenever a trigger level for any contaminant is exceeded. An additional consideration for upgrading to higher PPE levels for highly flammable materials is to ensure 10% of the LEL is not exceeded. For example, 10% of the LEL for gasoline (1.1 volume %) is 1,100 ppm. This is 3.7 times the PEL of 300 ppm. Since even a half face organic vapor respirator provides a protection factor of 10, the limiting condition is explosivity.

Air Monitoring Plan

The air monitoring plan is developed to address PPE trigger levels, LEL, fenceline monitoring, and medical monitoring requirements using available instrumentation. The plan must include direct reading instruments and chemical detector tubes to determine the proper PPE levels and when to cease operations such as drilling in the event potentially explosive atmospheres occur as described above. The plan should also address the use of direct reading instruments and chemical detector tubes for fenceline monitoring to protect the public. In these cases, appropriate public exposure criteria must be identified. These will generally be significantly lower than the IDLH or PEL criteria for on-site personnel.

The following discusses air monitoring considerations for personal or area sampling with pump flow or passive monitors with the appropriate adsorption media to verify instrument results.

Sample protocols are designed within laboratory workload and financial restraints. This approach favors selection of materials present in large quantities. It discriminates against substances present in relatively small quantities, unless the health hazard of even infrequent exposure is deemed overriding.

Personal samples should be taken, even in the absence of direct instrument readings indicating contaminants. This sampling will verify the lack of contamination or provide additional information on the nature of the contamination undetected by the direct reading instruments. The *NIOSH Occupational Exposure Sampling Strategy Manual* [11] suggests selective monitoring of high-risk workers; specifically, monitoring those workers who are closest to the source of contaminant generation. The rationale for this procedure is that the possibility of a significant exposure varies directly with distance from the source. If the high-risk workers are not exposed significantly, then monitoring high-risk workers conserves resources that would otherwise be necessary to monitor workers further removed from the contaminant source.

In multi-substance environments, where simultaneous exposures are anticipated and where the contaminants must be collected on a number of different media, it may be necessary to sample more than one worker in each operation. Because it is not usually possible to draw air through different sampling media using a single portable battery-operated pump, it requires several days to measure the exposure of a specific individual using each of the media [12, 13]. Repetitive sampling of more than one worker in each operation is recommended. One way to overcome this problem is to collect multiple area samples on pieces of heavy equipment. While technically not a personal sample, heavy equipment operators remain at the vehicle operators position throughout most of the workshift and usually are employed in the active materials handling part of the site. Samples collected very close to the breathing zone are reasonably representative of personal exposure and these multi-media samples yield as much information as several personal samples [14].

Sampling should continue throughout the cleanup, unless it can be demonstrated that the site contaminants are homogeneously distributed and that consistent exposures would be anticipated.

Air monitoring at cleanups is not subject to the uncertainties inherent in emergency response actions because background information is usually available to identify prospective contaminants. For planned sampling visits to evaluate suspected chronic hazards, examine the available background data to select the site contaminants to be measured. Information sources include the site assessment and remedial investigation reports. These reports provide information on drum samples, contaminant volumes, and the degree and extent of groundwater and soil contamination.

From this information determine the class of contaminants (e.g., pesticides, petroleum hydrocarbons, etc.) and the quantities and concentrations of each. This allows ranking of contaminants by hazard potential and grouping by sample media (e.g., general hydrocarbons on charcoal, amines on silica gel, etc.).

The physical state of a contaminant must also be considered. Many contaminants such as PCBs, PNAs, or pesticides should be measured as both particulate-bound contaminants and as vapors. The volatile component is collected on a solid adsorbent and the non-volatile component is collected on a filter. More than two dozen methods have been developed by NIOSH [15, 16] which make use of a dual media sampling system to efficiently collect both the particulate and vapor portion of a single contaminant, e.g., MOCA. Measurement techniques that analyze only the vapor phase of a substance may fail to identify significant exposure to toxic contaminants if the substance is primarily particulate or particulate bound. Some of the sampling media and analytical techniques that have been used during NIOSH studies at hazardous waste sites are listed in Table 5-3.

Table 5-2. Estimated Volume of Chemicals [12] Triangle Chemical Site Bridge City, TX		
Number of Drums	**Contents**	**Volume (gallons)**
260	Solvents	10,400
60	Acids	3,600
90	Bases	3,600
175	Alcohols	7,000
85	Ether	3,400
250	Empty	0
	TOTAL	28,000

	Table 5-3. Estimated Frequency of Chemicals [12] Triangle Chemical Site Bridge City, TX	
Category	**Compounds**	**Relative Abundance**
Solvents	Dichlorobenzene Toluene Trichlorethylene Xylenes Methylethylketone Orthodichlorobenzene	37%
Acids	Cresylic Acid Hydrochloric Acid Hydrofluoric Acid Surfactant (pH 1) Nitric Acid Phosphoric Acid	13%
Bases	Ammonium Hydroxide Caustic (pH 12) Diethanolamine Methylethylamine	13g
Alcohols	Butanol p-Decyl-phenol Ethanol Glycols Rust tem 200 Methanol p-Nonylphenol	25%
Ethers	Ether	12%
		100%

DIRECT READING INSTRUMENTS

Underground miners were among the first to become aware of the need for a device to detect the presence of hazardous gas concentrations. In their environment the gases could include methane, carbon dioxide, carbon monoxide, oxygen deficiency, and others. Of these gases, methane has often been present in mines in sufficient quantities to explode. Since it is not a systemic toxicant and has no warning odor, explosive levels can accumulate before a worker realizes the potential risk. With high methane concentrations, any source of ignition, including those in the original miner's lamps, could readily set off an explosion. It is in this setting that the use of the first "combustible gas indicator," the Davie's Lamp, provided a significant step forward in mine safety. The visible characteristics of the flame of the Davie's Lamp could inform the experienced user of much more than just the presence of methane. Refinements of the Davie's Lamp are still in use today.

A variety of instruments for measuring combustible gases and vapors are currently marketed. However, most are based upon one of five common sensor systems: catalytic combustion, photoionization, flame ionization, solid state, and infrared. These are described below and include descriptions of the general operating principles, performance characteristics, and sensor limitations.

Catalytic Combustion

This sensor type literally measures the contaminant by combustion. Air containing the contaminating gases flows over a sensor heated above the ignition temperature of the gas. The gas is ignited and oxidized to carbon dioxide and water. Higher temperatures in the sensor chamber develop as higher concentrations of contaminant gas are ignited. The increase in temperature is measured by a platinum resistance thermometer. As the temperature increases, the resistance of the thermometer increases resulting in a imbalance in the Wheatstone bridge circuitry.

The encapsulation of a platinum resistance thermometer in a ceramic bead coated with a palladium oxide catalyst results in combustion reactions occurring at the significantly lower temperature of 500°C compared to the original hot wire combustible gas indicator. This results in a much more stable zero condition and the encapsulation provides a degree of protection against shock such as accidentally dropping the probe. If the sensor is properly designed, oxidation on the catalytic surface will be diffusion controlled (this will occur even if the sample is drawn past the sensor by pump or aspirated flow) and all flammable gases will be oxidized regardless of other reaction kinetics [17].

The signal produced is generally a linear function of the concentration of the combustible gas or vapor present up to 80 percent LEL. When expressed as a percentage of the lower explosive limit, instrument response is relatively independent of the specific contaminant for most hydrocarbons [18]. This is because the product of the heat of oxidation and the lower explosive level is a constant for the commonly encountered hydrocarbons [17].

As the concentration approaches the lower explosive limit, the instrument will reach a maximum level (peg-out). It will stay at this level until the concentration reaches the upper explosive level (UEL). As the concentration rises above the UEL, the response will decrease due to the lack of oxygen to support combustion. This is shown in Figure 5-1.

These instruments should be relatively unaffected by changes in humidity, however, several users have reported humidity effects. These effects are generally in a positive direction (meter reading is greater than known concentration).

Although these instruments will respond to chlorinated hydrocarbons, a product of combustion is hydrochloric acid which corrodes the sensor and greatly reduces sensor lifetime. Organic lead compounds such as found in leaded gasoline may poison the sensor.

Strengths:
- General purpose detector for most combustible hydrocarbons.
- Linear response to 80 percent LEL.
- Indicates total combustibles present.
- Relatively unaffected by temperature and humidity changes.

Weaknesses:
- Nonspecific.
- Requires oxygen (air) for operation.
- Not recommended for chlorinated hydrocarbons or tetraethyl lead containing compounds.

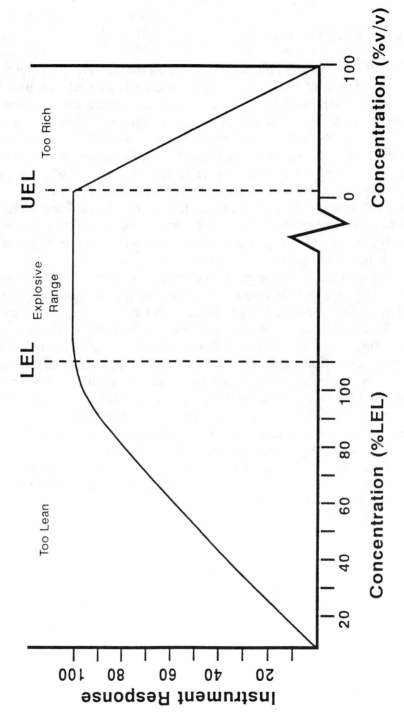

Figure 5-1. Catalytic combustion detector response

Photoionization Detector

The PID ionizes contaminants in the air stream with ultraviolet light. The ionized molecules are collected at the negatively charged electrode. The ion current is measured, electronically processed and presented as a meter readout. The PID ionizes molecules with ionization potentials below the electron voltage of the bulb. A smaller percentage of molecules with ionization potentials above the bulb voltage will also be ionized. See Figure 5-2. Typical bulb voltages are 10.2 electron volts (eV), 10.6 eV, and 11.7 eV.

The signal produced varies with contaminant and is not necessarily linear with concentration and tends to flatten out at higher concentrations. This is shown in Figure 5-3. It is most sensitive for molecules with a large number of pi electrons in the electron shell. This includes benzene and other benzene ring compounds such as toluene and xylene.

High humidity decreases the PID sensitivity. Since the magnitude of this effect varies with the instrument, consult the manufacturer. UV energy does not ionize oxygen but oxygen does absorb some UV energy. As a result, the PID will indicate a greater contaminant concentration at lower oxygen levels. This is unlikely to present a problem except under extreme oxygen deficient atmospheres. This effect can be minimized by calibrating the PID with a oxygen concentration similar to the atmosphere to be measured. A more likely error is during the calibration of the PID. The PID calibrated with a nitrogen based (i.e., no oxygen) calibration standard will indicate erroneously low contaminant concentrations in the atmosphere to be measured.

A similar signal decrease effect was reported in the presence of biogenic methane. Signal decreases of 30% at 0.5% methane and 90% at 5% methane were observed [19]. Significantly higher readings with an FID or catalytic combustion instrument compared to PID readings is indicative of a methane interference.

Strengths:
- Good general purpose detector.
- Durable and reliable.
- Wide common use.
- Common contaminant ionization potentials are readily available in the NIOSH Guide to Hazardous Chemicals [4].

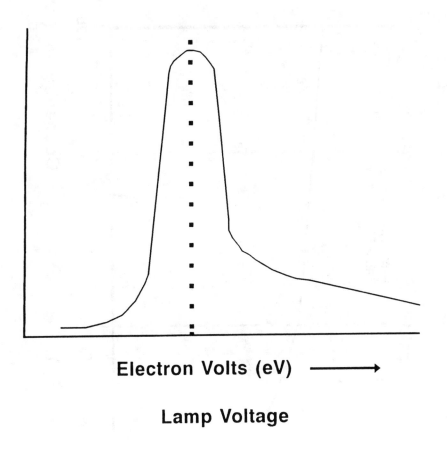

Electron Volts (eV) ⟶

Lamp Voltage

Figure 5-2. Photoionization potential

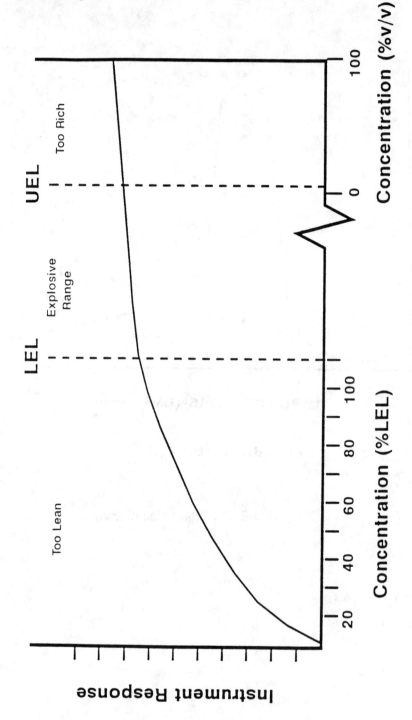

Figure 5-3. Photoionization detector response

Weaknesses:
- Nonspecific.
- Response varies with contaminant.
- Affected by humidity.
- Affected by methane.
- Higher bulb voltages (<10.6 eV) are associated with greater instability and greater baseline drift.

Flame Ionization Detector

A hydrogen flame ionizes contaminants in the airstream. The ions are collected at one electrode resulting in an ion current. This current is electronically processed producing a signal proportional to the level of contaminant present. The signal produced is generally a linear function of the concentration of the combustible gas or vapor present up to 80 percent LEL. FID sensitivity increases with increasing carbon number.

Since the FID is a combustion process it does require oxygen to operate. However, if calibrated for anticipated oxygen levels, it should function properly at levels above the oxygen based IDLH level. At lower oxygen levels, a separate air source can be used.

As the concentration approaches the lower explosive limit, the instrument will reach a maximum level (peg-out). It will stay at this level until the concentration reaches the upper explosive level (UEL). As the concentration rises above the UEL, the instrument flames out due to the lack of oxygen necessary to support combustion in the hydrogen flame. This is shown in Figure 5-4.

These instruments are relatively unaffected by changes in humidity.

Although these instruments will respond to chlorinated hydrocarbons, a product of combustion is hydrochloric acid which corrodes the sensor and greatly reduces sensor lifetime.

Strengths:
- General purpose detector for most combustible hydrocarbons.
- Linear response to 80 percent LEL.
- Indicates total combustibles present.
- Relatively unaffected by temperature and humidity changes.

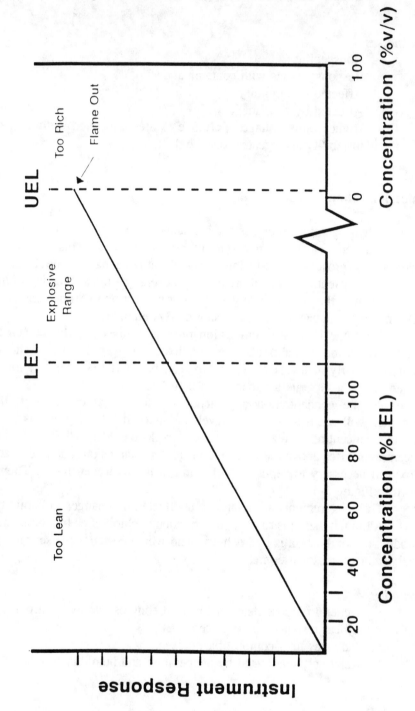

Figure 5-4. Flame Ionization Detector Response

Weaknesses:
- Nonspecific.
- Requires oxygen (air) for operation.
- Not recommended for chlorinated hydrocarbons.

Infrared Detector

Infrared (IR) energy is absorbed by molecules in the contaminated airstream. The absorbed energy is measured by a detector, electronically processed, and presented on a meter readout. The IR source is usually a nichrome wire. The IR energy is focused through an IR transparent window, and bounced between mirrors to the IR detector. By focusing the mirrors, paths from 0.75 meters to 20.25 meters are possible. However, the longer the pathlength, the greater the energy dissipation.

Specifically, IR energy is absorbed by the bending and stretching of molecular bonds. This produces a very compound specific IR fingerprint. However, most detectors limit the detection to a single wavelength which is common to many compounds within a class of compounds. For example, the detector could measure the bending or stretching of the carbon-hydrogen double bond in a benzene ring. This wavelength will detect all benzene ring containing compounds.

The signal produced is compound dependent and likewise dependent on all interferences. It is relatively unaffected by contaminant concentration. While the response should be theoretically linear with concentration in accordance with Beer's Law, in practice the response tends to drop off as shown in Figure 5-5. Lower concentrations are measured by increasing the pathlength between the IR source and the detector. The longer the path, the more likely the energy will interact with the molecules.

The IR detector is affected by humidity in two ways. First, the most common IR transparent windows are made of sodium chloride (glass absorbs IR energy) which is very hygroscopic. High humidity can fog the windows requiring expensive replacement. Silver bromide windows are relatively immune to humidity effects. However, these windows are much more expensive than the sodium chloride windows. Silver bromide is strongly affected by ammonia vapors which cause fogging requiring replacement.

In addition to equipment effects, water vapor absorbs IR energy. This absorption can be in the same region as the contaminant of interest. The effect of this interference depends upon the contaminant and concentration of interest. However, since water vapor present in relatively high concentrations, it is best to select a wavelength which is not affected by water vapor.

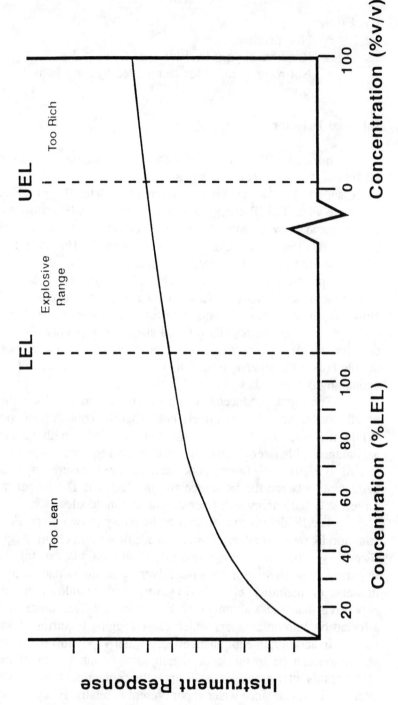

Figure 5-5. Infrared detector response

Strengths:
- Can be used in oxygen deficient atmospheres
- Can be tuned to respond to specific components

Weaknesses:
- Relatively nonspecific in multicomponent atmospheres. This weakness can be overcome to a large extent by Fourier Transform Infrared (FTIR) [20]. However, at this time these instruments are considerably more expensive than the more common filtered IR systems.
- Influenced by high humidity.

Solid State

Solid state semiconductors can be used to detect combustible gases and other compounds. The contaminant gas reacts on the surface of the sensor bead, producing a change in conductivity of the semiconductor which is measured electronically. The change in conductivity is the result of changes in electron distribution in the semiconductor and not due to thermal effects such as occur in catalytic and hot wire detectors.

For n-type sintered tin oxide semiconductors, the contaminant gas is adsorbed and reacts on the detector surface with previously adsorbed oxygen ions producing typical oxidation products such as carbon dioxide and water. The removal of the oxygen ions from the sensor surface releases electrons to the semiconductor metal resulting in a measurable increase in conductivity. The output is then read as a function of the electronic concentration of the contaminant gas that is present. To increase the surface reaction rate, the sensor is heated, usually using a platinum coil. This temperature (e.g., 200°C) is generally less than the temperature of catalytic or hot wire devices [17]. This lower temperature provides long term zero stability and prevents the sensor from poisoning by compounds which decompose at higher temperatures. However, at these temperatures, several reactions can proceed in addition to the surface adsorption reactions. These are:

Direct burning: The direct burning process is similar to that of the catalytic sensors. It requires oxygen to proceed and heats the sensor. The response increases the conductivity providing a positive response. Since combustion is involved, a flashback arrestor is required to isolate the hot sensor from the explosive atmosphere when high concentrations are measured.

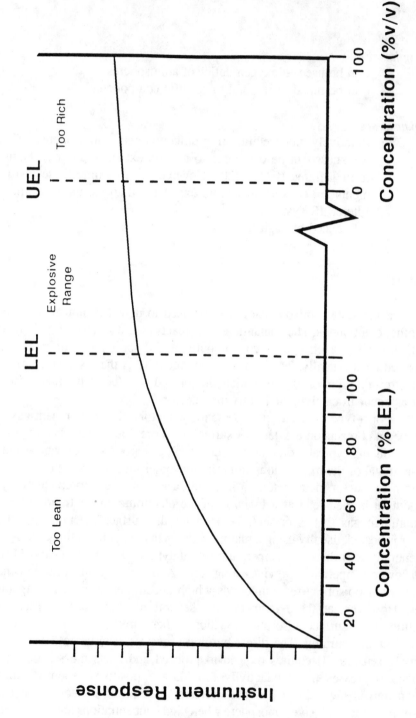

Figure 5-6. Solid state detector response

Oxidation: This reaction is similar to burning, but has been limited here to that occurring at temperatures below the ignition temperatures. This process is also exothermic.

Reduction: This term is applied to the reduction of the semiconductor material to the metallic state. Such a change also reduces resistance since the metals are more conductive than their oxides.

Absorption: The physical absorption of the contaminants by the bead results in some release of heat and therefore some instrument response.

Absorption: This molecular process is parallel to absorption.

Thermal effects: The high thermal conductivity of some 'hydrocarbon gasses tends to cool the sensor which results in a decrease in conductivity. This is normally negligible, but can be observed. This action can typically show up during a search for gas leaks. First there is a gradual rise in response until a momentary dip is observed where a sudden surge of the combustible gas is met. For survey type work the transient observed can be evidence for the source of the leak, and the change in instrument sensitivity does not affect the evaluation.

Hydrocarbons, halogenated hydrocarbons, alcohols, ethers, ketones, esters, nitro and amine compounds produce a measurable change in conductivity. Several inorganic gases including ammonia, carbon monoxide, hydrogen, hydrogen cyanide, hydrogen sulfide, nitrogen oxide, and water can also be detected. The sensitivity to water can be a problem in high humidity atmospheres. Water vapor is required for operation as the instrument will not operate in "bone dry" environments. As the humidity increases, instrument sensitivity and response also increase.

This sensor type measures all contaminants that react on the surface and is very sensitive to small concentration changes. However, the response produced may vary greatly among contaminants and is a function of the contaminant, the sensor, and the surface reactions. A meter indication is an indication of contamination, not necessarily explosivity; unlike the catalytic combustion sensor which produces a composite signal indicative of the total combustible concentration.

Response to propane was reported at 1000 ppm, less than a twentieth of its LEL of 22000 ppm (2.2%). Carbon monoxide is detectable at 50 ppm (LEL, 12.5%). This sensor is also sensitive to hydrogen sulfide at low concentrations. This combination of sensitivities makes it possible to use it as a multiple sensor for the gases that are typically found in sewage treatment processes and related manholes.

At and above the LEL, the sensor response is relatively flat. Therefore, it may not be possible to determine if the atmosphere is at the LEL, in the explosive range, or above the UEL. This is shown in Figure 5-6.

When this sensor is poisoned, the sensor must be replaced. Poisoning is indicated when the sensor does not respond to known combustibles.

Strengths:
- Can be tailored for use for a variety of contaminants, including inorganics.
- Can be used in oxygen deficient atmospheres (except totally inert).

Weaknesses:
- Response near and above the lower explosive limit is relatively flat.
- Not recommended in high humidity atmospheres (> 70%).
- Response is unpredictable (although generally positive) in multicomponent mixtures due to the variety of reactions that can occur.

INSTRUMENT SELECTION AND USE

Considerations for Instrument Selection

A flowchart outlining the steps in selecting and using combustible gas or health survey meters is shown in Figure 5-7. The first and most important step in selecting and using a combustible gas or health survey meter is to determine the agent to be sampled and the identification of any possible interferences, including water from high humidity. Next, determine if the atmosphere to be sampled is likely to be at or above 10% of the LEL. The following discussions depend on the initial assessment.

Lower Explosive Limit Measurements

Oxygen should always be measured prior to confined space entries or anytime high vapor or low oxygen concentrations are expected. Instruments based upon combustion principles require oxygen to properly quantify the sampled atmosphere.

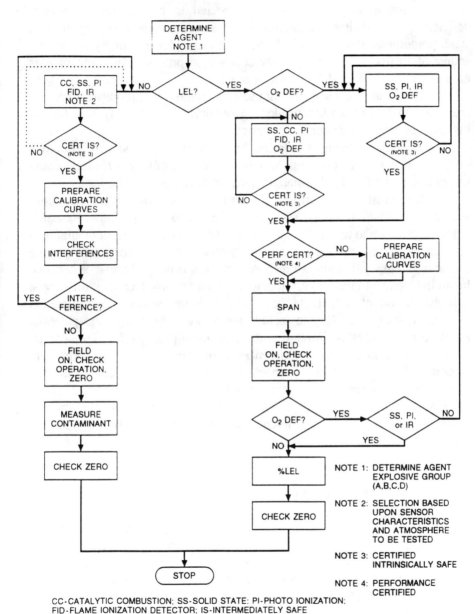

Figure 5-7. Instrument selection flowchart [30]

If the atmosphere is, or is suspected to be, potentially oxygen deficient (e.g., inerting operations), select an instrument based upon solid state, photoionization, or infrared operating principles, or supply an outside source of air (oxygen) to support the combustion process. These instruments are not strongly affected by a lack of oxygen.

Any instrument selected for use in potentially hazardous atmospheres must be certified by an independent laboratory as intrinsically safe for the highest category atmosphere to be tested.

If an instrument is selected based upon a combustion principle, oxygen concentrations can be used to correct combustible gas readings using information supplied by the manufacturer or developed by the user.

Is the instrument performance certified by an independent laboratory such as the Canadian Safety Association (CSA) or Factory Mutual Research (FM)? In addition to testing for intrinsic safety, some independent laboratories also check to ensure the instrument meets certain performance criteria including accuracy, linearity of response, etc. If it is not performance certified by an independent laboratory, validate the manufacturer's calibration curves. It is also important to calibrate the instrument to the vapors to be sampled at the conditions of sampling to include temperature, humidity, and potential interferences present. A simple way to determine if potential interferences are unimportant is to add the interference vapors and observe the instrument response. If no effect is observed, the potential interferences are not important. If interferences are determined to be important, efforts must be taken to eliminate the interferences with filters, or to use instrumentation either not affected by the interferences or capable of separating the components.

Health Survey Measurements

Select the instrument with the best operating characteristics for the atmosphere to be measured. This selection should consider optimum instrument response for the contaminant of interest and minimum response from potential interferences. Although intrinsic safety certification is not a requirement for health survey instruments due to the lower concentrations expected, a certified instrument is recommended if there is any possibility of encountering potentially hazardous atmospheres. In addition, certain certifications (e.g., CSA, FM) ensure instruments meet certain accuracy and other operating criteria.

Prepare calibration curves for the compounds to be measured, for the concentrations expected, and for similar environmental conditions (primarily temperature and humidity) for the atmosphere to be measured. Users of one combustible gas indicator found the instrument calibration had to be performed in humid air (greater than 50% relative humidity (RH)) to achieve agreement with the manufacturer's calibration data. Lower humidity resulted in decreased instrument response. In addition, because it is not unusual to obtain different instrument readings on different scales, ensure calibration readings are obtained for the same atmosphere on different instrument scales.

Check for possible interferences from other chemicals likely to be in the atmosphere to be sampled. Simply inject into the test chamber or sampling bag quantities of other chemicals likely to be encountered. Note any instrument response. Care and judgement must be exercised to determine if any observed effect is sufficient to negate the instrument's use. If the interference is great, alternate instruments using different operating principles should be investigated. If other instrumentation is either not available or determined to be ineffective, knowledge of the degree and direction of the interference may still allow use of the instrument. However, care must be exercised in interpreting the readings and documenting the results. In all cases, follow-up sampling with an approved method is recommended.

A properly calibrated infrared instrument was used to monitor ethylene oxide from a hospital sterilizer. During the sterilization cycle, a period when no ethylene oxide was expected, a sudden increase in instrument was observed. This response was traced to the use of a bactericidal cleaning compound used to mop the floor. Additional investigation of the same operation, revealed that water vapor absorbs near, and interferes with, the ethylene oxide peak chosen to eliminate the known Freon 12 interference, also present in the sterilization operation. Since no other peak was available in the infrared region, a portable gas chromatograph was selected to perform the evaluation.

Instrument Use

Prior to using any combustible gas or health survey instrument, ensure the instrument is in proper operating condition. As a minimum the following should be checked:

1. Ensure the batteries are functioning by using the battery selection position on the meter. Refer to the manufacturer's instructions.
2. Ensure the sampling lines are in good condition, free of leaks and visual damage to include cracking or nicks. Also check the

fittings to ensure a proper air tight connection through the sampling train.

3. Visually inspect all in-line filters and driers. Ensure manufacturer's recommended preventive maintenance is performed.

4. Set the instrument to read the proper concentration using the manufacturer's recommended span gas [21, 22].

5. In the field, turn the instrument on and allow sufficient warm up time as noted by a stable zero baseline. Ensure the instrument is zeroed in a contaminant free atmosphere or use zero gas. Care must be used to ensure the zero gas is the same as the atmosphere to be sampled with only the contaminant(s) removed. For example, zero gas may be pure nitrogen or may be extremely low in humidity. Use of the zero gases can result in improper instrument zero and cause instrument reading error. An appropriate filter can also be used. However, ensure through laboratory experiments the filter use does not alter instrument response either due to pressure differentials or possible water (humidity) removal. Once zeroed, check instrument operation using a known flammable or contaminant source. A permanent marker (alcohol based) is a suitable source.

6. For all confined space entries or any atmosphere in which oxygen deficiency cannot be ruled out, the oxygen concentration must be measured. This may be accomplished using the oxygen sensor of the combustible gas meter if so equipped, (Figure 7), or a separate oxygen meter. If a oxygen concentration is less than 19.5% or greater than 21.5% oxygen by volume, care must be taken in interpreting readings from instruments based upon combustion principles. These instruments will read low in oxygen deficient atmospheres and high in oxygen enriched atmospheres. Corrections may be made based upon calibration curves prepared at different oxygen concentrations. Although instruments based upon solid state, photo ionization, and infrared are generally unaffected by oxygen content, oxygen concentration must be determined prior to any entry into the sampled atmosphere.

7. Measure the concentration starting with the highest (least sensitive) instrument scale. Increase the instrument sensitivity by selecting a lower scale until a reading is obtained. Correct the instrument reading using the manufacturer's or user developed calibration curves.

8. At the completion of measurements, and periodically throughout the measurement period, the instrument should be re-zeroed using zero gas, and the span checked and readjusted if necessary. In addition, periodically check the instrument with a known flammable source (e.g., alcohol based permanent marker) to ensure the instrument is operating.

Limitations

The following are common limitations the user should recognize and consider while operating a combustible gas indicator.

Combustible gas indicators are used to detect the presence and concentration of a combustible gas or vapor or a composite of the gases present. They generally cannot differentiate between various substances. If calibrated for a single gas or vapor, it can be relied upon for accurate determinations of that substance in the environment, provided there are no other combustible or interfering gases or vapors present in that environment.

Catalytic or hot wire combustible gas indicators should not be used for, or in the presence of halogenated hydrocarbon gases or vapors. The thermal decomposition products generated by these substances will corrode the sensor and alter its sensitivity and integrity.

A combustible gas indicator or hydrocarbon detector must be selected for the purposes intended. If it is to evaluate health exposure to toxic gases or vapors which are combustible, the sensitivity of the instrument must be greater than if the instrument is to be used for the determination of potential fire hazard levels.

If a potential exists for a hazardous atmosphere (10% LEL), ensure the instrument selected is certified by an independent laboratory as intrinsically safe for the atmosphere to be tested. This will ensure the instrument will not ignite the sampled atmosphere.

The sensitivity and accuracy of combustible gas indicators are affected by a wide range of conditions. These include the presence of dust, humidity and temperature extremes. For these reasons the instrument should be calibrated under conditions similar to conditions expected in the environment to be sampled.

Do not interchange parts between two instruments of different manufacturers or different models. If parts of two identical instruments (model and manufacturer) are interchanged, the instrument must be recalibrated before it is used.

Any instrument that requires repair work that replaces the flame arrestor or that breaches the intrinsic safety of the device should be sent to the manufacturer for testing and recertification of its safe use for the purpose intended.

A combustible gas indicator or hydrocarbon indicator should be tested and field calibrated with a known gas or vapor concentration (e.g., with span gas) before each use. The instrumentation should be calibrated in conditions similar to that expected in the field (e.g., similar temperature and humidity). In addition, if a long sampling line is needed in the field, the same length of line should be used during the calibration check. The instrument should also be tested for operation at the sample location. A permanent marker (alcohol based) or butane lighter can be used for this purpose.

Instruments may exhibit "zero drift." It is important to check and reset the "zero" reading in a clean environment on a frequent basis. If the instrument is taken into a mine or other environment where vapors are always present, a sample of clean or zero air should be carried with the instrument to facilitate frequent zeroing adjustment. This clean or zero air must be contaminant free but similar to the sample environment in all other aspects. For example, pure nitrogen zero air may result in a different reading when exposed to normal air which includes oxygen. A zero air filter which removes the contaminant may also be used.

DETECTOR TUBE SELECTION AND USE

The selection of detector tubes follows the same general logic as the selection of direct reading instruments. Select a detector tube which will measure the specific contaminant of interest. The manufacturer's literature will identify known interferences and whether the interferences are positive or negative. Usually these interferences will be positive and will be similar in chemical structure (e.g., benzene, toluene, and xylene) and will also be likely found in conjunction with the chemical of interest at the hazardous waste site. While this will tend towards the conservative application of PPE, it is more specific than the direct reading instrument. Detector tubes are used in accordance with the manufacturer's directions. One note of caution, do not mix detector tubes from one manufacturer with a detector tube pump from another. Detector tubes are matched with the pump with specific flow rates, often unique to the manufacturer's pump.

PERSONAL SAMPLING

Personal sampling methodologies are similar to general industrial hygiene sampling. Once the contaminants of interest are identified, use the OSHA Field Operations Manual [23] to determine the proper sampling media and flowrates.

HAZARDOUS ATMOSPHERE CLASSIFICATION

Locations containing, or potentially containing, explosive concentrations of vapors, gases, or dusts, are classified according to the degree of hazard. This classification scheme is defined in Article 500 of the National Electric Code (NEC) [24] which is found in the National Fire Protection Agency (NFPA) publications.

Class

There are three hazardous atmosphere classes; Class I, Class II, and Class III. Class I includes all atmospheres containing or potentially containing explosive gases or vapors. Class II includes those atmospheres containing or potentially containing explosive dusts. Class III includes those atmospheres containing or potentially containing explosive fibers.

Division

Within each Class, there are two divisions, Division 1 and Division 2. In Division 1, a flammable material is continuously or usually present. In Division 2 locations, flammables are only present under accident conditions.

Group

Hazardous locations are further classified by group. The groups are A through D for vapors and gases, and E through G for dusts and particulates. Group designations for specific materials are given in NFPA publication 497M, "Classification of Gases, Vapors and Dusts for Electrical Equipment in Hazardous (Classified) Locations" [25].

Gases and Vapors: Group A is the most hazardous (most flammable or explosive) while Group D is the least hazardous. Representative chemicals in each of the Groups are:

Group A: Acetylene
Group B: Hydrogen, ethylene oxide
Group C: Ethylene, carbon monoxide
Group D: Methane and most common hydrocarbons

Dusts and Particulates: The groups for dusts and particulate are specified for particular dusts and particulate as follows:

Group E: Combustible metal dusts regardless of resistivity, or other combustible dusts having a resistivity of less than ohm-centimeters or greater. Examples include aluminum, tin, and iron.

Group F: Carbon black, charcoal, coal or coke dust having more than 8 percent total volatile material or atmospheres having a resistivity greater that ohm-centimeters but equal to or less than ohm-centimeters.

Group G: Combustible dusts having a resistivity equal to or greater than ohm-centimeters. Examples include corn, rice, and other agricultural dusts.

Use of Hazardous Location Classifications

Instrumentation must be selected on the basis of the most hazardous atmosphere classification. For example, in measuring a potentially explosive atmosphere of ethylene oxide, one would select an instrument which was certified intrinsically safe for Class I, Division 1, Group B. In practice, instruments certified for use in gas and vapor hazardous atmospheres are certified for the most hazardous atmosphere and include all the lower classifications. For example, an instrument certified for use in Class I, Division 1, Group A, would be labeled for use in Class I, Division 1, Groups A, B, C, and D.

Although Group D contains methane, this certification is not the same as the Mine Safety and Health Administration 2G certification. The 2G certification is for use in methane atmospheres only. Methane requires a much greater ignition energy than the other members of Group D. Therefore, although methane is in Group D, instrumentation certified safe for use in methane atmospheres, may not be safe for use in atmospheres containing other Group D chemicals.

INSTRUMENT CERTIFICATION

Intrinsic Safety

Instruments selected for use in potentially hazardous atmospheres must be certified by an independent testing laboratory to ensure the instrument is intrinsically safe. As defined by the NFPA in Article 500 of the NEC:

> "Intrinsically safe equipment and wiring shall not be capable of releasing sufficient electrical or thermal energy under normal or abnormal conditions to cause ignition of a specific flammable or combustible atmospheric mixture in its most easily ignitible concentration." [24]

In other words, the equipment shall not be capable of igniting a explosive mixture under normal or fault conditions.

There are two basic testing programs. One tests only for intrinsic safety. A user can be assured the instrument is safe to operate in the atmosphere for which it is certified. The second program includes testing for performance also. The user is then assured the instrument is not only safe to use but that it will perform to documented performance criteria as well.

Intrinsic Safety Testing

The basic testing standard for intrinsic safety is ANSI/UL 913-1988 [26]. This standard was written by Underwriters Laboratories and adopted by the American National Standards Institute. It specifies the conditions for testing equipment for intrinsic safety. These conditions include evaluation of circuits for sources of spark ignition, maximum temperature, possible fault conditions, and testing under normal and fault conditions in hazardous atmospheres. The test atmospheres are representative gases at concentrations within the explosive range. The representative gases are:

Groups A and B: Hydrogen
Group C: Ethylene
Group D: Propane

Performance Testing

In addition to intrinsic safety testing, instruments may also be tested by independent laboratories for performance. The primary performance standard is ANSI/ISA-S12.13, Part 1-1986 [25]. This standard was written by the Instrument Society of America and adopted by the American National Standards Institute. It specifies the conditions for testing instrument performance. Areas tested include:

Accuracy: The instrument must indicate the true test concentration within + 3 percent of full scale gas concentration or + 10 percent of the applied gas concentration, whichever is greater.

Temperature Variation: The instrument sensing element will be subjected to temperatures of 0°C and 50°C and the meter indication should be vary from the test concentration by more than +5 percent of the full-scale gas concentration.

Concentration Step Change: When exposed to a test atmosphere of 100 percent of full-scale concentration, the instrument must respond to 60 percent of full scale within 12 seconds. When removed from this concentration, the instrument response should decline below 50 percent of full scale within 20 seconds and below 10 percent within 45 seconds.

Humidity Variation: Instruments are tested at 10 and 90 percent relative humidity after calibration at 50 percent relative humidity. The meter output should not vary more than + 10 percent of full-scale concentration from the 50 percent relative humidity concentration indication. Air Velocity Variation: The instrument response should be within +10 percent or 5 percent of the static concentration indication when exposed to a velocity of 5 + 0.5 meters per second.

Additional Tests: Instruments are also tested for vibration, electromagnetic interference, and long-term storage.

Certification Programs

Factory Mutual Research (FM): FM considers all combustible gas instruments as life support equipment requiring certification for performance in addition to intrinsic safety. Their performance tests are published in FM publication "Approval Standard, Combustible Gas Detectors" and are similar to ANSI/ISA S12-13, Part 1- 1986 [26]. Their intrinsic safety tests are similar to ANSI/UL 913-1988 [27]. Instrumentation successfully passing both the intrinsic safety and performance tests are approved by FM for use in the specified hazardous locations. This approval is indicated by the marking shown in Figure 5-8.

Canadian Safety Association (CSA): CSA approval is essentially the same as FM. Their approval marking is shown in Figure 5-9.

Underwriters Laboratories (UL): UL has two different testing approvals listing and classification. Information on UL listing and classification is as follows:

Classification: Instruments are checked to ensure they operate according to the manufacturer's instructions and are tested for intrinsic safety using the ANSI/UL 913-1988 protocol. Instruments which successfully pass these tests are listed as safe for use in specified hazardous locations.

Listed: In addition to intrinsic safety testing, UL also performs instrument performance testing. This testing may be to ANSI/ISA 12-13, Part 1-1986 or other criteria as specified by UL. The approval marking is the same as for the classified approval but the words will specify "Listed for Use In" performance testing criteria. The user must contact the manufacturer or UL to determine the exact performance criteria [28]. The approval marking is shown in Figure 5-10.

National Recognized Testing Laboratories (NRTL): Since UL and FM were the only laboratories providing intrinsic safety testing services when OSHA first wrote standards, OSHA regulations required certification by FM and UL. As a result of additional laboratories with testing capabilities, OSHA has developed the NRTL program. OSHA reviews the capabilities of laboratories to perform intrinsic safety testing (or other specific testing). OSHA requires intrinsic safety testing to an appropriate standard. Although not specified, most testing laboratories use ANSI/UL 913-1988. Laboratories successfully passing this review are recognized by OSHA as NRTLs [29]. This recognition is published in the Federal Register and laboratories are authorized to use NRTL in advertisements. As of June 1990, ETL, FM, MET, and UL are the only NRTLs for intrinsic safety.

MET Electrical Testing Laboratories: MET performs intrinsic safety testing in accordance with ANSI/UL 913-1988. Their approval marking is shown in Figure 5-11.

ETL: ETL performs intrinsic safety testing in accordance with ANSI/UL 913-1988. Their approval marking is shown in Figure 5-12.

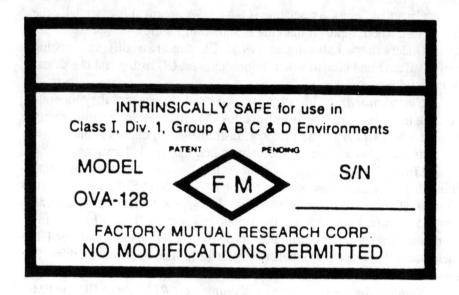

Figure 5-8. Factory Mutual approval markings [30]

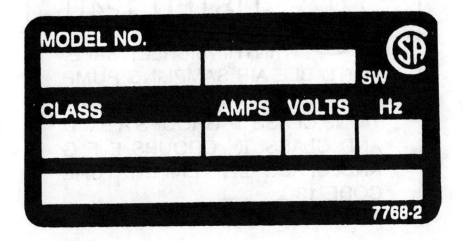

Figure 5-9. Canadian Safety Association approval marking [30]

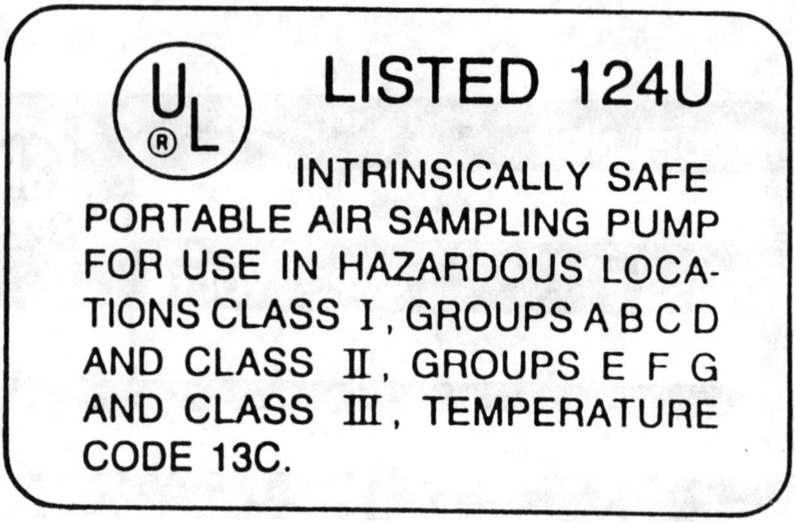

Figure 5-10. Underwriters Laboratory listed approval marking [30]

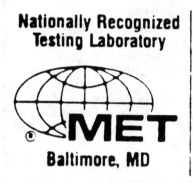

Figure 5-11. MET approval marking [30]

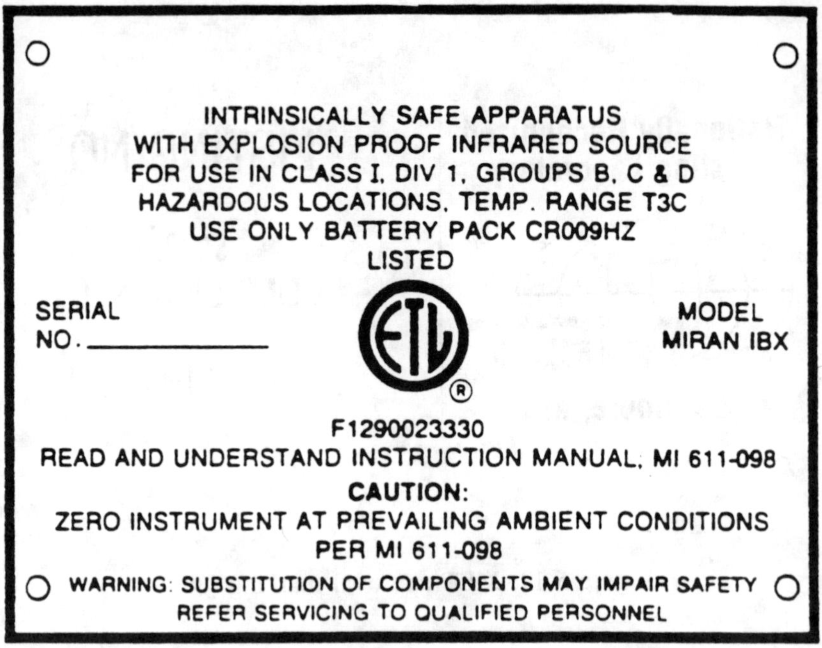

INTRINSICALLY SAFE APPARATUS
WITH EXPLOSION PROOF INFRARED SOURCE
FOR USE IN CLASS I, DIV 1, GROUPS B, C & D
HAZARDOUS LOCATIONS, TEMP. RANGE T3C
USE ONLY BATTERY PACK CR009HZ
LISTED

SERIAL
NO. _____

MODEL
MIRAN IBX

F1290023330
READ AND UNDERSTAND INSTRUCTION MANUAL, MI 611-098
CAUTION:
ZERO INSTRUMENT AT PREVAILING AMBIENT CONDITIONS
PER MI 611-098
WARNING: SUBSTITUTION OF COMPONENTS MAY IMPAIR SAFETY
REFER SERVICING TO QUALIFIED PERSONNEL

Figure 5-12. ETL approval marking [30]

LABELS

Instruments meeting the approval standards for intrinsic safety are marked with the independent testing laboratory's approval marking. This marking also includes the specific hazardous locations applicable to the approval (e.g., Class I, Division 1, Groups B, C, and D). Instrument users must ensure the instrument is approved for use in hazardous atmosphere to be measured.

REFERENCES

1.   Costello, R. J. and M. V. King. "Worker Inhalation Exposure Monitoring During Removal of Hazardous Waste From a Superfund Site" paper presented at the American Industrial Hygiene Association, Philadelphia, PA, May 22, 1983.
2.   Costello, R. J., and M. V. King. "Protecting Workers Who Cleanup Hazardous Waste Sites," *Amer. Ind. Hyg. Assoc. J.* 43:12-17 (1982).
3.   US Department of Labor, Title 29 Code of Federal Regulations, Part 1910.120. Hazardous Waste Operations and Emergency Response, USDOL, Washington, DC, (1989).
4.   NIOSH Pocket Guide to Chemical Hazards. US Department of Health and Human Services, National Institute for Occupational Safety and Health (1990).
5.   ACGIH. "1992-1993, Threshold Limit Values for Chemical Substances and Physical Agents and Biological Exposure Indices," American Conference of Governmental Industrial Hygienists, Cincinnati, OH (1992).
6.   Levine, S.P., Turpin, R.D. and M. Gochfeld. "Protecting Personnel at Hazardous Waste Sites: Current Issues", *Appl. Occup. Environ. Hyg.* 6(12) 1007-1013.
7.   U.S. Department of Labor, Title 29 Code of Federal Regulations, Part 1910.146, Permit Required Confined Spaces, USDOL, Washington, DC, (1993).
8.   Smith, J.M. and H.C. Van Ness, *Introduction to Chemical Engineering Thermodynamics, Third Edition*, McGraw-Hill, New York (1975)
9.   *TOMES Plus*, Micromedex, Inc., 1993.
10.   *AIHA Engineering Field Reference Manual*, AIHA, Akron, OH (1982).
11.   Leidel, N. A., K. A. Busch, and J. R. Lynch. "Occupational Exposure Sampling Strategy Manual," NIOSH (1977).
12.   Costello, R. J. "U.S. Environmental Protection Agency Triangle Chemical Site, Bridge City, Texas," NIOSH, Health Hazard Evaluations Determination Report HETA 83-417-1357, (1983).
13.   Costello, R. J. and J. Melius. "Technical Assistance Determination Report, Chemical Control, Elizabeth, New Jersey, TA 80-77," The National Institute for Occupational Safety and Health, (1981).
14.   Costello, R. J., B. Froenberg, and J. Melius. "Health Hazard Evaluation Determination Report, Rollins Environmental Services, Baton Rouge, Louisiana, HE 81-37," The National Institute for Occupational Safety and Health, (1981).

15. Hill R. H., and J. E. Arnold. "A Personal Air Sampler for Pesticides," *Arch. Environ. Contam. Toxicol.*, 8:621-28 (1979).

16. Taylor, D. G., Ed. NIOSH Manual of Analytical Methods 2nd. ed., The National Institute for Occupational Safety and Health, (1977).

17. Cullis, C.F. and J.G. Firth. *Detection and Measurement of Hazardous Gases*. Heinemann, London.

18. Personal Communication with Industrial Scientific Corporation Technical Staff (May, 1993).

19. Nyquist, J.E., Wilson, D.L., Norman, L.A., and R.B. Gammage. "Decreased Sensitivity of Photoionization Detector Total Organic Vapor Detectors in the Presence of Methane", *Am. Ind. Hyg. Assoc. J.* 51(6):326-330 (1990)

20. Levine, S.P., Li-Shi, Y, Strang, C.R., and X. Hong-Kui. "Advantages and Disadvantages in the Use of Fourier Transform Infrared (FTIR) and Filter Infrared (FIR) Spectrometers for Monitoring Airborne Gases and Vapors of Industrial Hygiene Concern", *Appl. Ind. Hyg.*, 4(7):180-187 (1989).

22. Organization Internationale de Metrologie Legale, Guide to Portable Instruments for Assessing Airborne Pollutants Arising from Hazardous Wastes, OIML D 22 (1991

23. U.S. Department of Labor, OSHA Field Operations Manual. USDOL(OSHA), Washington, DC (1990).

24. Article 500, *National Electrical Code*, NFPA -70, Hazardous (Classified) Locations, National Fire Protection Association.

25. *NFPA 497M, Classification of Gases, Vapors and Dusts for Electrical Equipment in Hazardous (Classified) Locations 1986*. National Fire Protection Association.

26. UL/ANSI. ANSI/UL 913-1988. Standard for Intrinsically Safe Apparatus and Associated Apparatus for Use in Class I, II, and III, Division 1, Hazardous (Classified) Locations", Underwriters Laboratories, Inc. (1988).

27. ANSI/ISA. ANSI/ISA-S12.13, Part I-1986. Performance Requirements, Combustible Gas Detectors. Instrument Society of America (1986).

28. Factory Mutual Research. "Approval Standard, Combustible Gas Detectors", Factory Mutual Research. (1989)

29. Factory Mutual Research. "Approval Standard for Intrinsically Safe Apparatus and Associated Apparatus for Use in Class I, II, and III, Division 1, Hazardous (Classified) Locations", Factory Mutual Research (1988)

30.   *AIHA Manual of Recommended Practice for Combustible Gas indicators and Portable, Direct Reading Hydrocarbon Detectors, Second Edition*, AIHA, (1993).

31.   U.S. Department of Labor, Title 29 Code of Federal Regulations, Part 1907 and 1910. Safety Testing or Certification of Certain Workplace Equipment and Materials; Final Rule. USDOL, Washington, DC, (1988).

6

COMPATIBILITY TESTING

Timothy G. Prothero, B.A.
Mark A. Puskar, Ph.D.

The stockpiling or dumping of waste chemicals in drums has been a widespread practice throughout the United States. At one-quarter of all abandoned waste sites major drum-related problems, including handling, integrity, characterization, and disposal exist [1, 2]. Bulk recontainerization (bulking) of hazardous materials located in drums, labpacks, tanks, and holding ponds, has become the most time- and cost-effective solution to handling the waste. The potentially hazardous incompatibilities must be known before co-mingling wastes for worker safety. Potential hazards that can result from improper mixing of chemicals include fire, explosion, violent splashing or reaction, polymerization, and corrosive or toxic gas generation.

Bulking involves removing the hazardous materials from the drums, labpacks, tanks, and holding ponds and combining compatible wastes into larger transportable containers [3]. When mixed together, many chemicals can produce potentially hazardous effects such as fires, explosions, violent reactions, and the release of toxic dusts, mists, fumes, and gases. Therefore, chemical wastes must first be tested for compatibility before they are bulked and incompatible chemicals must be segregated [4].

Chemical compatibility testing is not as extensive as the complete characterization of each individual drum of waste by standard laboratory testing procedures (e.g., RCRA Series, GC/MS, Emission Spectrography). There are several useful guidelines for developing field testing protocols. The American Society for Testing and Materials (ASTM) has several useful standards. Several textbooks on qualitative spot tests are useful for developing field testing protocols. The government has developed some guidelines concerning chemical compatibilities. These guideline "References" are listed at the end of this chapter [20-28]. Complete chemical characterization would be far too costly and time consuming for the purposes of hazardous waste cleanup. Compatibility testing, followed by bulking compatible drum contents into large containers appears to be the most cost- and time-effective method of preparing the waste for transportation to an approved disposal facility. Therefore, the second goal of compatibility testing is to generate enough knowledge of the characteristics of the waste to develop a hazardous waste classification for the shipping manifest which will be acceptable to the site manager, state or federal agency, transporter, and receiver of the waste.

This chapter will discuss the importance of compatibility testing, the general steps involved, and the limitations of compatibility testing. In general, compatibility testing involves performing a group of simple chemical tests (e.g., water solubility, pH, flammability) following a flowchart scheme which ultimately classifies the material into general categories. A comprehensive field compatibility protocol will include tests for several potential hazards including: flammability tests, pH, tests for oxidizers, water and air reactivity tests, gas generation, heat generation, polymerization potential. Even a comprehensive field testing protocol will have limitations. One example is the reaction rate. Oxidation/reduction reactions may be slow in generating sufficient heat for ignition; an example is the combination of motor oil and certain kitty litter brands. Field conditions, including drafts and temperature, also interfere with test performance. Therefore, because of potential interferences with field compatibility tests, field cleanup personnel must be alert to chemical reactions during cleanup operations [3, 5-12].

IMPORTANCE OF COMPATIBILITY TESTING

The importance of compatibility testing is evident after examining situations where proper compatibility testing was not performed prior to handling of potentially hazardous waste.

On April 21, 1980, a massive explosion and fire occurred in Elizabeth, New Jersey, at a hazardous waste site owned by the Chemical Control Corporation. Of the 45,000 drums present at the site, more than 20,000 were consumed. During the initial site investigation which had been underway for 12 months prior to the fire, no compatibility testing and drum segregation had been performed. The post-fire cleanup cost millions more than the pre-fire estimates [13, 14].

In January of 1982, workers were unloading chemical wastes from a tank truck at the Liquid Disposal Incineration, Inc., in Utica, Michigan. Deadly hydrogen sulfide gas was generated when a mislabeled sulfide waste from the tank truck mixed with acid in the receiving vessel. Two workers died and six others required hospitalization. Compatibility testing had not been performed on the incoming waste [15].

Field Analyses Plan (FAP)

A meticulous plan of action must be developed before testing chemicals in the field. The Field Analyses Plan must be in writing, and prepared by a qualified and experienced chemist after careful consideration of:

- the site conditions, including availability of field laboratory, temperature control, safety fume hoods, protection from explosive/flammable vapors, etc.;
- known and suspected waste types and hazards; and
- how the wastes are "packaged;" for example, are the wastes in drums, lagoons, tanks, or are all wastes diluted or mixed into environmental media such as water or soil?

A Field Analyses Plan emphasizing known and suspected site hazards must also include potential, yet unsuspected, hazards. For example, when planning field tests for an abandoned metal working plant site, hazardous polymerization screening must still be included despite metal working plants, such as tube mills and welding shops, not typically working with polymerizable compounds. Composite samples of similar or identical characteristics can be screened for polymerization instead of testing each sample. Table 6-1 offers suggestions for a FAP.

Table 6-1. Example Contents of a Field Analysis Plan	
1	Purpose of Plan, objectives, and safety precautions and protocols
2	List of known and suspected hazards/wastes
3	Testing procedure for compatibility of mixing wastes
4	Fire/explosion potential testing procedures
5	Air/water reactivity testing procedures
6	Tests for potential to generate toxic gases
7	Solubility, flame tests and physical screening for characterization of wastes
8	Oxidizer testing
9	pH testing
10	Special tests as needed for treatment or disposal of wastes
11	Procedures to inform workers about results of tests

Field analyses must be done by qualified chemists following standard laboratory safety protocols. Detailed discussions of laboratory safety practices are beyond the scope of this chapter.

The chemist must be familiar with, and closely follow, standard laboratory safety practices and laboratory hygiene plans. The analyst must use appropriate personal protective equipment including, but not limited to, protective gloves, goggles, face shield, heavy rubber laboratory apron, and arm protectors. A protective fume hood should be used. All tests must be done in a safe (non-flammable and non-toxic) atmosphere.

COMMON CHARACTERISTICS OF COMPATIBILITY METHODS

Although the above incidents exemplify the importance of compatibility testing, a universally accepted compatibility testing procedure does not exist. The contractor that is awarded the site cleanup contract is given a suggested scheme to follow. The only requirements are that these proposed protocols provide analytical data, compatibility testing results and are environmentally sensitive during removal and disposal of hazardous waste from the site [8]. The scheme chosen for a specific remedial action site is based on the following factors:

(1) The general kinds of waste materials suspected to be present on-site as determined by the initial site screening.
(2) The criteria chosen by the governmental agency supervising the cleanup.
(3) The preferences of the prime contractor and their experience with compatibility testing.
(4) The criteria of the disposal facility to which the waste will ultimately be sent.

The groups listed below have all developed compatibility schemes. These schemes separate the waste into as few as ten categories [9, 12] and as many as 41 [3]:

1. USEPA, Office of Research and Development, Municipal Environmental Research Laboratory (MERL) [3].
2. Samsel Services Company, Cleveland, Ohio [9].
3. Environmental Response Team, USEPA [10].
4. O. H. Materials Co., Findley, Ohio [12].

5. U.S. Army Corps of Engineers [8].
6. ASTM, scheme developed by committee D-34 [7].
7. Chemical Manufacturers Association, Inc. [11].
8. NIOSH, Occupational Safety and Health Guidance Manual [16].
9. USEPA, HAZCAT.

The basic *procedure* in compatibility testing involves subdividing the liquids into general disposal categories, given the following assumptions:

1. A large number of drums exist on-site, and simple overpacking with complete laboratory analysis (GC-MS) is not time- or cost-effective.
2. An on-site facility is available with proper room, equipment, and experienced personnel to perform the analytical tests.
3. The waste contains a complex mixture of solids and liquids.

Compatibility testing is only one step in the handling of drum wastes on a remedial action site. Figure 6-1 diagrams the role that compatibility testing plays during drum handling.

Although each compatibility scheme is unique, most follow a similar flowchart. Figure 6-2 is the flowchart of the scheme used by O. H. Materials Co. Note that incompatible wastes such as radioactive, air and water reactive, PCB, sulfide, and cyanide wastes are identified by compatibility testing, but are usually not bulked prior to disposal. These highly hazardous wastes are repacked or overpacked, depending on the condition and size of their original container, and disposed separately.

The basic steps in compatibility testing occur in three stages of drum handling: 1) testing performed prior to drum opening; 2) testing performed during drum handling; and 3) testing performed on collected samples. The tests generally performed in each of these stages are discussed below.

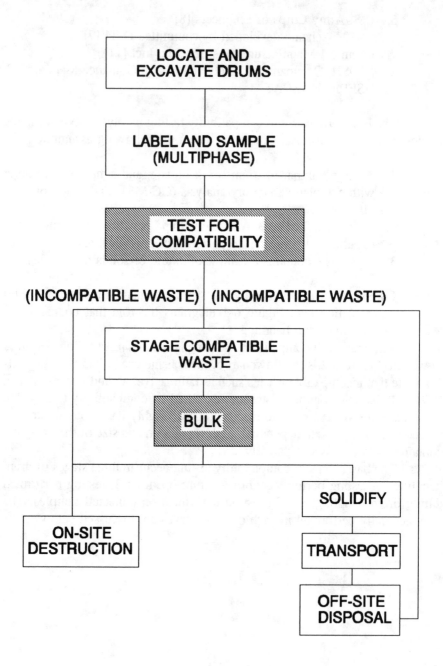

Figure 6-1. Flow diagram of drum handling operations during site remedial action.

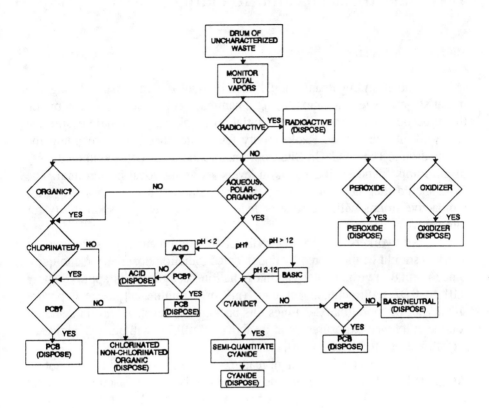

Figure 6-2. Compatibility testing for characterization of hazardous wastes.

TESTING PERFORMED PRIOR TO DRUM OPENING

Radioactive Wastes

The sampling team should identify radioactive wastes during the initial stage of site evaluation, using a gamma survey instrument. Following this procedure and performing the initial air monitoring will help ensure the safety of site personnel. Radioactivity levels are checked by scanning the closed drums. The OSC (On-Site Coordinator) should be notified immediately of all drums found having radiation levels above the local background. The OSC should then determine the appropriate handling and disposal steps for radioactive drums with the state or federal agency having responsibility for radioactive wastes.

All workers performing radioactive drum handling, sampling, or analysis should be monitored by documented radiation dosimetry techniques. Since normal environmental gamma radiation background is approximately 0.01 to 0.02 milliroentgen per hour (mR/hr.), routine employee exposure should not be more than 2-3 times this background level. At no time should routine employee exposures be at or above 10 mR/hr. without the advice of a qualified health physicist [10] .

The absence of instrument readings above background should not be interpreted as the complete absence of radioactivity. Radioactive materials emitting low-level gamma, alpha, or beta radiation may be present, but for a number of reasons may not cause a response on the portable instrument. However, unless they are airborne, these radioactive materials should present minimal hazard. Reanalysis for radioactivity during sample compatibility testing is recommended. See Chapter 14, Radiation Safety for more details.

TESTING PERFORMED DURING DRUM SAMPLING

Physical Screening

At abandoned waste sites, unknown wastes can be organized into streams through a combination of physical screening, compatibility testing, and laboratory analyses. Wastes with identical physical characteristics can be grouped for compatibility screening because they are likely candidates for bulking or mixing. Table 6-2 gives example physical parameters to use for characterizing unknown wastes [3].

Table 6-2. Physical Characterizations of Wastes	
Color	Describe color(s) of waste in decreasing order of prominence
Turbidity	Transparent, translucent, or opaque
Viscosity	Estimate in terms of common products, examples: Low (water); medium (motor oil); high (honey or molasses)
Physical State	Liquid, semi-solid, solid, powder, granular, mixed phasing
Layering	How many layers and physical characteristics of each

Explosives/Air Reactives

After radioactive testing has been performed and all radioactive drums have been separated, the remaining drums are staged and opened for sampling. Drum opening, sampling, and staging protocols are shown in the process flow diagram in Figure 6-1, and detailed in the literature [8, 11] and must be *strictly* followed.

The objective of taking total vapor concentrations values just inside the bung hole is to assist in determining whether or not the headspace has a potentially explosive atmosphere. The limitations and operating characteristics of the monitoring instrument must be recognized and understood. Instruments such as the photoionization detectors (PID) and the organic vapor analyzer (OVA-FID) have unique sensitivities and specificities to identical substances, and proper calibration when dealing with "unknowns" is impossible. Also, dangerous gases/vapors undetectable by photo and flame ionization detectors may be present. Such gases would include: phosgene, hydrogen cyanide, chlorine gas, and liquid/solid particulates.

The next compatibility test performed on opened drums is air reactivity. This is performed by visual observation during sampling. Any sample taken from a drum containing a solid which ignites or emits fumes or gases is considered air reactive and is immediately resealed and separated [9]. Also, any drum found containing metal submerged in liquid should be immediately segregated and considered air reactive. Additional sampling should be done to identify the type of metal. The most common elements found disposed in this manner are phosphorus (air reactive) and sodium (water reactive).

TESTING PERFORMED ON COLLECTED SAMPLES

Water Reactivity/Solubility

Radioactive, air reactive, and explosive testing are performed prior to and during sampling. One of the first compatibility tests performed on the collected samples should be water reactivity/solubility. This simple test can generate a host of information on the uncharacterized waste.

The characteristics of reactivity, as defined in the RCRA regulations (40 CFR 261.23), are exhibited if a representative sample of the waste has any of several properties, including:

(1) it reacts violently with water;
(2) it forms potentially explosive mixtures with water;
(3) when mixed with water, it generates toxic gases, vapors, or fumes in a quantity sufficient to present a danger to human health or the environment.

The compatibility methods call for a small volume (1 mL for highly reactives to 10-mL for non-reactives) of liquid waste to be added to water and the mixture observed for water miscibility, temperature exotherm, precipitation, and/or gas formation. If any of these occur, the waste is classified water reactive. Following this definition, acids and bases are initially classified as water reactive. They will later be separated by pH measurements. A major interference of this test is that certain water reactive materials may require a reaction time, catalyst, or heat before reactions occur. While potentially dangerous, this test can be relatively safe if precautions against explosions and toxic vapors hazards are taken. Unknown organic vapors, hydrogen cyanide, hydrogen sulfide, chlorine, ammonia, and hydrogen gases could be generated in small amounts.

Another scheme [9] only classifies materials which evolve gases, fumes, or ignite as water reactive. Materials which produce a temperature change are not considered to be water reactive unless the water approached boiling temperature. Following this definition, acids and bases are initially separated from water reactives. Water reactive drums should be isolated and sheltered from the elements. However, because of the danger of explosion and fire, indoor storage is not recommended. Table 6-3 presents solubility characteristics of selected compounds [29].

Table 6-3. Solubility Characteristics of Selected Compounds				
Compound	**Water**	**Ether**	**HCl**	**NaOH**
Salts of Acids, Bases	Soluble	Insoluble		
Alcohols, Esters, Ethers	Soluble	Soluble		
Hydrocarbons, Aliphatic or Aromatic	Insoluble	Soluble		
Amines, Amino Acids	Insoluble		Soluble	
Acids, Anhydrides	Insoluble			Soluble
Phenols	Insoluble			Soluble
Nitriles	Insoluble	Insoluble	Insoluble	Insoluble

Organics/Inorganics

When a liquid sample from an uncharacterized waste drum is placed in water and is nonreactive, it will either be soluble or insoluble in the water. If it is insoluble, it will either sink or float (becomes the top or bottom phase).

Samples that are soluble in water are strong suspects for inorganic classification. The solubility of these samples is determined in hexane, and if they are soluble in the hexane they are classified as nonhalogenated organics (polar). If they are insoluble in the hexane, they are classified as inorganic liquids.

Organics/Halogenated Organics

Samples that are insoluble in water and are the top phase are classified as organic liquids. Two schemes [3, 11] check the vapor concentration above the sample at this point with either a PID or a OVA-FID to determine if the organic liquid should be classified as volatile or not. A value of 12000 ppm is recommended to classify an organic sample as volatile.

Samples that are insoluble in water and are the bottom phase are classified as halogenated organics. This procedure for determining halogenated organics is essentially a procedure designed to determine gross halogen content, not parts per million as required by law for PCBs. Further tests to confirm the presence of halogens using either a copper loop flame test [12], halogenated organic GC-ECD scan [18], potentiometric titration [11], and total organic halogen (TOX) have been suggested.

Analysis of all drums classified as organic for PCBs [8] must be conducted to determine if ultimate disposal is possible in a non-PCB approved incinerator (for liquids) or landfill (solids and soil). This testing procedure, semi-quantitative from a hexane extraction by gas chromatography [11], should be conducted prior to drum bulking so isolation of PCB-contaminated containers and/or a change in bulking sequence can be inserted to avoid further PCB contamination. The PCB analysis can be conducted on composited samples, to save time and money; however, it would be expedient to not composite more than ten drums per sample. Any drums determined to be> 50 ppm PCB are classified as PCB-contaminated wastes.

Flammability

Although a standard flashpoint test would furnish helpful information about the unidentified waste, this analytical method becomes impractical when dealing with large numbers of drums on a remedial action site. For example, if a test could be performed every 20 minutes, it would take approximately three man-years to analyze 20,000 mono-phasic drums. Thus, simple flammability techniques have been developed to separate flammables from nonflammables.

For solid unknowns, a small sample (20 to 50 mg) is transferred on a steel spatula into an open flame. If the material is a liquid, a stainless steel loop holding a drop of the unknown is employed [9]. If the sample ignites violently at some point in the heating, it is classified as an explosive. If the material burns with the flame, it is considered flammable and organic. Exceptions to this guideline are inorganics such as phosphorus and sulfur;

however, their characteristics during burning may be used to distinguish them from organics. Also, clear halogenated organics, such as chloroform or carbon tetrachloride, test as inorganics in the flame test. If the material chars or turns black, it is suspected of being organic. If the material does not burn, it is considered inorganic. The first screen test requires only one drop of a representative sample on a spatula or forceps. As that drop is brought close to a flame, observe whether the flame seems to "jump" out at the drop. That happens because sample vapors are ignited; the sample is flammable. If the sample will ignite only when the drop is at the flame, then there has been no formation of flammable vapors, but the sample is combustible. When the drop must be heated by the flame before igniting, the waste is combustible with a high flash point. If the drop of sample is flammable, or "pops" or explodes, do not test with larger sample amounts. Table 6-4 provides some interpretations of the flame type that might be observed with this test [4].

Table 6-4. Flame Tests	
Flame Type	**Interpretation**
Almost smokeless	Low chain organics
Bluish flame	Compounds with lots of oxygen
Dark smoke	Halogenated
Sooty smoke	Aromatic
Boils without igniting	Aqueous
Chars without igniting	Inorganic

The above test may result falsely in the negative from the small amount of sample used, or the susceptibility to air drafts, or difficulty to see the flame. A larger amount may be tested after the initial test indicates that there are no undue hazards in further testing. Place between 1 to 5 g or mL of sample in a non-flammable container such as a metal weighing dish or a crucible cover. Holding the dish with long forceps, bring the dish to a blue, bunsen burner flame slowly. Alternately, the dish may be held in place by a laboratory apparatus stand while the burner is moved slowly to the dish. Observe the actions of the flame and sample. A sample that ignites before or when the burner flame touches the dish is considered to have positive flammability potential. A sample that does not ignite after 15 seconds in the burner flame is considered to have negative flammability potential [23].

Another scheme [10] suggests placing a 2-5 ml representative sample in a disposable beaker. The beaker is placed in a large sandbox and a propane torch is slowly passed over the unidentified waste. If a flame is observed, the waste is classified as flammable. A nonflammable classification is assigned to the waste after the torch has passed over the waste several times. Certain disposal facilities may require confirmation flashpoint testing to be conducted on all spot-tested samples which were classified positive.

Most observers will be able to make a distinction between organics, inorganics, and free metals using a flame test. Because of the dangers of explosions or fires with these types of flammability testing, safety requirements must be strictly followed. Indoor flammability testing should be performed in explosion-proof high-flow hoods. Fire extinguishers and safety showers must be immediately available. A field quality control program would be useful to verify field observations. Several compounds of known flash points can provide the field analyst with points of reference for his or her observations. The quality control program is especially important when interpretations of the flame and smoke types are desired.

pH

To guard against explosive exothermic reactions and evolution of deadly gases (cyanide, sulfide) caused by the commingling of caustic and acidic wastes, pH measurements are taken to separate potentially dangerous drums. The pH of each sample, previously classified as water soluble, is determined using either an electronic pH meter with temperature compensation adjustment and appropriate electrodes, or indicator strips (pH paper) covering the pH range of interest. Both have disadvantages when used on "dirty" samples containing organic layers, sludge, or concentrated solutions. For instance, standard pH electrodes are easily fouled and require constant cleaning, recalibration, and regular replacement. Most colorimetric indicators and papers are easily obscured by grease, sludge, or opaque solutions.

A pH meter can determine the pH of a representative sample to within 0.1 of a pH unit. The pH meter must be calibrated by using at least two standard buffer solutions. Clean the pH electrode gently before and after each use. Dip the electrode into sufficient sample to immerse the electrode's sensing element. Record the pH. Clean the electrode. Repeat the process on several samples of the same material until the readings differ by 0.1 pH unit [26]. Interfering chemicals may even cause false color changes. These interferences are limited by the use of multiband pH paper which contains reaction zones and a series of indicator colors fixed for reference. After the strip has been exposed to the waste, the color comparison of the reaction zone and the indicator color is made "assuming" that both have been affected in the same way by the waste.

The greatest concern with the commingling of acids and bases is the generation of deadly cyanide and sulfide gases. Cyanide and sulfide wastes are usually buffered at a pH of 10 in order to remain in aqueous solution. This important fact has been used to define acids and bases for compatibility purposes. Caustic wastes are defined as those with a pH above 10, and acidic wastes are defined as those with a pH below 10 [10]. Following this definition, the accidental release of sulfide or cyanide gas during drum bulking is greatly reduced.

Other schemes [8, 9, 11] separate the wastes into three or four categories depending on the pH value. Wastes with pH values less than 2 are classified as acids; between 2 and 7 are classified as acidic aqueous solutions; between 7 and 12 are classified as basic aqueous wastes; and greater than 12 are classified as bases.

Wet methods [11], and the use of ion-selective electrodes [12], are used to determine the presence and concentration of cyanide and sulfide in bases. All drums tested positive are separated from the bases. Additional staging safeguards, including barriers, are recommended to reduce the risk of accidental mixing of cyanide/sulfide bases with acids.

The method of defining acids and bases and selecting analytical methods should be based on the future analytical tests required to meet the criteria set by the approved disposal facility accepting the waste. Many disposal facilities require base and acid reactivity testing prior to acceptance. This method can be found in the *Federal Register*, 40 CFR 261, Subpart C [25]. The hazardous wastes regulations under RCRA (40 CFR 261) regulate as hazardously corrosive those acidic compounds with pH from 0 to 2, and those basic compounds with pH from 12.5 to 14 [25].

Strong acids and (sulfide- and cyanide-free) bases identified can be blended on-site for neutralization. These reactions will be highly exothermic and should not be attempted without adequate safeguards [11] including real-time sulfide/cyanide air monitoring systems and bulking chamber temperature monitors. On-site neutralization may significantly lower disposal costs of waste acids and bases.

Screening for Sulfides or Cyanides

Acidify a small amount of a representative sample in a test tube to screen for sulfides or cyanides in a material. Then test the gases evolved for the presence of the toxic gases. Please note that proper safety precautions must be taken to avoid exposure to the toxic gases.

Testing for sulfide may be done by acidifying 5 to 10 g of sample in a large test tube or small beaker with hydrochloric acid. A wet strip of lead acetate paper over the top of the tube or beaker will react with hydrogen sulfide to change the paper color to brown or black. An alternate test method for sulfides is to acidify the sample with a phosphoric acid solution in a beaker. The air above the test solution, inside the beaker, is pumped through a gas detector tube selected for its sulfide sensitivity. A color change in the gas detector tube is an indication of the presence of sulfides in the sample [27].

Four field tests for cyanide are published by ASTM. As with the tests for sulfides, cyanide in wastes can be tested by acidifying a sample and testing for cyanide in the evolved gases. Cyantesmo test paper, or gas detector tubes, can be used to detect cyanide in the gases over the acidified samples. A distinct color change is considered a positive test result. Two other test methods involve using specific reagents to produce color changes in the test solutions. One solution will detect cyanides amenable to chlorination; the other is an indicator of free cyanide and many complex cyanides [28].

Oxidizers/Reducers

Compatibility testing procedures have been developed for analyzing and classifying drums containing oxidizing or reducing agents, including wet methods, test papers, and portable instrumentation methods.

The wet methods [9] include a colorimetric determination of organic peroxides in solid organic unknowns using titanium sulfate as a yellow color indicator and a colorimetric determination of inorganic oxidizers in solids or liquids using manganous chloride as a black or brown indicator. Test papers have had the widest acceptance due to their quickness and simplicity [3, 12]; however, the authors are unaware of any documentation of their ability to determine oxidizers and reducers in complex waste samples.

A potentiometric determination of the redox potential of drum samples through the use of a portable battery-operated instrument has been developed and tested [10]. The unique features of this method is its ability to perform redox measurements not only in aqueous but also organic matrices, such as are found on hazardous waste sites. The entire procedure requires only a few minutes and can be performed by inexperienced operators in the drum staging area. The test is very sensitive and a reaction with only a small portion of an oxidizing agent will give a positive test.

The method involves using an electrolyte solution to generate a known redox potential and then measuring the change in the potential when an unknown waste is added to the electrolyte. Ferrous ammonium sulfate, as a standard electrolyte, is used for oxidation readings. Potassium chromate is substituted for reduction measurements.

Two minor problems have been encountered with this field procedure: electrode probe clogging and electrolyte freezing at sub-O C temperatures. The clogging problem is identical to the pH electrode clogging problem and can be resolved by proper cleaning of the probe between samples. The cold weather, however, causes the probe electrolyte to freeze. This problem is resolved by conducting the tests inside an on-site laboratory.

Another oxidizer screening test is relatively simple. A small sample is placed on a piece of potassium iodide starch paper. A positive test result is indicated by the appearance of a blue color change in the paper. Obviously, dark and opaque samples might mask the color change and give false negative results. A drop of liquid sample on the starch paper is enough for this test. To test solid and semi-solid samples, mix a small amount of sample into a similar amount of water. Apply a drop of the water to the starch paper [6].

Use known oxidizing compounds for the quality control program. Compounds selected on the basis of their widely different oxidizer potentials will acquaint the analyst with the sensitivity of the test.

Labpacks

Labpacks are 55-gallon drums which contain small volume containers of waste chemicals. Most are unlabeled chemical reagents discarded by laboratories. Proper disposal of this type of container presents a unique and hazardous clean-up problem. The chemicals stored in many of these small containers are incompatible. Usually, these containers were not packed in absorbent material prior to original disposal, so breakage and chemical mixing during drum handling is common. For this reason, these drums are considered primary ignition sources for fires during remedial action.

Compatibility testing is performed by chemists conducting visual inspection of the containers, without opening, and attempting to classify them. If crystalline material is observed in the neck of any bottle, it is handled as shock sensitive, due to the potential presence of picric acid or similar materials. Shock-sensitive containers are repacked in absorbent material, and repacked not more than five to a drum, and shipped to a disposal facility or detonated on-site. The containers with markings that can be identified and trusted (a purely subjective judgement) are segregated into similar compatibility categories and repacked in absorbent material [17].

The repacking protocol for unidentifiable containers is set by the facility accepting them for final disposal. This usually involves separating the unknowns into solids and liquids, and the liquids into single- and multi-phased.

A compatibility scheme for labpacks has been tested which identifies expected chemicals among unlabeled materials, segregates the remaining unlabeled materials into one of six disposal groups and destroys or neutralizes the excepted materials sufficiently to permit landfill disposal. This method [9] involves opening, sampling, and performing classic compatibility testing on each container.

Another suggested scheme for the disposal of labpacks calls for opening each container with a high velocity, low mass projectile (a 0.22 caliber bullet) [19]. This safely accomplishes two things: the container (almost exclusively glass bottles) are remotely opened by fracture from the bullet impact, and the contents are collected and rendered stable in an absorbent material. Advantages to this method include simplicity over remote control detonation, minimal set-up, low-technical procedure, low visibility compared to detonation, and low cost; however, this procedure would be impossible in a populated location. In highly populated locations, this scheme has been adapted by opening each container by running it over with a bulldozer, and then performing RCRA testing on the contaminated soil.

Compatibility Screening Prior to Mixing Wastes

Before mixing wastes for shipment or disposal, those wastes must be screened for mutually compatibility. Typical mixing hazards include fire, explosion, violent reaction, splashing, heat or toxic gases generation and violent polymerization [20].

Representative samples of the wastes are mixed under controlled conditions. The test mixture is carefully monitored for any adverse reaction [21].

Compatibility screening requires determination of which wastes will be mixed, what volume of each, and in what order will they be combined. Mix 1 to 2 mL of representative samples of the wastes into a stainless steel vessel which is thermometrically monitored. Mix those samples in the same sequence in which the wastes will be mixed. A common laboratory safety guideline illustrates the importance of performing the compatibility screen test by mixing the samples in identical order as the wastes. The laboratory safety guideline notes that acid must always be added acid to water for safety sake; violent reactions may occur when water is added to acid. Potentially hazardous reactions might be missed if the samples are not mixed in the same order as the wastes. Carefully note any heat generation, or other adverse reactions. Stop testing immediately when any adverse reaction is noticed [21].

Once the screen test is completed without adverse reactions, the testing may continue using larger amounts of samples. The resulting amount of the tested representative samples should be about 150 mL. Again, stop the test when any reaction is observed. Mixing the samples in equal amounts increases the sensitivity of the test.

Another approach to compatibility screening involves testing samples of unknown wastes against known chemicals. Table 6-5, from 40 CFR 264 Appendix IV, shows potentially incompatible waste types. An unknown material can be characterized into a compatibility scheme by mixing very small samples of unknown wastes with similar amounts of known materials.

Table 6-5. Potentially Incompatible Wastes

Group 1-A	Group 1-B
Acetylene sludge Alkaline caustic liquids Alkaline cleaner Alkaline corrosive liquids Alkaline corrosive battery fluid Caustic wastewater Lime sludge and other corrosive alkalies Lime wastewater Lime and water Spent caustic	Acid sludge Acid and water Battery acid Chemical cleaners Electrolyte, acid Etching acid liquid or solvent Pickling liquor and other corrosive acids Spent acid Spent mixed acid Spent sulfuric acid
Potential consequences of mixing Groups 1-A and 1-B: Heat generation; violent reaction.	
Group 2-A	Group 2-B
Aluminum Beryllium Calcium Lithium Magnesium Potassium Sodium Zinc powder Other reactive metals and metal hydrides	Any waste in Group 1-A or 1-B
Potential consequences of mixing Groups 2-A and 2-B: Fire or explosion; generation of flammable hydrogen gas.	
Group 3-A	Group 3-B
Alcohols Water	Any concentrated waste in Groups 1-A or 1-B Calcium Lithium Metal hydrides Potassium Other water-reactive waste
Potential consequences of mixing Groups 3-A and 3-B: Fire, explosion, or heat generation; generation of flammable or toxic gases.	

Table 6-5. Potentially Incompatible Wastes	
Group 4-A	Group 4-B
Alcohols Aldehydes Halogenated hydrocarbons Nitrated hydrocarbons Unsaturated hydrocarbons Other reactive organic compounds and solvents	Concentrated Group 1-A or 1-B wastes Group 2-A wastes
Potential consequences of mixing Groups 4-A and 4-B: Fire, explosion, or violent reaction.	
Group 5-A	Group 5-B
Spent cyanide and sulfide solutions	Group 1-B wastes
Potential consequences of mixing Groups 5-A and 5-B: Generation of toxic hydrogen cyanide or hydrogen sulfide gas.	
Group 6-A	Group 6-B
Chlorates Chlorine Chlorites Chromic acid Hypochlorite Nitrates Nitric acid, fuming Perchlorates Permanganates Peroxides Other strong oxidizers	Acetic acid and other organic acids Concentrated mineral acids Group 2-A wastes Group 4-A wastes Other flammable and combustible wastes
Potential consequences of mixing Groups 6-A and 6-B: Fire, explosion, or violent reaction.	

Instead of preparing a test with all seven combinations listed, other tests in this chapter are more appropriate in classifying some reactivity groups in Table 6-5. For example, pH is a fast and easy method to classify wastes in groups 1-A, 1-B, 2-B, part of group 3-B, 4-B, 5-B, and parts of groups 6-A and 6-B. Wastes that fall into other reactivity groups from Table 6-5 can be identified by tests discussed in this chapter.

To determine the polymerization potential of a waste, mix a small sample of the waste into a similar amount of triethylamine on a ceramic spotplate. Please note the potential for violent reaction and take appropriate safety precautions. Observe any reaction including gelling, fuming, gas evolution, burning or charring. Only if no reaction was observed, should larger amounts be used in a test tube, about 5 mL each of sample and reagent. Do not hold the test tube. Again, observe for any chemical reaction. Any chemical reaction is a positive indication of incompatibility [21].

A field quality control program can be established by periodically testing compounds of known composition and compatibility. Demonstrations of incompatible reactions under controlled conditions are commonplace in chemistry classes. For example, the reaction of a small piece of sodium in water is commonly used for safety lectures.

Limitations of Compatibility Testing Procedures

It should be understood that the compatibility methods discussed are designed to detect acute incompatibility only. Reactions which require heat or other catalyzing effects for initiation will not be detected by these tests [8].

Mixtures are only identified as far as it is necessary to place them into one of the disposal groups. Since these procedures are not designed to identify specific compounds, there are a number of types of materials for which these procedures are not applicable. The identification of highly toxic or carcinogenic materials, such as dioxin, which should not be landfilled is beyond the scope of these procedures. Although these procedures may be employed to segregate total unknowns into disposal groups, additional specific tests must be performed to determine the presence and concentration of materials that cannot be landfilled [9]. This problem may be controlled for by incinerating all nonsoil wastes in a Class B facility; however, this solution is not cost-effective.

The need to test-mix the wastes on a small scale, prior to drum bulking, is emphasized even if the compatibility tests indicate compatibility. A major problem with the test mixing, and thus compatibility testing, is obtaining a homogeneous sample from each uncharacterized drum, especially when working with multi-phased drums containing both liquids and solids. Even after the unknown drums are mixed, the clean-up personnel are unable to estimate the short-term (minutes to hours) or long-term (days to weeks) effects of mixing and recontainerizing unknown materials [3].

Very little data exists that document the effectiveness of compatibility schemes in separating unknown wastes. The data that does exist details major classes that cannot be identified, including isocyanates, epoxides, nitriles, and polymerizable materials. In addition, a need exists for a sound quality-control criteria for compatibility testing [3].

No methods have been proposed for the screening of pathogenic or infectious materials. These may be present in the uncharacterized drums, especially labpacks.

Although compatibility testing is generally detailed enough for disposal purposes, its use from an industrial/environmental hygiene standpoint is limited. Since no other assays are performed (unless expensive GC-MS is ordered for legal purposes), very little information exists, particularly on drum content, that is useful from a toxicological standpoint. For example, when a drum is categorized non-halogenated organic, no other data is generated to determine if the drum contains a slightly toxic compound toluene (TLV 100 ppm, 8.7 g/kg LD50), a moderately toxic chemical benzaldehyde (TLV None, 1g/kg LD50), a highly toxic chemical parathion (TLV 0.0lmg/m3, 2mg/kg LD50), or a mixture of all three.

A greater knowledge of drum material composition would permit the tailoring of worker and community protection strategies to those specific materials. To meet these needs, however, classic compatibility test procedures (spot tests) have become more and more complex. Consequently, they have lost their time- and cost-effectiveness and become prone to positive and negative interferences [3].

A need exists for an analysis procedure that can potentially fill the gap between compatibility testing and expensive GC-MS. This procedure should:

(1) Furnish chemical information beyond that which is obtainable via compatibility testing, (i.e., identification of the primary constituents of uncharacterized drum samples);
(2) be rapid enough to complete 100-200 samples with a 24-hour turnaround;
(3) be cost-effective with respect to compatibility ($30/sample) and simple GC-MS ($750/sample) testing.

Research continues in the development of new compatibility testing procedures, which attempt to meet the criteria listed above; however, until a new method is developed and tested following proper peer review, the classical spot-test methods are recommended as the only alternatives.

SUMMARY

This chapter addressed the role that compatibility testing plays during the waste characterization and bulking phase of a remedial action. The classical spot-test methods were discussed in depth, and proposed unique methods were outlined. Major safety problems encountered and proposed safety protocols were detailed.

The limitations of compatibility testing was addressed, pointing out the need for a quality-control protocol. A criteria based on the need for fast, cheap, but high quality compatibility testing was given against which to judge future proposed methods.

REFERENCES

1. Wetzel, R., et al. "Drum Handling Practices at Abandoned Sites," Management of Uncontrolled Hazardous Waste Sites Conference, Washington, D.C., 1982. Bennett and Bernard, eds., Silver Spring, Maryland, Hazardous Waste Control Research Institute, 1982.
2. Neely, N., et al. "Remedial Action at Hazardous Waste Sites. Survey and Case Studies." EPA 430-9-81-005. SCS Engineers, Covington, KY for USEPA Municipal Environmental Research Laboratory, Cincinnati, OH, 1981.
3. Wolbach, C. D. "Protocol for Identification of Reactivities of Unknown Wastes," Management of Uncontrolled Hazardous Waste Sites Conference, Washington, D.C., December 1983. Bennett and Bernard, Eds., Silver Spring, MD, Hazardous Waste Control Research Institute, 1983.
4. Federal Register, 40 CFR, Part 260, May 19, 1980.
5. "Hazardous Material Incident Response Operations Training Manual," U.S. EPA Office of Emergency and Remedial Response, Hazardous Response Support Division, June 1982.
6. "Hazardous Material Response Manual," U.S. Coast Guard, Environmental Coordination Branch, Draft Document, May 1982.
7. "Guide for Determining the Compatibility of Hazardous Wastes," ASTM D-34.04.04, Draft 3, June 10, 1982.
8. "U.S. Corps of Engineers/U.S. EPA Hazardous Waste Site Remedial Action Guidelines," RFP for Chem-Dyne Site, Hamilton, OH, January 1983.
9. Hina, C. E., et al. "Techniques for Identification and Neutralization of Unknown Hazardous Materials," Management of Uncontrolled Hazardous Waste Sites Conference, Washington, D.C., 1983, Bennett and Bernard, Eds., Silver Spring, MD, Hazardous Waste Control Research Institute, 1983.
10. Turpin, R. D., et al. "Compatibility Testing Procedures for Unidentified Hazardous Wastes," Management of Uncontrolled Hazardous Waste Sites Conference, Washington, D.C., 1981, Bennett and Bernard, eds., Silver Spring, MD, Hazardous Waste Control Research Institute, 1981.
11. Mayhew, J. D., G. M. Sodaro, and D. W. Carroll. *A Hazardous Waste Site Management Plan*, (Washington, D.C.: Chemical Manufactures Association, 1982.

12.   "Compatibility Testing for Characterization of Hazardous Waste," O. H. Materials Co. (1983).

13.   Finkel, A. M., and R. S. Golob. "Implications of the Chemical Control Corp. Incident," Management of Uncontrolled Hazardous Waste Sites Conference, Washington, D.C., 1981, Bennett and Bernard, eds., Silver Spring, MD, Hazardous Waste Control Research Institute, 1981.

14.   "Hazardous Waste Sites: National Priorities List," U. S. EPA, U.S. Government Printing Office (1983).

15.   Clinical Outpatient Notes, Occupational Health Clinic, The University of Michigan, September 22, 1982.

16.   "Occupational Safety and Health Guidance Manual," NIOSH, Appendices A-C1, Draft Copy (1983).

17.   Wyeth, R. K. "The use of Laboratory Screening Procedures in the Chemical Evaluation of Uncontrolled Hazardous Waste Sites," Management of Uncontrolled Hazardous Waste Sites Conference, Washington, D.C., December 1981, Bennett and Bernard, eds., Silver Spring, MD, Hazardous Waste Control Research Institute, 1981.

18.   "Lab Pack Disposal Procedures," U.S. EPA (1983).

19.   "Request for Modification to Approved Work Plan for Handling Lab Packs," O. H. Materials Co. (1983).

20.   Title 40 C.F.R. Part 264 Appendix V - Examples of Potentially Incompatible Waste, July 1, 1992.

21.   Annual Book of ASTM Standards, Volume 11, ASTM-D 5058-90, Standard Test Method for Compatibility Screening Analysis of Waste, American Society for Testing and Materials, Philadelphia, 1992.

22.   Annual Book of ASTM Standards, Volume 11, ASTM-D 4979-89, Standard Test Method for Physical Description Screening Analysis of Waste, American Society for Testing and Materials, Philadelphia, 1992.

23.   Annual Book of ASTM Standards, Volume 11, ASTM-D 4982-89, Standard Test Method for Flammability Potential Screening Analysis of Waste, American Society for Testing and Materials, Philadelphia, 1992.

24.   Annual Book of ASTM Standards, Volume 11, ASTM-D 4981-89, Standard Test Method for Screening of Oxidizers in Waste, American Society for Testing and Materials, Philadelphia, 1992.

25.   Title 40 C.F.R. Part 261 Subpart C - Characteristics of Hazardous Waste, July 1, 1992.

26.   Annual Book of ASTM Standards, Volume 11, ASTM-D 4980-89, Standard Test Method for Screening of pH in Waste, American Society for Testing and Materials, Philadelphia, 1992.

27.   Annual Book of ASTM Standards, Volume 11, ASTM-D 4978-89, Standard Test Method for Screening of Sulfides in Waste, American Society for Testing and Materials, Philadelphia, 1992.

28.   Annual Book of ASTM Standards, Volume 11, ASTM-D 5049-90, Standard Test Method for Screening of Cyanides in Waste, American Society for Testing and Materials, Philadelphia, 1992.

29.   Feigl, Fritz and V. Anger, (R. E. Oesper, translator), Spot Tests in Organic Analysis, Seventh Edition, Elsevier Scientific Publishing Company, New York, 1975, pp. 48-51.

MEDICAL SURVEILLANCE FOR HAZARDOUS WASTE WORKERS

James M. Melius, M.D.

Designing a medical surveillance program for workers is a difficult task [1]. While available industrial hygiene data indicate that these workers usually have very low levels of exposures to the multiple chemicals commonly present at a hazardous waste site, there is a significant potential for these workers to be exposed for short periods of time to higher levels during waste cleanup activities. These short term exposures are unlikely to be identified or quantified by industrial hygiene monitoring at these sites. These potential exposure situations also provide the rationale for much of the protective equipment and work practice programs described elsewhere in this book.

The other obvious difficulty with designing medical surveillance programs for workers at hazardous waste sites is the potential for exposure to multiple toxic substances, many of which may not be identified prior to the cleanup activity beginning nor during the cleanup process. This possible ignorance must always be considered in developing protective programs and in the design and operation of the medical surveillance program.

Finally, the design of a medical surveillance program for these workers also differs from many other situations in another important aspect. Most medical surveillance is predicated on the occurrence of a significant degree of exposure to specific toxic substances. The medical testing is designed for health effects that could potentially occur from that level of exposure to that specific toxic substance. Combining the usual medical screening recommendations for each chemical to which the hazardous waste worker could be exposed would produce a costly, unwieldy list of screening recommendations that would be of doubtful effectiveness.

The following recommendations for a medical program for workers are based on the established health hazard for those workers, a review of the available data on their exposures, current OSHA standards [2], and available information on medical programs for these workers. Currently, a variety of approaches are being taken which is appropriate given the variety of hazardous waste sites in this country. This chapter is intended not to provide a general program applicable to all hazardous waste site programs, but rather to show the basic steps in designing medical programs for different hazardous waste cleanup operations (see Exhibit 7-1). The medical recommendations are intended for a program under the direction of a physician trained in occupational health or with considerable experience in conducting occupational health programs. These recommendations also are based on the assumption that workers will be adequately protected by the use of engineering controls and work practices as delineated elsewhere in this book. The recommendations are presented in four parts: preemployment screening, periodic screening, provisions for episodic and emergency medical care, and recordkeeping.

PREEMPLOYMENT SCREENING

The Occupational Safety and Health Administration has promulgated their final regulations covering hazardous waste operations [2]. These regulations require medical screening for all employees engaged in hazardous waste operations who a) are or may be exposed above permissible exposure limits for 30 days or more a year, b) wear a respirator for 30 days or more a year, c) are injured due to overexposure from an emergency incident involving hazardous substances or health hazards, and d)members of hazardous materials response teams. The Occupational Safety and Health Administration (OSHA) respirator standard (29 CFR 1910, Part 134), also states that no employee may be assigned to a task that requires the use of a respirator unless it has been determined that the person is physically able to perform under such conditions. This latter standard should be kept in mind while determining which employees should receive preemployment examinations.

The major focus of preemployment examinations should be to ascertain whether the worker is physically fit to perform the assigned work [3]. This work often involves physically strenuous activity (moving 55-gallon drums, etc.) and, in addition, requires the worker to wear personal protective equipment (respirators, protective suits, etc.). Wearing this equipment poses an added physiological burden on the worker, particularly when working in high ambient temperatures [4]. Unfortunately, there is no accurate method of quantitatively measuring this added physiological burden at the present time.

The preemployment screening should therefore include a medical history and physical examination to determine if the worker will be able to handle strenuous work while wearing personal protective equipment. The medical history should ascertain information on past illnesses and chronic diseases (particularly asthma, pulmonary disease, and cardiovascular disease), and include a review of symptoms (especially dyspnea on exertion, other chronic respiratory symptoms, chest pain, and heat intolerance). Other characteristics which may make an individual more susceptible to heat stroke, such as obesity and little physical exercise, should also be ascertained.

The physical examination should focus on the pulmonary and cardio-vascular system. Depending on the results of the medical history and physical examination, and on the worker's age, further medical testing, such as a chest X-ray, pulmonary function testing, and an electrocardiogram may be useful in ascertaining the person's ability to perform strenuous work while wearing a respirator and other protective equipment. These additional tests, however, need not be done for everyone. The medical history and exam by themselves may disqualify some individuals. Little information would be gained from these additional tests for a young, healthy, nonsmoking worker. On the other hand, pulmonary function testing and an electrocardiogram may prove quite useful in evaluating an older worker with a long history of cigarette smoking.

Based on the medical history, physical examination, and appropriate further tests, the examining physician must then make a decision on the worker's ability to perform the required work while wearing protective equipment. Unfortunately, there is very little sound guidance in the literature on which to base this decision [3]. Prospective employees with severe lung or heart disease should obviously be excluded; however, there are no clear-cut guidelines for an asymptomatic worker with modest reduction in pulmonary function. Usually in these instances the medical assessment must be based on an overall assessment of the person's medical examination. Current research on the physiological burden involved in wearing respirators and protective clothing, and on the effects of reduction in pulmonary function and respirator tolerance, should help provide better guidance for these assessments in the future.

Another major purpose of preemployment testing is to ascertain the worker's ability to work in hazardous environments (i.e., is the worker unusually susceptible to specific chemical exposures?). Since exposures at hazardous waste sites are multiple and often unpredictable, other than serious medical conditions which would disqualify a worker by the above criteria or a history of severe asthmatic reaction to a specific chemical, specific medical testing would not be effective for this purpose.

The final purpose of preemployment medical screening is to establish baseline data to better evaluate the effects of subsequent toxic exposures. This baseline testing may include both medical screening tests and biological monitoring tests. The latter (e.g., blood lead level) may be useful for ascertaining preexposure body burdens of specific substances to which the worker may be exposed and for which reliable tests are available. Given the problem in predicting significant exposures for these workers, there are no clear guidelines for prescribing certain tests. Alternative approaches range from doing no testing to conducting an extensive battery of biochemical and biological monitoring. A more rational approach would include baseline testing selected according to the past history of the workers (previous medical and occupational history) and on some assessment of the predominant and significant exposures which the worker may experience.

The most common potential chemical exposures for workers at a hazardous waste site are solvents. Although some solvents have specific toxicity (e.g., leukemia can result from benzene exposure), the most common medical effects from solvent exposure are neurotoxic and hepatotoxic. Other than history and physical examination, routine preemployment screening tests for neurotoxic effects are not readily available. Liver enzyme tests are commonly used in testing for hepatotoxic effects, but their sensitivity and specificity for detecting the effects from low- level exposures to multiple solvents are unknown and probably low [5]. Their utility in preemployment or periodic screening is questionable, and if used care has to be taken especially because of the high rate of "false positive" tests. Likewise, the value of other commonly used preemployment biochemical tests (BUN, calcium, etc.) or other baseline laboratory testing is also questionable.

An alternative approach to baseline testing would involve a situation where a specific significant exposure for the hazardous waste worker is known and biological or biochemical monitoring of that exposure is well established. For example, long-term cleanup of a polychlorinated biphenyl (PCB) waste facility could be monitored with preemployment and periodic serum PCB testing [6]. Lead, cadmium, arsenic, and organophosphate pesticides are additional examples of substances for which this approach could be appropriate. Given the common use of respirators and protective clothing for workers at hazardous waste sites, usual industrial hygiene monitoring will not provide an accurate indication of the worker's actual exposure (i.e., through the respirator and protective clothing). Therefore, in situations where a hazardous waste worker may be exposed over a sufficient period of time to a substance which can be monitored by available biological monitoring techniques, preexposure and periodic biological monitoring for that substance may provide very useful information on the actual exposure for that worker or group of workers.

A related approach would involve drawing preemployment blood specimens and freezing serum for later testing if environmental monitoring indicates significant exposures to an agent amenable to such monitoring (e.g., PCB, some pesticides).

PERIODIC SCREENING

The frequency and content of periodic screening of hazardous waste workers will depend on the nature of their work. In general, these examinations should take place at least yearly. The OSHA regulations allow the physician to extend this to two years but not longer. Termination examinations are required unless the employee has been examined within the previous six months. The screening should include an interval history and physical examination. The medical history should focus on changes in health status, illnesses, and possible work-related symptoms occurring since the last screening examination. The examining physician should have some knowledge of the worker's exposure during that period of time. This information should include any exposure monitoring done at the worker's job site. This could be supplemented by self-reported exposure histories or more general information on the potential exposures at the hazardous waste sites where the employee has worked. Additional medical testing would depend on the available exposure information and on the medical history and examination results. This additional testing should be specific for the possible medical effects of the worker's exposure. The application of a large batch of medical tests in an attempt to cover all of the possible medical effects of the multitude of potential exposures facing the worker is not very useful. Such testing may only lead to problems due to the occurrence of elevated values due to other factors or to chance (i.e., false positives).

More frequent monitoring may be appropriate for significant exposures at specific sites (e.g., PCB, lead, etc.) as described in the preceding section. The schedule for this monitoring would depend on the degree and type of exposure and the duration of work at the job site. Periodic review of the screening results can help determine the appropriate frequency.

ACUTE OR EPISODIC MEDICAL CARE

Provisions for acute medical care need to be developed for each hazardous waste site. This should include provisions for emergency first aid at the site. Key employees at the site should have some formal first aid training, particularly in dealing with explosion and burn injuries, with heat stress, and with acute chemical toxicity. Appropriate first aid equipment also needs to be available at the site.

Arrangements for evacuating injured or ill personnel need to be available, including transportation to a nearby hospital. These arrangements should include assisting the hospital in preparing for medical occurrences. Preparation can avoid unnecessary delays in treating injured or ill workers due to inappropriate concerns about chemical contamination of the hospital (this has actually occurred after a fire at a hazardous waste facility). The medical care facility should be informed about the nature of potential exposures at the site, the specific details on the incident involving the ill or injured worker, and about the worker's medical history. These arrangements are particularly important when specific medical treatment is required for a toxic exposure (e.g., cyanide, organophosphate pesticides).

In addition to the provisions for a medical emergency, a mechanism to provide episodic medical care for hazardous waste workers needs to be arranged. This may be difficult, particularly if the worker is not close to the home office of the employer or is working in a rural area. Nevertheless, it is important to ensure that any possible symptoms or illnesses are properly evaluated in the context of the worker's exposures at the site and that other illnesses do not put the worker at greater risk due to the requirements of working with hazardous waste. Arrangements need to be made for the treating physician to have access to the worker's medical records. Depending on the situation, this can be done by keeping the medical records (or a copy) at the hazardous waste site (with appropriate provisions for security) or at a nearby hospital.

Another important group of workers who may be exposed at hazardous waste sites is emergency response personnel. These workers may encounter significant acute exposures in responding to fires or other emergencies. Proper preparation can help prevent serious exposures in these situations. Prior to the hazardous waste site cleanup, the fire department and other emergency response personnel need to be informed on potential hazards from incidents at the site. Procedures to limit these exposures and to assure the availability of appropriate protective equipment can be made. Arrangements also need to be made for decontamination or disposal and replacement of fire fighting equipment used at the site. In the event of significant exposure for any of these workers, arrangements need to be made for appropriate medical or emergency care, including informing the medical care provider of possible exposures at the site.

RECORDKEEPING AND PROGRAM REVIEW

Recordkeeping is an important part of any medical surveillance program. For hazardous waste workers, this may be difficult due to the multiple locations where they may work over a period of time. Current OSHA regulations require that medical records on exposed workers be maintained for 30 years after they leave employment (45 FR 35212). The results of medical testing and full medical records must also be available to the workers, their union representatives, and OSHA inspection staff. Informing workers about their exposures and medical testing is particularly important in helping them to take appropriate precautions and for informing their other or subsequent medical care providers of their exposures as a hazardous waste worker. Occupational accident and illness records must also be maintained and reported yearly to OSHA.

A successful health and safety program should include periodic reassessment of its effectiveness. This will involve reviewing medical records; therefore, these documents should be well maintained. Each accident or illness should be promptly evaluated to determine the cause of the incident and to implement appropriate changes in the health and safety procedures for the site. This activity is particularly important in conducting a program for hazardous waste sites where the nature of the work and the variety of potential occupational exposures require good compliance with work procedures (e.g., respirator use) to maintain an effective health and safety program.

Periodic review of the results of medical surveillance testing is also important in maintaining the effectiveness of the medical surveillance program. This review should attempt to critically evaluate the efficiency of specific medical surveillance testing, particularly in the context of information on the exposures or potential exposures at hazardous waste sites. Industrial hygiene and environmental data may suggest the need for adding specific medical tests to the surveillance program. The director of the medical surveillance program should also review the potential exposures at new hazardous waste sites to determine if additional medical testing is required for the workers at that specific site.

CONCLUSION

The design and conduct of a medical program for hazardous waste workers is a difficult task. These workers are potentially exposed to thousands of toxic substances, often in situations where identification or quantification of these exposures is not possible. The medical program for these workers must provide a baseline of preemployment and periodic screening, yet remain adaptable to the exposures at specific sites. Most important, this program must be integrated with the industrial hygiene program, personal protective equipment program, and safety procedures for the site. Together these programs can provide a safe and healthful workplace in what initially appears to be an unsafe workplace—a hazardous waste site.

Exhibit 7-1. Medical Program for
Hazardous Waste Workers

PREEMPLOYMENT SCREENING

A. Recommended

1. Medical history and physical examination with selective medical testing (e.g., chest X-rays, pulmonary function testing, EKG) to determine worker's fitness to work while wearing protective equipment.
2. Preemployment or (preexposure) baseline biological monitoring for specific exposure at a hazardous waste site (e.g., PCB).

B. Optional

1. Freezing a preemployment serum specimen for later testing.
2. Other routine baseline tests—blood count, liver enzyme tests, etc.

PERIODIC SCREENING

A. Recommended

1. Yearly medical history and physical examination with appropriate medical testing selected on the basis of this examination and on the worker's exposure history.
2. More frequent screening based on exposure to specific hazards (e.g., organophosphate pesticides, PCBs) or individual health factors.

B. Optional

1. Yearly testing using routine medical tests (e.g., blood count, liver function tests, etc.).

ACUTE MEDICAL CARE

A.   Recommended

1. Provisions for emergency first aid at the site.
2. Provisions for hospital transportation, and for informing the hospital about exposures at the site, particularly if specific medical treatment is available for a toxic exposure (e.g., cyanides).
3. Mechanism for episodic health care with evaluation of possible site-related illness.

RECORDKEEPING AND PROGRAM REVIEW

A.   Recommended

1. Maintenance and access to medical records in accordance with OSHA regulations.
2. Recording and reporting of occupational injuries and illnesses.
3. Periodic review of the medical surveillance program including integration with available exposure information about the hazardous waste sites where the workers are employed.
4. Review of specific site safety plans to determine if special testing is required for the workers at that site.

REFERENCES

1.   Melius, J. M. , and W. E. Halperin. "Medical Screening of Workers
at Hazardous Waste Disposal Sites," in *Hazardous Waste Disposal:
Assessing the Problem*, J. Highland, Ed. (Ann Arbor : Ann Arbor
Science Publishers, 1982).

2.   Occupational Safety and Health Administration. Hazardous Waste
Operations and Emergency Response; Final Rule; 29 CFR Part 1910.

3.   Hoffman, B.H. and Jones, D.W. "Evaluating Physical Fitness for
Hazardous Waste Work," in *State of the Art Reviews in Occupational
Medicine: Hazardous Waste Workers*, M. Gochfeld and E. Favata,
Ed. (Philadelphia: Hanley & Belfus, Inc., 1990)

4.   Favata, E.H., Buckler, G., and Gochfeld, M. "Heat Stress in Hazardous Waste Workers: Evaluation and Prevention, in *State of the Art
Reviews in Occupational Medicine: Hazardous Waste Workers*, M.
Gochfeld and E. Favata, Ed. (Philadelphia: Hanley & Belfus, Inc.,
1990)

5.   Hodgson, M.J., Goodman-Klein, B., and Van Theil, D.H. "Evaluating
the Liver in Hazardous Waste Workers," in *State of the Art Reviews
in Occupational Medicine: Hazardous Waste Workers*, M. Gochfeld
and E. Favata, Ed. (Philadelphia: Hanley & Belfus, Inc., 1990)

6.   Chase, K.H. and Shields, P.G., "Medical Surveillance of Hazardous
Waste Site Workers Exposed to Polychlorinated Biphenyls (PCBs),
in *State of the Art Reviews in Occupational Medicine: Hazardous
Waste Workers*, M. Gochfeld and E. Favata, Ed. (Philadelphia:
Hanley & Belfus, Inc., 1990)

8

SITE LAYOUT AND ENGINEERED CONTROLS

Lynn P. Wallace, Ph.D., P.E., D.E.E.

Hazardous waste site management will directly affect the health and safety of not only personnel who work at the site, but also those in surrounding environments. On-site activities at hazardous waste sites usually include the investigation, handling, treatment, and transportation of hazardous materials. Personnel, equipment, and previously uncontaminated areas may become contaminated by spilled toxic materials or harmful airborne dusts and vapors if proper controls are not established and maintained. Proper site management will render contaminants harmless or will contain them.

Hazards must be eliminated or isolated to protect workers and others from injury, illness, or death, and to protect surrounding environments.

This chapter discusses site management as it relates to: 1) *site layout* through the establishment of work zones, and 2) *engineered controls.*

SITE LAYOUT

The manner by which the site is physically arranged and laid-out to accomplish the remedial objectives is one of the most important aspects of site management. The establishment of *controlled* work zones at hazardous waste sites is the basis of good site layout. (See Figure 8-1.)

A properly laid-out and managed site will have excellent materials handling operations and control over every entry and exit of personnel, equipment, and materials. Such control significantly increases the safety of personnel on-site and decreases the migration of contaminants from the site. An EPA Standard Operating Guide (SOG) for Establishing Work Zones [1] offers the following:

"One of the basic elements of an effective site control program is the delineation of work zones at the site. This delineation specifies the type of operations that will occur in each zone, the degree of hazard at different locations within the site, and the areas at the site that should be avoided by unauthorized or unprotected employees. Specifically, the purpose of

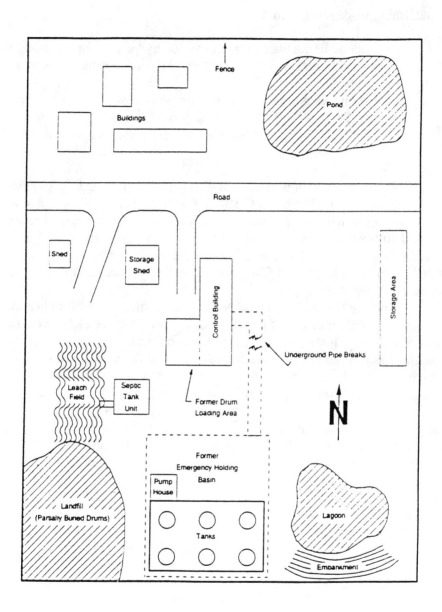

Figure 8-1. Sample Site Map.

establishing work zones is to:

- Reduce the likelihood that workers or equipment will accidentally spread hazardous substances from the contaminated areas to the clean areas;
- Confine work activities to the appropriate areas, thereby minimizing the likelihood of accidental exposure; and
- Facilitate the location and evacuation of personnel in the event of an emergency."

The shape and topography of the site and the existing physical facilities, such as buildings, pits, tanks, stacks of barrels, fences, roads, overhead power lines, ponds, etc., that are located on-site or adjacent to the site will influence or control the establishment of work zones. All such physical facilities should be identified, located and mapped as part of the initial site investigation. (See Chapter 2, Federal Government Programs and Information Gathering.)

Since no two sites are the same, this information is vital for planning the best physical arrangement for activities and functions at each particular site. Similarly, information on the types and locations of existing and potential hazards should be known so that a safe and functional layout can be accomplished. All such information should be included on a site map and must be used in developing the master control plan.

In addition to identifying the on-site location of all waste piles, physical barriers, hazards, and special problems on the site map, working areas must be identified. Specific areas are needed for sampling, staging, detoxifying, processing, bulking, treating, loading, transporting, storing, decontaminating, and numerous support functions. Some of these activities, like detoxification and staging can take place in areas that are not free of contamination. Other activities, like storing containers of decontaminated materials or most support functions, must take place in areas that are clean and free from contamination. All such areas must be identified and considered in the site layout plan and should be located on the site map.

The site map is a very important tool to be used both in planning and in executing the control plan. It is a visual tool to compliment written plans or orders and must be updated as changes occur. Clear plastic overlays can be used to easily make changes and show current information on all posted maps.

The site map must be easily understood by all personnel and visitors if it is to be of maximum value. Every effort should be made to ensure that the information contained on the map is both current and accurate.

One key to a successful site operation is total control of the entrance and exit of all materials, equipment, and personnel. The site plan must therefore consider the location of existing and potential routes for entering and leaving the site, especially emergency access routes. Separate routes for personnel and equipment must sometimes be included. All such routes and locations should be clearly marked on the site map.

CONTROL ZONES

The recommended method to prevent or reduce the transfer of contaminants and maintain control is to delineate zones or specific areas on each site where prescribed operations occur or are planned. The site must then be operated to insure that only those operations which are prescribed occur within a designated zone. Control of access points for entrance and exit to each of the zones or specific areas is the key to site-control as was discussed previously in this chapter. Movement of personnel and equipment between zones and onto the site itself are then limited to the access points. This will help keep contaminants within specified areas on-site and thus reduce the potential for spreading contamination.

A site may be divided into as many zones as necessary to minimize exposure to hazardous substances. The three zones or control areas most frequently identified and designated at hazardous waste sites [2] are (see Figure 8-2):

- Zone 1: Exclusion Zone (or "hot zone")
- Zone 2: Contamination Reduction Zone (CRZ)
- Zone 3: Support Zone (or "clean zone")

The use of a three-zone system, access control points, and exacting contamination reduction procedures provides a reasonable assurance against the translocation of contaminating substances and is highly recommended. A description of the purpose and layout of each zone follows.

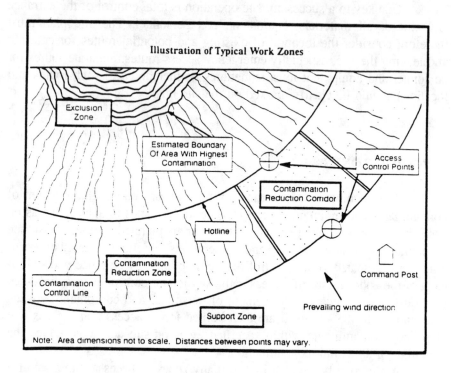

Figure 8-2. Illustration of Typical Work Zones

Zone 1: Exclusion Zone

The Exclusion Zone is laid out to include all of the areas on-site where contamination is known or suspected to occur, and all of the areas where the processing of hazardous wastes is planned. The boundaries are initially established from information obtained during preliminary site investigations. (See Chapter 2, Federal Government Programs and Information Gathering) Such information should include site records, visual observations, and instrument readings indicating the presence of possible contaminants. Organic or inorganic vapors or gases, harmful particulates in air, combustible gases, radiation, and the results of water and soil samples are used as indicators of the presence of possible contaminants. Other factors to consider when locating Exclusion Zone boundaries include the distance needed to prevent fire or explosion from affecting personnel and equipment outside the zone, the physical area necessary to conduct the various operations which directly involve the hazardous materials, and the potential for contaminants to be wind-blown from the area. (For hazardous materials incidents, the boundary of the Exclusion Zone is established by surveying the immediate environs of the incident to determine where the hazardous substances are located, noting where leachate or discoloration are visible, and determining drainage patterns.)

In order to separate the Exclusion Zone from the rest of the site, the outer boundary of the Exclusion Zone must be clearly marked. This outer boundary is known as the "hotline" and is physically marked on-site and clearly shown on the site map.

The "hotline" should be established up-wind of operations and separated from Exclusion Zone operations by sufficient distance to account for unexpected venting of materials such as during a fire or explosion and to protect entering personnel.

Access to and from the Exclusion Zone should be restricted to designated access control points at the "hotline". Such access points are used to regulate the flow of personnel and equipment into and out of the contaminated area and to verify that site control procedures are followed. Separate entrances and exits should be established to separate personnel and equipment movement into and out of the Exclusion Zone.

Once the boundaries and access points of the Exclusion Zone have been determined, they should be physically secured and well-defined by visible landmarks. It is recommended that physical barriers such as chains, fences, earth-berms, ditches, or barricades be erected around this zone to designate its location and to control access to and from it. Signs must be posted and the use of bright-colored flagging or other visual material to draw attention to its location are very helpful and will probably be required.

The Exclusion Zone may be subdivided into different areas of contamination based on the known or expected type and degree of hazard or the incompatibility of waste streams. If the Exclusion Zone is subdivided in this manner, additional demarcation and access control points may be necessary to ensure minimal personnel exposure.

Hazardous wastes at uncontrolled sites are either treated and disposed of on-site or are prepared for safe shipment to an approved disposal site. In either case, the work of opening, sampling, emptying, bulking, mixing, detoxifying, treating, solidifying, filling, staging, and associated handling of hazardous materials, is done within the Exclusion Zone. Liquid and solid residues from the decontamination processes located in the Contamination Reduction Zone, and any other contaminated material from the site, are brought to the Exclusion Zone for treatment and disposal. If the wastes are to be properly confined so as not to spread contaminants, then all such functions must be controlled and contained within this zone.

The Exclusion Zone must be laid out to allow multiple operations. Some remedial functions will occur simultaneously and others will occur sequentially. For example, there may be drum sampling, drum moving, drum staging and monitor-well drilling all going on simultaneously, while bulking, solidifying, and loading would all be preceded by other operations. Site layout must be planned to assist in accomplishing the goals and sequences of the remedial actions which will be required at each particular site.

During remedial actions in the Exclusion Zone, adequate space must be provided for: (This is not intended to be an all inclusive list.)

- Sampling and identifying wastes, including remote drum opening operations.
- Moving wastes. There must be room to maneuver waste handling equipment without bumping or spilling other wastes.
- Storing wastes. Wastes must be stored only with other wastes which are compatible. This may require several separate storage areas. Wastes are stored until they are treated and/or removed.
- Bulking wastes. Emptying the contents of drums or small containers into tanks or other large containers for processing or removal. There may be several bulking areas depending on waste compatibility and the volume of operations.
- Treating wastes. There must be room for each of the treatment processes which are to be used on-site. Some processes may have

much larger space requirements than others, such as ponds, mixing basins, incinerators, reactor vessels, explosion pits, etc.
- A space buffer in case of fire or explosion
- Storing and treating contaminated run-off or surface water.
- Entrance and exit corridors for both equipment and personnel.
- Demolition of structures, tanks, or equipment and storage of the residue until their treatment and/or removal.
- Excavation of buried wastes, including room for the excavation to take place and storing both the excavated soil and wastes.
- Equipment storage for loaders, backhoes, drum grapplers, trucks, pumps, hoses, etc.
- Fire fighting or other emergency equipment to operate.
- Well drilling equipment to drill monitoring wells or test holes.

During subsequent operations, the location of zone boundaries may be moved or modified as required to meet program, operational, or environmental changes. Zone boundaries must be made to serve the purposes of the remedial actions taking place on-site.

As the name implies, all personnel and equipment are to be excluded from this zone unless they have specific permission of the on-site coordinator or site manager *and* are properly protected by the prescribed level of personal protective equipment (PPE). Prescribed levels are based on site-specific conditions which include the type of work to be done, the hazards that might be encountered, the physical condition of the worker, and environmental conditions such as weather. (See Chapter 9, Personal Protective Equipment.)

Entry and exit control points must be clearly established along the "hotline" at the periphery of the Exclusion Zone to regulate the flow of personnel and equipment into and out of the zone and to verify that the procedures established to enter and exit are followed.

Because many different activities can occur at the same time within the Exclusion Zone, different levels of protection are often justified. For example, the task of collecting samples from open containers might require one level of protection, while a walk-through air monitoring task or an observer task may require a different level of protection. The level of protection is determined by the measured concentration of substances in the work area, the potential for contamination while performing the task, the known or suspected presence of highly toxic substances, and perceived hazards—chemical and physical—of the site.

It is important that levels of protection be established commensurate with the actual or perceived hazards and not based on worst case scenarios that may not pertain to that particular site or site conditions. It may seem easier to designate one level of protection for everyone rather than worry about controlling several different levels in one zone. However, the assignment, when appropriate, of different levels of protection within the Exclusion Zone generally makes for a more flexible, effective, and less costly operation, while still maintaining a high degree of safety.

Where different levels are permitted, areas within the zone must be conspicuously marked to identify the limits of each area and clearly labeled as to what levels of personal protective equipment are required for each area. This is not only important for the workers within the zone, but it is vital for any emergency response personnel who may be required to enter the Exclusion Zone.

Zone 2: Contamination Reduction Zone

The Contamination Reduction Zone is laid out to surround the Exclusion Zone and provide a buffer or isolation area to separate contaminated areas from uncontaminated or clean areas. This zone provides a transition area to assure that the physical transfer of contaminating substances on personnel and equipment does not occur, or is limited to acceptable levels.

Contamination reduction is accomplished by a combination of factors including control of access, decontamination procedures, distance between zones, work functions, and zone restrictions. If on-site contamination is physically contained within the Exclusion Zone boundaries, then the Contamination Reduction Zone will begin and remain a non-contaminated area, except where decontamination activities occur.

Contamination Reduction Corridors, which are access control points between the Exclusion Zone and the Support Zone, will need to be established. (See Figure 8-2.) These corridors for both personnel and equipment should consist of an appropriate number of decontamination stations necessary to address the contaminants at a particular site.

As operations proceed, the Contamination Reduction Zone will remain an effective transition area only if it is properly maintained and managed. Some minor contamination may occur, but on a relative basis, the amount of contaminants should decrease from the "hotline" and not be detected at the Support Zone boundary. Any contamination that does occur should be removed and returned to the Exclusion Zone for treatment.

At the boundary between the Exclusion Zone and the Contamination Reduction Zone, and along the Contamination Reduction Corridors, decontamination stations are established for personnel and equipment as required. The decontamination stations serve as control points to contain the contamination within the Exclusion Zone. Chapter 11, Contamination Reduction/Removal Methods, outlines requirements and procedures and gives necessary details on setting up and operating decontamination stations.

Access to the Contamination Reduction Zone from the Support Zone must also be controlled. The Contamination Control Line marks the boundary between the Contamination Reduction Zone and the Support Zone. Personnel and equipment must be allowed to enter only through designated control points and only when authorized. Personnel entering the Contamination Reduction Zone from the Support Zone must wear the personal protective equipment prescribed for this zone. The decontamination area always requires some level of protection.

Personnel should leave any contaminated protective equipment at the decontamination station when leaving the Contamination Reduction Zone. Personnel and equipment entering this zone from the Exclusion Zone will go through the decontamination stations and will leave all contaminated equipment and clothing at the stations. They must still maintain the specified level of protection required for this zone while passing to the Support Zone.

This means that the control or safety plan must address all activities and functions that take place at a remedial site and prescribe the personal protective equipment that will be used for each activity or function. The planning and execution of the plan to assure compliance are important steps to insure that the operation will be conducted safely commensurate with the actual problems of each function or activity.

Zone 3: Support Zone

To establish a proper Support Zone, the specific hazards and the degree of potential personnel exposure at the site must be considered. Site characterization is the basis for developing the site health and safety plan (HASP), and provides needed information to identify site hazards, select proper personal protective equipment, and implement safe work practices. The Support Zone must be located in clean or non-contaminated areas outside of the Contamination Reduction Zone, usually in the outermost portions of the site and sometimes in areas separated from the site. *It is important to remember that the absence of sampling results should not be considered evidence that an area is clean* [3].

The Support Zone is generally located within an established site security perimeter, however some support activities such as personal vehicle storage and some emergency care facilities may be located outside of the security perimeter. Since support functions may be located in several different parts of the site, security must be maintained at required areas of the Support Zone. Contaminated personal clothing, equipment, and samples are not permitted in this zone, but are left in or taken to the decontamination stations in the Contamination Reduction Zone.

Support functions such as the command post, medical station, equipment and supply center, laboratory facilities, equipment storage, training or briefing rooms, observation tower or platform, and administrative functions, etc., are normally located within this zone. This does not mean that observation facilities, laboratory facilities, equipment storage, or first aid facilities cannot or are not located elsewhere, but only indicates that the Support Zone is set up to provide support functions in a clean area.

Care must be exercised in locating each and every facility on-site. Site inspections have revealed that the level of contamination, based on air monitoring results, was greater in one support laboratory than was measured in the Exclusion Zone [4]. This, of course, may not always be the case, but it points out that planning and control are necessary in locating *all* activities on-site if a safe and efficient operation is to be maintained. Laboratories and other facilities that handle grossly contaminated samples or conduct tests that could release airborne contaminants, should be located within the Contamination Reduction Zone or the Exclusion Zone.

Personal protective equipment is not usually required within this zone. Normal work clothes are appropriate. Emergency respiratory protective equipment should be available in case of an explosion, fire, or unexpected occurrence, but this would be for an emergency action and not for normal operations. All personnel working in the Support Zone should receive instruction in the use of such emergency equipment and in proper evacuation procedures in case of a hazardous substance emergency.

The location of the command post and other support facilities in the Support Zone depends on a number of factors. They include:

- Accessibility, topography, open space available, location of highways and railroad tracks, location of available emergency routes, or other limitations.
- Wind direction, preferably the support facilities should be located up-wind of the Exclusion Zone. Shifts in wind direction and other conditions may dictate that the initial selection of certain support functions was not correct and they may have to be moved to a greater distance from work areas than was originally anticipated.
- Resources such as telephone and power lines, water, adequate roads for moving materials and equipment, and shelter.

Other functions that may be located in the Support Zone include the communications area, the staging area for supplies and equipment, a wind direction indicator visible to all, a visitor briefing area or facility traffic control and site security control headquarters, medical center, and other auxiliary functions that support a complex operation.

Some operations such as those provided by local police and fire departments may not be located within the Support Zone, but still must be considered in site layout. For example, sufficient room must be provided for access and maneuverability of special equipment (fire engines), and water sources must be identified for fire fighting operations. Access routes must be provided and kept unobstructed for ambulances or emergency vehicles.

The location and operation of all functions at hazardous waste sites is dictated largely by what the function does or is supposed to do. If the operation is clean or must be kept clean, it should be located in the Support Zone. If it is an operation that involves sampling or handling of contaminated materials it should be located in either the Exclusion Zone or Contamination Reduction Zone.

It is conceivable that the Support Zone may inadvertently become contaminated after site remediation begins. For example, changes in the wind speed and direction, temperature, and rainfall may result in exposures different from those experienced during initial on-site surveys. It is important that the integrity of the Support Zone be maintained throughout response operations. The Support Zone *must remain clean*! This may require periodic monitoring of the Support Zone. Proper zone siting and strict use of site controls will help minimize the transfer of contamination into this clean area. In the event that contamination has occurred, the boundaries of the work zones should be reevaluated and, if appropriate, realigned [2, 3].

AREA DIMENSIONS

The distance between various on-site functions must all be site-specific. The size of each zone or work area must also be based on the conditions at each site and not on some standard formula. Considerable judgment is needed to ensure that the distances between zone boundaries and distances between activities within zones are large enough to provide room for the necessary operations. The distances must also be great enough to prevent the spread of contaminants and eliminate or significantly reduce the possibility of injury due to explosion or fire.

The following criteria should be considered in establishing area dimensions and boundary distances:

- Physical and topographical features of the site, including the exterior dimensions of the site itself.
- Weather conditions.
- Field and laboratory measurements of air contaminants and environmental samples.
- Air dispersion calculations.
- Potential for explosion and flying debris.
- Physical, chemical, toxicological, and other characteristics of the substances.
- Clean-up activities required.
- Potential for fire both on-site and to surrounding areas.
- Area needed to conduct operations.
- Decontamination procedures
- Dimensions of actual contaminated areas.
- Potential for exposure.
- Accessibility to support services (e.g., power lines, roads, telephones, shelter, and water).
- Duration of cleanup activities.

Boundaries should not be considered permanent but should be thought of as flexible and moveable as the demands of the site change.

CONTAMINATION CONTROL

The project manager, team leader, or on-site coordinator is responsible for control of all on-site activities. The safety officer only assists, but should have the authority to stop an operation if it is found to be life-threatening. A site will only be as safe as those who are in control are willing to make it safe. Contamination will only be contained if control measures are planned and implemented.

Procedures must be established to assure that the clean zone remains clean. This is done through utilizing proper clean-up and mitigation methods in the Exclusion Zone and proper decontamination methods in the Contamination Reduction Zone. It is also done by controlling entrances and exits of all zones as indicated earlier, and in providing the facilities and separation necessary to safely accomplish the work.

An elevated observation tower and/or strategically located video cameras provide useful methods to observe safety procedures, work progress, and work procedures. During an emergency, having visual observation capabilities can be very helpful. This method can also be used to observe ways to improve existing procedures, and visitors can be given a visual tour of the site without having to enter restricted areas or be trained in the use of personal protective equipment.

To verify that site control procedures and existing boundary locations are preventing the spread of contamination, a monitoring and sampling program should be established. Zones should be regularly monitored to provide the necessary data from which to make management decisions. Operations should involve reasonable methods to determine if contaminated material is being transferred between zones, to assist in modifying zone or site boundaries, and to modify site safety or control plans as required. All such monitoring must be kept within the capacity of the analytical support functions available or it will be of limited or no value in making rapid decisions. Where applicable, direct reading instruments can be used to monitor vapor, gases, and particulates in the air. Some data on contaminants in water can be obtained rapidly but normally most analyses for water and soil take several days to obtain results.

The use of a three-zone system, access control points and corridors, effective clean-up, and exacting decontamination procedures provide a reasonable assurance that contaminating substances can be controlled. Much of the information presented in this chapter is based on a "worst case" situation. Less stringent site control and decontamination procedures may be utilized if more definitive information is available on the types of substances involved and the hazards present. The necessary information can be obtained through air monitoring, instrument surveys and sampling, and technical data concerning the characteristics and behavior of the material on-site that must be handled. Experience gained from previous remedial work is very valuable in assessing the conditions and dangers associated with this type of work. Most decisions are judgmental and rely on the ability and experience of the decision-maker in cooperation with the monitoring or enforcement authority.

Each site is different, hazards are different, conditions are different, personnel are often different, and the regulatory agency is sometimes different. The site layout procedures given in this chapter must be adapted to the unique situation at each individual site.

ENGINEERED CONTROLS

Occupational safety and health professionals consider the use of engineered safeguards that contain, isolate, or remove the hazard from the worker to be superior to the use of personal protective equipment that attempts to isolate the worker from the hazard. This approach works well in industrial settings where ventilation systems and physical barriers are employed to isolate or remove the hazard and leave the worker in a safe environment. This approach is considerably more difficult to accomplish at hazardous waste sites because of the outdoor conditions that normally exist at such sites and because the operations are usually of much shorter duration than in industrial settings. Nevertheless, it is still a better policy to control the hazard by isolation, processing, containment, and removal in conjunction with proper worker protection than to rely solely on protecting the worker. When the hazards are controlled, all personnel are protected. If personal protective equipment is the only protection provided, it requires independent effort by each worker involved, and may not be as effective.

Engineered safeguards to isolate hazards from workers can include remote handling devices such as hydraulic drum handlers, sparkless drum openers, pneumatic bung openers for drums, explosion or fire pits, berms of earth to form barriers between wastes and workers, explosion shields, explosion containers, and drum overpacks.

Many hazardous or potentially hazardous conditions on-site can be eliminated or significantly reduced by employing engineered controls. Unsafe conditions, such as rutted or bumpy roads for forklifts carrying hazardous chemicals, sharp objects that could rip protective clothing, inadequate warning devices to warn of backing equipment, fire and explosion hazards, inadequate illumination in closed areas or at night, excess noise levels, confined spaces without proper ventilation, and buried or overhead electrical cables are all examples of potential causes of accidents or injuries at hazardous waste sites. Effective engineering can help prevent such accidents.

Remote or robot controlled drum handling or drum opening devices, protective berms or embankments, sparkless tools, vacuum pumps and tanks, overpack drums, and controlled drainage areas are examples of engineered controls that can be used to isolate or control hazardous materials handling activities and thus reduce human exposure to hazardous substances.

Selection of alternate processes or activities can also provide an engineered safeguard for personnel. If the suggested treatment procedure for a particular waste was incineration and there was a danger of explosion of a waste stored nearby, an alternate process of chemical mixing, solidifying with inert materials, and containerizing might provide a solution with less risk to personnel. All such alternate approaches should be considered during planning and operation to assure that the best possible alternative is used commensurate with the problem.

Engineered safeguards, alternate processes, special equipment, and engineered construction techniques can and should be used whenever possible at a hazardous waste site.

SITE PREPARATION

Prior to undertaking response activities, time and effort must be spent in preparing a site for clean-up activities to ensure that response operations are efficient and that personnel safety is effective. Because of the real and potential hazards involved in site preparation, personnel should place high priority on safety measures during all site preparation activities.

Before on-site response or remediation activities begin, the following site preparation activities should be performed:[3]

- Construct roadways to provide a sound roadbed for heavy equipment and vehicles and arrange traffic patterns to provide ease of access and to ensure safe and efficient operations;
- Eliminate physical hazards from the site to the greatest extent possible, including;
  - ignition sources in flammable hazardous areas;
  - exposed of underground wiring and low overhead wiring that may entangle equipment;
  - sharp or protruding edges (e.g., glass, nails, torn metal, etc.) that may puncture protective clothing and equipment or inflict puncture wounds;
  - debris, holes, loose steps or flooring, protruding objects, slippery surfaces, or unsecured railings, that can cause falls, slips, or trips or obstruct visibility;
  - unsecured objects, such as bricks and gas cylinders near the edge of elevated surfaces such as catwalks, roof tops, and scaffolding, that may dislodge and fall on workers;

- Install skid-resistant strips and other anti-skid devices on slippery surfaces;
- Construct operation pads for mobile facilities and temporary structures, loading docks, processing and staging areas, and decontamination pads;
- Provide adequate illumination for work activities. Equip temporary lights with protective guards to prevent accidental contact; and
- Install wiring and electrical equipment in accordance with the National Fire Code.

ISOLATION AND CONTAINMENT BARRIERS

Containment of materials can often be achieved by the construction of berms and dikes of suitable on-site soils, or in rare cases, imported soils. Liners may be required to contain the liquids if porous soils are used. Liners can also help to reduce the amount of contaminated soil that may require disposal. Such barriers will contain spills and releases of liquids or solids; however, splashing liquids, liquids under pressure, and gases may not be adequately contained. Trenches can be constructed to collect or divert spills and releases of liquids or contaminated water for later treatment and disposal, e.g., leachate and contaminated runoff. Dispersion of wastes to both on-site and off-site areas can thereby be controlled.

Access to contaminated areas or potential areas of contamination can be controlled by exclusion barriers such as chains, fences, trenches, or earth-berms to keep people and vehicles out, thereby preventing inadvertent entry into hazardous areas. Signs are required by law to be posted at hazardous waste facilities. Streamers, flags, ribbons, or other visual warning can alert persons to hazard areas and reduce accidental entry into such areas.

SPECIAL EQUIPMENT

Equipment can be selected, developed, or modified to reduce direct contact of workers with wastes and containers during handling and transport of materials. Remote or robot operated equipment is now being developed for hazardous waste operations. Recent surveys of hazardous waste sites has identified the frequency of occurrence of various material such as metals,

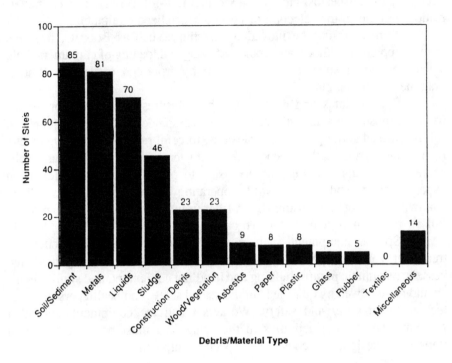

Figure 8-3. Frequency of occurrence for types of
debris/materials found on 100 hazardous waste sites.

sludge, paper, asbestos, etc. [11]. (See Figure 8-3.) This type of character-ization will aid in the selection of needed specialized equipment.

Containers can be moved by machines such as Bobcats, forklifts, drum grapplers, backhoes, and cranes. Moving and loading of containers, bulk solids and small spills can be achieved by front-end loaders, backhoes, draglines, Bobcats, etc.

Splash plates or shields and cab enclosures can prevent or reduce worker exposure to spills, splashes, and releases under force, e.g., liquids and solids released under pressure, explosions, forceful rupture of containers, etc. In extreme cases, total cab enclosures with temperature controls and self-contained air supplies could be necessary to provide total protection from vapors, solids, and liquids while operating in hazardous areas. Some contractors are routinely using HEPA filter from asbestos hardware to provide full air filtration systems for sealed cabs.

Special equipment such as reactor vessels for on-site chemical treatment, tanks or ponds for wastewater treatment, vacuum pumps and vessels, pneumatic pumps, bulking and handling equipment, and similar items should be reviewed by qualified engineers and safety and health personnel for technical suitability and safety. Workers using the equipment and other personnel performing activities in the same area must be protected from improperly designed or constructed special equipment.

WARNING ALARMS AND DEVICES

Emergency alarms should be provided to alert personnel of emergen-cy conditions such as fire, dangerous weather conditions, accidents, material releases, etc. All personnel should be familiar with the different alarms, signals, and warnings established for different types of emergencies.

For operations where vehicles or equipment must backup, and for loaders carrying containers in front which partially block visibility, the use of warning devices is advisable and in most cases required. Flashing lights and audible warning devices such as beepers or horns are necessary to alert workers who may not be watching or whose vision and hearing may be reduced because of their personal protective equipment.

Certain hazardous conditions such as vapor and oxygen concentrations can be monitored by devices which will give an audible alarm when concentrations reach a pre-set level. Use of these devices in enclosed spaces is particularly advisable. Heat and smoke detectors can be used to alert workers and off-site response groups to fires and potential fire conditions.

Such devices should be used whenever workers are involved in activities adjacent to the potential hazardous conditions. Heat and smoke detectors can signal fire departments and trigger alarms when personnel are not working such as evenings and weekends. For further discussion of emergencies, see Chapter 13, Contingency Plans.

AIR POLLUTION CONTROL

Control or minimization of the concentrations of air contaminants such as mists, vapors, and particulates can be achieved several ways. Using devices to collect or draw off the contaminants from the work area, application of water or other appropriate liquids, encapsulation of the wastes, dispersion and dilution of contaminants, proper handling of wastes and debris, permissible controlled releases at specified intervals or under controlled conditions, and selection of alternative treatment methods which reduce generation of air contaminants.

Gas collection systems such as passive gas trenches, passive trench barriers, and active gas extraction wells [5] are designed to control gas migration through soils and subsequent releases to the air or to other areas containing buried hazardous wastes. If necessary, filters, flares, or other methods can be used to treat gases vented from these types of systems.

Ventilation systems consist of air moving devices, hoods or vents, ductwork, and air cleaning devices (when appropriate). Such systems can either collect the contaminants at the source using canopy hoods or enclosures (i.e., local ventilation), or dilute the level of contaminants by exhausting the air through appropriately placed vents (i.e., general ventilation). The air flow is usually supplied for these systems by intrinsically safe fans. Fans can be located to either draw air into the system by negative pressure or force air into the system by positive pressure. General ventilation basically reduces or dilutes contaminants while local ventilation is designed to prevent any exposures to workers.

Mobile on-site laboratories are equipped with hoods to prevent exposure to lab workers. Most sites are not conducive to the application of large ventilation systems. If ventilation systems are required or if they can be cost-effective, they should be designed by qualified safety engineers or industrial hygienists.

Exhausts from ventilation systems can either be released (based on proper dispersion models) or treated by applicable pollution control devices such as electrostatic precipitators, bag house systems, etc. This decision should be based on the concentration of contaminants in the exhaust stream and the potential hazards of each pollutant. Treatment residues must be disposed of in accordance with applicable regulations. Any major use of ventilation systems for contaminant control should carefully consider the safety, effectiveness, practicality and costs of such systems.

The use of general ventilation by forced air to aid in the dispersion of contaminants in the working area, to aid in worker comfort in hot weather, or to add warmth during cold weather should be carefully monitored and controlled so as not to disperse contaminants to other locations on-site or off-site. Properly located exhaust stacks can make good use of normal dispersion for dilution of contaminants providing exhaust levels do not exceed acceptable limits [6].

Wetting down road surfaces serves to reduce the amount of dust generated and assists in compaction of the road surfaces [7]. Dust controls should be employed using water sprays and other suitable liquids. Contaminated road dusts can be reduced by wise use of wetting agents and liquids, applied by water wagons or similar mobile applicators.

Liquid sprays and curtains can be used to reduce dust during transfer, handling, and packaging of bulk wastes and wastes with particle sizes capable of air dispersion such as powders and finely ground compounds. For some wastes, this may require the use of special wetting agents to aid in adherence or adsorption to the particles. The wetted materials must be collected, contained, and disposed of in accordance with applicable regulations to prevent redispersion [8]. Similar wetting of waste piles, working areas, and containers can serve to reduce dust during materials handling operations and clean-up activities as long as the wetting agents are compatible with the wastes. Care must also be taken to avoid using too much water and spreading pollutants by the run-off.

Reduction of airborne contaminants can also be achieved by the clean-up of debris and containment of wastes. This can be accomplished by using appropriate cover materials such as tarps, caps or sealants, and containers such as drums, overpacks, covered tanks, and dumpsters with closable lids. This normally involves common sense and good housekeeping practices. However, the selection of appropriate materials for caps and sealants is a technical decision.

Surface and reburial can be used to control hazardous gas and dust emissions for extended periods of time or as permanent remedial actions [5, 9]. Short-term or temporary controls such as the use of tarps and containers mentioned above, are more applicable to clean-up operations involving off-site disposal. Contaminated tarps must be disposed of by incineration or burial if they cannot be decontaminated.

The cost of providing control of air pollutants and protecting worker health and safety should be a major consideration in the selection of acceptable alternative remedial actions. Unfortunately, it is often difficult to obtain accurate estimates for increased costs associated with protecting workers' safety and health [10]. Efforts should be made to select methods and procedures for tasks at remedial action sites that reduce exposures by minimizing generation of dusts, vapors, and mists.

CONTAMINATED SURFACE WATER CONTROL

Exposure of workers to contaminated water and migration of contaminated water to clean work areas or off-site areas can be prevented or minimized by diverting rain run-off away from wastes, and collecting storing and treating the contaminated water that is generated. Dikes, berms, drainage pipes, ditches, and contour grading are some of the engineered controls which are used to keep surface water from flowing onto hazardous waste locations. Similar devices or controls are used to direct contaminated run-off water coming from the site to collection basins and ponds for pre-treatment and/or transfer to on-site treatment facilities, or to off-site treatment and disposal facilities [5, 9]. Sites where surface water control/containment is expected should have this topic addressed in original work plans. Use of packaged filtration units with sand and carbon, and pre-established action levels for discharge can be a very cost-effective site management device. In areas of insufficient water for fire protection, rain or surface water that is kept from entering the site is a possible source for this purpose. Run-off water or leachate from the site should not be used for fire control.

DEBRIS/MATERIALS CONTROL

Debris is defined as any unused, unwanted, or discarded solid or liquid that requires staging, loading, transporting, pretreating, treatment, and/or disposal on a hazardous waste site. The largest quantities of materials requiring handling and engineered controls are soil/sediments followed by metals, liquids and sludges [11]. (See Figure 8-3.)

The wide variety of chemicals found on hazardous waste sites may lead to handling problems because of factors such as high corrosivity (resulting in a need for corrosion-resistant equipment), shields on heavy machinery or highly toxic volatile compounds, which require special personal protective equipment. Additional handling problems may arise from reactions occurring because of the complex mixtures of chemicals found on-site. In addition to debris, other materials (e.g., soil, sludge, asbestos, and various liquids) must be handled [11].

These problems compound the selection and use of engineered controls needed to handle the large quantities and varieties of debris/materials resulting from hazardous waste remedial actions. The problems also require that equipment usage/modification/fabrication is sometimes site specific and often involves trial and error.

Most of the equipment used for excavation and removal work at hazardous waste sites is standard heavy duty construction equipment. Selection of excavation equipment depends on the quantity and physical properties of the debris and materials present. Valuable performance data on such equipment at hazardous waste sites are available in an EPA publication - "Survey of Materials-Handling Technologies used at Hazardous Waste Sites" [11]. This book is a valuable resource for understanding what has worked at previous sites to avoid making mistakes that could be avoided when considering engineered controls for a large majority of debris and materials that require handling at such sites.

Despite the site-specific nature of hazardous waste remediation, similar conditions are often found at many sites (i.e., landfills, battery breaking operations, sludge piles, etc.). This results in similar techniques and standard operating procedures (SOP) being used at different sites for materials-handling. The following are site-specific solutions to problems found at hazardous waste sites involving equipment that was required at several sites [11]. Similar conditions will probably exist at future hazardous waste operations so the lessons learned may be helpful.

- Hydraulic systems may have to be modified to adapt a backhoe for drum handling (grappler).
- Rubber or foam tires may be required instead of pneumatic tires at sites with large quantities of sharp metal/glass objects.
- Splash shields will be required and must be installed on heavy equipment.
- Large bulldozers may be required to winch smaller dozers up and down the steep grades of asbestos or other tailing piles.
- Propane-powered instead of diesel powered loaders may be required to reduce fumes, especially in enclosed areas.

- Heavy equipment may require special attention to avoid failure due to weather (e.g., cracked hydraulic lines from cold, tractability during icy conditions, metal fatigue from digging frozen soil).
- A drum crusher may be required instead of a backhoe to crush drums.
- Rolloff boxes may be converted into treatment chambers for wastes such as cyanide-contaminated film chips. These units can be very effective containment devices for drum piercing activities and provide considerable explosive protection.

Engineers and operators involved in selecting, designing and operating engineered controls to increase efficiencies and the effectiveness of materials handling operations are expected to be innovative and creative in accomplishing their tasks. The more that can be learned from past efforts and the more we understand the nature of the material that must be handled, the better we can get the job done in a safe manner.

REFERENCES

1.   "Standard Operating Guide (SOG) for Establishing Work Zones" - DRAFT - Office of Emergency and Remedial Response, U. S. EPA, Pub.#9285.2-04A, September, 1992.
2.   "Establishing Work Zones at Uncontrolled Hazardous Waste Sites," Office of Solid Waste and Emergency Response, U.S. EPA, Pub.#9285.2-06FS, April, 1991
3.   "Standard Operating Safety Guides," Office of Emergency and Remedial Response, U. S. EPA, Pub.#9285.1-03 PB92-963414, June, 1992.
4.   Costello, R. J., C. Geraci, P. Eller, and R. Ronk. "Health Hazard Evaluation Determination Report IA 82-40, Triangle Chemical Site, Bridge City, Texas," National Institute for Occupational Safety and Health, Cincinnati, OH, 1983.
5.   Walsh, J. J., and D. P. Gillespie, "Selecting Among Alternative Remedial Actions for Uncontrolled Hazardous Waste Sites," U. S. EPA, Cincinnati, OH, 1982.
6.   "Documentation of Threshold Limit Values," 4th Rev. Ed. - 1980, with 1982 changes and editions, ISBN 0-9367 12-12-9, American Conference of Governmental Industrial Hygienists, Cincinnati, OH, 1982.
7.   Church, H. K., *Excavation Handbook* McGray - Hill Book Co., New York, 1981.
8.   *Fundamentals of Industrial Hygiene* (National Safety Council [NSC], Chicago, 1971.)
9.   Rogeshewski, P., H. Bryson, and K. Wagner, "Handbook for Remedial Action at Waste Disposal Sites", U. S. EPA Report 625/6-82-006, Cincinnati, OH, 1982.
10.   Lippitt, J. M., J. Walsh and A. D. Puccio, "Costs of Remedial Actions at Uncontrolled Hazardous Waste Sites: Worker Health and Safety Considerations," in Proceedings of Conference on Hazardous Wastes and Environmental Emergencies, Houston, TX, March 12-14, 1984.
11.   "Survey of Materials-Handling Technologies Used at Hazardous Waste Sites", Risk Reduction Engineering Laboratory, Office of Research and Development, U.S. EPA, PB91-921283, EPA/540/2-91/010, June, 1991.

9

PERSONAL PROTECTIVE EQUIPMENT

Arthur D. Schwope, M.A.
Christopher C. O'Leary, C.I.H., C.S.P.

A variety of known and unknown chemical and physical health hazards are potentially present on a hazardous waste site. Remedial action personnel must be properly protected to prevent short- and long-term disabilities related to these hazards. Engineering controls, administrative controls, good work practices, and personnel protective equipment (PPE) are the routes to such protection. Since the focus of this chapter is protection from chemicals, rather than physical hazards, the discussion is focussed on respirators and chemical protective clothing.

HAZARDS

A virtually infinite number of chemicals and chemical mixtures are potentially present on hazardous waste sites. These chemicals and chemical mixtures may be in the form of solids, liquids, and gasses, and they can range from benign to extremely toxic poisons and carcinogens. (See Chapters 4, Toxicology; and 6, Compatibility Testing and Material Handling.) They, furthermore, may be corrosive, explosive, flammable, or radioactive. Oxygen deficient confined spaces may also be present [1]. Although less common but of growing concern, potentially hazardous biologically active materials such as bacteria and viruses may also be present. Physical stresses on-site may include high noise (e.g., excavation machinery, drum crushing), rough surfaces, and cut and puncture threats. In addition, the climate, work load, and PPE may introduce heat or cold stresses. (See Chapter 10, Heat Stress in Industrial Protective Encapsulating Garments.)

Such hazards can produce a multitude of different health effects, including:

- temporary or permanent damage to the eyes, ears, skin, internal organs, or the nervous or circulatory systems
- carcinogenicity, mutagenicity, or teratogenicity
- loss of limbs, organs, or death

This chapter is focussed on PPE as a means for minimizing or eliminating deleterious health effects due to contact with chemicals. These health effects are dependent principally on the route of exposure, the duration of the exposure, and the toxicity of the chemical. The routes of exposure may be ingestion, inhalation, and skin contact. Upon skin contact, there may be damage to the skin itself as well as absorption into the body where other effects may occur. For any given exposure, the effects may also vary from individual to individual [2, 3].

TYPES OF PPE

At a typical site, personal protective equipment is an essential component of a sound worker protection program. Chemical protective equipment (CPE), which is a subset of PPE, includes respirators, gloves, boots, aprons, goggles, face shields, hoods, and coveralls. In extreme situations, CPE is comprised of self-contained breathing apparatus and a full-encapsulating, gas-tight ensemble. Virtually all types of chemical protective equipment is fabricated from synthetic materials (i.e., plastic and rubber). Such materials have been developed to resist degradation by and absorption of chemicals. As will be discussed later, chemical protective clothing (CPC) from a wide variety of such materials of construction is available. The challenge to those persons responsible for worker safety and health is to select the most appropriate material for the hazards involved. For example leather gloves and boots are to be avoided where there are potential chemical hazards since leather readily absorbs many chemicals, posing a health hazard to the wearer. Leather is also very difficult to decontaminate. Hard hats and safety footwear should be worn in conjunction with chemical protective clothing [4].

Eye, ear, and face PPE can include safety glasses or goggles, ear muffs, ear plugs, and faceshields. Tinted safety glasses and goggles are available for welding and burning applications. Goggles can be gas-tight to prevent gases and vapors from contacting the eyes or vented to allow for good ventilation, depending on the application. Faceshields protect the entire face and in some cases the neck region from liquids and solid objects. Good fitting eye, ear, and face protection is critical to providing protection, as well as not introducing additional hazards. Equipment from several manufacturers may be required in order to assure that every worker has a good fit for each item. Poorly fitting ear plugs will not attenuate the noise, and loosely fitting safety glasses or goggles may create an additional hazard during strenuous fast-paced work. The advantages and limitations of these protective devices should be fully defined and understood by the individual user [4, 5].

Hoods used in combination with hard hat, goggles, and respirators will adequately cover the back of the neck and head from spills and splashes of chemicals. Aprons and sleeves may be utilized, bearing in mind the limitations of their coverage.

Coverage of the body may be by one-piece (coverall-type) suits, two-piece ensembles (pants and shirt/jacket), and encapsulating ensembles. Each of these types of garments is available in both reusable, single-use (i.e., disposable) and limited-use forms [5].

Encapsulating suits provide a self-contained internal environment for the wearer. All parts of the body, including head, hands, and feet are enclosed. These suits must be equipped with a supplied-air system to provide the user with a fresh air source. Fully-encapsulating suits can be chemical resistant, as well as heat-resistant, thus permitting personnel to work in dual-hazard environments.

In addition to protecting the body, single- and multi-component suits prevent contamination of the individual's street and underclothing [6]. This reduces the potential for spreading the hazard to lunch and smoking areas, offices, automobiles and homes.

On waste sites, gloves and respirators are considered the key items of personal protective equipment. Gloves should permit an individual to handle equipment and materials while providing a highly resistant barrier between hazardous chemicals and the skin. The effectiveness of gloves in providing a barrier has become an important issue in recent years. Chemical resistance and permeability of glove materials and other clothing materials such as butyl rubber, neoprene, and natural rubber, etc., are discussed later in this chapter.

In selecting and using PPE, one should seek to balance the needs of:

- protection
- worker productivity
- worker comfort
- cost

Briefly, the goal is to provide just the right amount of protection—no more and no less than is warranted by the hazard. By so doing, one minimizes the negative effects on worker productivity and comfort typically associated with protective equipment as well as the cost. The cost of PPE extends far beyond its purchase price and includes the costs associated with training the worker in the use of the PPE, lost productivity due to don and doff time as well as hindered mobility, dexterity, communications, vision, etc., decontamination, maintenance and storage, and disposal.

The remainder of this chapter focusses on respirators and chemical protective clothing.

RESPIRATORS

The purpose of respiratory protective equipment on a hazardous waste site is to prevent the inhalation of hazardous gases, vapors or particulates by the wearer. Since the type of respiratory protection needed for these classes of hazardous agents may differ in both design and function, the selection of the correct type of respirator must be made on the basis of the specific hazard against which protection is needed. Accordingly, it is necessary that some sort of hazard characterization be performed to determine the identity and concentration of hazardous agent(s) present at the work site.

For the purposes of this discussion, respirators refer to those devices which are tested and approved by the National Institute for Occupational Safety and Health (NIOSH) for protection against airborne hazards, including oxygen deficiency. So defined, respirators are commonly divided into two groups according to the method by which protection is provided [6]. *Air-purifying respirators* refer to those devices which provide protection by removing contaminants from the air inhaled by the worker. *Atmosphere-supplying respirators* protect the worker by providing an alternative source of respirable air.

One other commonly used system for categorizing respirators classifies the devices according to the facepiece pressure relative to atmospheric pressure. *Positive pressure respirators* are designed so that a positive pressure is maintained inside the facepiece throughout the entire breathing cycle. This assures that any leakage associated with a poor face to facepiece seal will not result in the introduction of contaminated air into the facepiece. Conversely, *negative pressure respirators* are those in which the facepiece pressure drops below atmospheric at some point during the inhalation-exhalation cycle.

Air-Purifying Respirators

Air-purifying respirators utilize various air purifying elements to remove contaminants present in the work area. As shown in Table 9-1, air-purifying elements are color-coded according to NIOSH specifications, and are designated for use against specific chemicals or classes of chemicals [7, 8]. The mechanism by which purification occurs depends on the type of element and the contaminant against which protection is required. For example, air purifying elements for protection against solid and liquid particles function as mechanical filters, and remove the contaminant via one of the several filtration mechanisms. When protection against gases or vapors is needed, the element operates as an absorption media, and the gas or vapor is removed as it is absorbed onto the material in the cartridge. Finally, some air purifying elements operate by converting the contaminant into a less toxic substance, e.g., the catalytic conversion of carbon monoxide into carbon dioxide.

TABLE 9-1. Respirator Selection by Colors Assigned to Atmospheric Contaminants	
Atmospheric Contaminants to be protected against . . .	**Colors Assigned ***
Acid gases	White
Hydrocyanic acid gas	White with ½-inch green stripe completely around the canister near the bottom
Chlorine gas	White with ½-inch yellow stripe completely around the canister near the bottom
Organic vapors	Black
Ammonia gas	Green
Acid gases and ammonia gas	Green with ½-inch blue stripe completely around the canister near the bottom
Carbon monoxide	Blue

TABLE 9-1. Respirator Selection by Colors Assigned to Atmospheric Contaminants	
Atmospheric Contaminants to be protected against . . .	**Colors Assigned ***
Acid gases and organic vapors	Yellow
Hydrocyanic acid gas and chloropicrin vapor	Yellow with ½-inch blue stripe completely around the canister near the bottom
Acid gases, organic vapors, and ammonia gases	Brown
Radioactive materials, excepting tritium and noble gases	Purple (Magenta)
Particulates (dusts, fumes, mists, fogs, or smokes)	Canister color for contaminant as designated combination with any of the above, with ½-inch gray above gases or vapors stripe completely around the canister near the top
All of the above atmospheric contaminants	Red with ½-inch gray stripe completely around the canister near the top

*   Gray shall not be assigned as the main color for a canister designed to remove acids or vapors. NOTE: Orange is used as a complete body or stripe color to represent gases not included in this table. The user will need to refer to the canister label to determine the degree of protection the canister will afford.

The mechanism by which the air purifying element operates is important since it permits the user to understand many of the limitations associated with the use of air-purifying respirators. For example, the end of the useful service life for a mechanical filter is indicated by an increase in breathing resistance associated with filter loading. The end of service life for a chemical cartridge is indicated by the detection (i.e., odor, taste, irritation) of contaminated breakthrough.

Air-purifying respirators are available in several different facepiece configurations, including quarter-facepiece, half-facepiece, and full-facepiece models. The selection of the proper facepiece configuration for a particular work environment depends on the degree of protection required, as well as the need for protection against other types of chemical and physical hazards (e.g., impact, splash, or irritation protection).

The quarter-facepiece covers only the nose and mouth, resting on the bridge of the nose and the front of the chin. The half-facepiece fits around the perimeter of the lower face, providing protection for the nose and mouth but not the eyes. The full-facepiece, fits around the perimeter of the wearer's face, and provides respiratory protection, as well as impact and splash protection.

Each of the facepieces can be equipped with replaceable air-purifying elements as dictated by the environment against which protection is needed. Alternatively, the air-purifying elements may be mounted elsewhere (e.g., on the user's belt), and connected to the facepiece with a breathing tube. In addition, there are many respirators in which the facepiece is constructed of the air-purifying media, and which are discarded after use. These respirators are referred to as single-use, maintenance-free, or disposable respirators.

Each of the facepiece configurations provides a different level of respiratory protection. This difference is not a function of the air-purifying elements, since they are identical for the different facepiece configurations made by the same manufacturer. Instead, the difference is a result of the effectiveness of the seal of the facepiece to the face of the user. Assigned protection factor associated with each facepiece configuration are shown in Table 9-2 [6].

TABLE 9-2. Respirator Protection Factors[1]		
Type Respirator[2]	Facepiece Pressure	Protection Factor
I. AIR-PURIFYING		
A. Particulate[3] removing		
Single-use[4], dust[5]	−	5
Quarter-Mask, dust[6]	−	5
Half-Mask, dust[5,6]	−	10
Half- or Quarter-Mask, fume[7]	−	10
Half- or Quarter-Mask, High-Efficiency[8]	−	10
Full-Facepiece, High Efficiency	−	50
Powered, High-Efficiency all enclosures	+	X[9]
Powered, dust or fume, all enclosures	+	X[9]
B. Gas and Vapor-Removing[10]		
Half-Mask	−	10
Full-Facepiece	−	50
II. ASMOSPHERE-SUPPLYING		
A. Supplied Air		
Demand, Half-Mask	−	10
Demand, Full-Facepiece	−	50
Hose Mask Without Blower, Full-Facepiece	−	50
Pressure-Demand, Half-Mask[11]	+	1,000
Pressure-Demand, Full-Facepiece[12]	+	2,000
Hose Mask With Blower, Full-Facepiece	−	50
Continuous Flow, Half-Mask[11]	+	1,000
Continuous Flow, Full-Facepiece[12]	+	2,000
Continuous Flow, Hood	+	2,000
Helmet, or Suit[13]	+	2,000
B. Self-Contained Breathing Apparatus (SCBA)		
Open-Circuit, Demand, Full-Facepiece	−	20
Open-Circuit, Pressure, Demand, Full-Facepiece	+	10,000[14]

TABLE 9-2. Respirator Protection Factors[1]		
Type Respirator[2]	Facepiece Pressure	Protection Factor
Closed-Circuit, Oxygen Tank-Type, Full-Facepiece	–	50
III. **COMBINATION RESPIRATOR**		
A. Any Combination of Air-Atmosphere-Supplying Respirator	Use minimum protection factor listed above for type of mode of operation	
B. Supplied-Air Respirator and an SCBA		

Exception: Combination supplied-air respirators, in pressure-demand or other positive pressure mode with an auxiliary self-contained air supply, and a full-facepiece, should use the PF for pressure-demand SCBA.

NOTE: Table is not to be reproduced without the accompanying footnotes.

SOURCE: Pritchard, John A. (1977) *A Guide to Industrial Respiratory Protection.* U.S. Energy Research and Development Administration.

1. The overall protection afforded by a given respirator design (and mode of operation) may be defined in terms of its protection factor (PF). The PF is a measure of the degree of protection afforded by a respirator, defined as the ratio of the concentration of contaminant in the ambient atmosphere to that inside the enclosure (usually inside the facepiece) under conditions of use. Respirators should be selected so that the concentration inhaled by the wearer will not exceed the appropriate limit. The recommended respirator PF's are selection and use guides, and should only be used when the employer has established a minimal acceptable respirator program as defined in Section 3 of the ANSI Z88.2-1969 Standard.

2. In addition to facepieces, this includes any type of enclosure or covering of the wearer's breathing zone, such as supplied-air hoods, helmets, or suits.

3. Includes dusts, mists, and fumes only. Does not apply when gases or vapors are absorbed on particulates and may be volatized or for particulates volatile at room temperature. Example: Coke oven emissions.

4. Any single-use dust respirator (with or without valve) not specifically tested against a specified contaminant.

5. Single-use dust respirators have been tested against asbestos and cotton dust and could be assigned a PF of 10 for these particulates.

6. Dust filter refers to a dust respirator approved by the silica dust test, and includes all types of media, that is, both nondegradable mechanical type media and degradable resin-impregnated wool felt or combination wool-synthetic felt media.

7. Fume filter refers to a fume respirator approved by the lead fume test. All types of media are included.

8. High-efficiency filter refers to a high-efficiency particulate respirator. The filter must be at least 99.97% efficient against 0.3 μm DOP to be approved.

9. Currently in question.

10. For gases and vapors, a PF should only be assigned when published test data indicate the cartridge or canister has adequate sorbent efficiency and service life for a specific gas or vapor. In addition, the PF should not be applied in gas or vapor concentrations that are: 1) immediately dangerous to life, 2) above the lower explosive limits, and 3) cause eye irritation when using a half-mask.

11. A positive pressure supplied-air respirator equipped with a half-mask facepiece may not be as stable on the face as a full facepiece. Therefore, the PF recommended is half that for a similar device equipped with a full facepiece.

12. A positive pressure supplied-air respirator equipped with a full-facepiece provides eye protection but is not approved for use in atmospheres immediately dangerous to life. It is recognized that the facepiece leakage, when a positive pressure is maintained, should be the same as an SCBA operated in the positive pressure mode. However, to emphasize that it basically is not for emergency use, the PF is limited to 2,000.

13. The design of the supplied-air hood, suit, or helmet (with a minimum of 6 cfm of air) may determine its overall efficiency and protection. For example, when working with the arms over the head, some hoods draw the contaminant into the hood breathing zone. This may be overcome by wearing a short hood under a coat or overalls. Other limitations specified by the approval agency must be considered before using in certain types of atmospheres.

14. The SCBA operated in the positive pressure mode has been tested on a selected 31-man panel and the facepiece leakage recorded as less than 0.01% penetration. Therefore, a PF of 10,000+ is recommended. At this time, the lower limit of detection 0.01% does not warrant listing a higher number. A positive pressure SCBA for an unknown concentration is recommended. This is consistent with the 10,000+ that is listed. It is essential to have an emergency device for use in unknown concentration. A combination supplied-air respirator in pressure-demand or other positive pressure mode, with auxiliary self-contained air supply is also recommended for use in unknown concentrations of contaminants immediately dangerous to life. Other limitations, such as skin absorption of HCN or tritium, must be considered.

The assigned protection factor (APF) is an estimate of the degree by which the respirator will reduce the concentration of contaminant in the air. For a respirator with an APF of 10, it may be assumed that the respirator will reduce the contaminant concentration by a factor of 10 when used in the field. The figure assumes that properly selected and maintained respirators are being used by persons who have been properly fitted, trained, and medically-qualified, and that this use is occurring within the context of an effective respirator protection program, under the direction of a qualified program administrator. To the extent that one or more of these assumptions may not be true, it is not reasonable to expect that the APF will be achieved in actual practice.

The air-purifying respirators discussed thus far are classified as negative pressure respirators. Air is drawn into the facepiece by the negative pressure created by the inhalation of the user. Accordingly, to the extent that the face to facepiece seal is ineffective, contaminated air may leak inward while the facepiece pressure is less than atmospheric. However, through the use of the powered air-purifying respirator (PAPR), some degree of positive pressure protection may be afforded.

The PAPR is a respirator which uses a fan to pull air through the air-purifying elements and then blows the purified air into the facepiece. To the extent that the batteries are charged and the respiration rate of the user does not exceed the capacity of the fan to provide purified air, the pressure inside the facepiece will be positive throughout the inhalation/exhalation cycle, and any breaks in the facepiece will result in outward, not inward, leakage.

Currently, there is some disagreement about whether or not a positive pressure is maintained inside the facepiece throughout the inhalation/exhalation cycle. For this reason, NIOSH and others have suggested that the APF of 1,000 may be unrealistically high even for tight fitting facepieces, and recommend that users exercise caution when using PAPRs in high contaminant concentrations [9, 10].

The fact that PAPRs do not rely on a face to facepiece seal for effectiveness has resulted in the development of a number of innovative facepiece configurations. PAPRs are often used with loose fitting facepieces that are intended to provide protection to persons with facial hair, facial deformities, or other conditions that might otherwise prevent an acceptable face to facepiece seal.

Supplied-Air Respirators

Like air-purifying respirators, supplied air respirators can be further divided into those devices which maintain a positive pressure inside the facepiece and those which permit the facepiece pressure to fall below atmospheric pressure during the inhalation/exhalation cycle. These subcategories are referred to as *pressure-demand* and *demand* respirators, respectively. It should be noted that demand supplied air respirators are increasingly rare, and have been displaced in industrial and hazardous waste site use by pressure-demand models.

Demand supplied-air respirators are those systems in which the flow of air is triggered when the facepiece pressure falls below atmospheric as the user inhales. Air is introduced into the mask from an external source of breathing air, and the pressure inside the facepiece returns to atmospheric. As the user exhales, the flow of air is stopped, and a flap valve on the facepiece permits the exhaled breath to escape to the environment. Since the facepiece pressure is negative for at least part of the breathing cycle, inward leakage is possible in the event of an incomplete face to facepiece seal. Accordingly, the APFs protection factors for demand airline respirators are the same as for negative pressure air-purifying respirators of the same facepiece configuration. The demand supplied-air respirator does provide some incremental benefits over the air-purifying respirators, in that the breathing resistance is generally lower, and it can be used in oxygen deficient atmospheres so long as the level of oxygen does not render the environment Immediately Dangerous to Life and Health (IDLH).

Pressure-demand supplied air respirators are more common than the demand models, and provide far superior protection. The increased protection arises from changes in two components of the respirator - the exhalation valve and the air delivery valve. The exhalation valve in a *pressure-demand* respirator is spring loaded so that it will not open until the pressure inside the facepiece is above atmospheric. This permits the buildup of a positive pressure inside the facepiece that is intended to prevent inward leakage of contaminated air in the event of a facepiece seal failure.

The air delivery valve is modified so that entry of air starts not when the facepiece pressure becomes negative, as with the *demand* models, but when the facepiece pressure falls below a slight positive pressure preset that is above atmospheric, but below the pressure at which the exhalation valve opens. By introducing air at the lower positive pressure and permitting its escape at the higher pressure, the *pressure-demand* respirator maintains a consistently positive facepiece pressure. This feature permits the respirator to be used in heavily contaminated environments, up to 10,000 times the permissible exposure limit for a specific chemical.

The source of the breathing air is a second criterion used to classify supplied-air respirators. Airline respirators refer to those supplied-air respirator in which the source of breathing air is connected to the mask via an airline umbilical. The source of breathing air is most often a compressor or a cylinder of compressed breathing air. The design of the entire system is determined by the conditions under which the unit was certified by NIOSH. For example, airline respirators are certified by NIOSH as a complete system, including mask, regulator and airline, and require a source of breathing air of acceptable quality, pressure and volume. To the extent that any of these change, the airline respirator may not satisfy the conditions under which it was certified, and that certification may be voided. On a hazardous waste site, this may happen if the airline being used is too long, or if airline from one manufacturer is used with a respirator from another manufacturer.

A second concern for users of airline respirators is the quality of the breathing air. It is quite simple to purchase cylinders of Grade D breathing air and use that as the source, but many users prefer to use a breathing air compressor instead. Breathing air delivered by a compressor may become contaminated if the compressor itself is located in a contaminated environment. In addition, if the compressor is not one designed specifically to provide respirable quality air, it may be lubricated with a petroleum based lubricant which may, if overheating occurs, release carbon monoxide into the respirable air. When using this type of compressor, it is necessary to monitor the air stream for carbon monoxide, and stop using the equipment if it is detected. Filtration and monitoring systems equipped with audible alarms are commercially available for use with mechanical compressors, and their use is highly recommended.

The second type of supplied-air respirator is the Self-Contained Breathing Apparatus (SCBA) in which the source of breathing air is a small cylinder integrated into the respirator itself and carried by the user. This design obviously imposes limits on the duration of use of the equipment, and is much heavier than an airline model, however, the benefits of increased mobility are important in many applications. The most commonly used SCBA are equipped with cylinders which permit a nominal duration of either 30 or 60 minutes, although actual use is often shorter if the wearer is operating at a moderate-to-high activity level.

SCBA can be further categorized into closed-circuit devices and open circuit devices. The units described above, in which the breathing air is exhaled into the external environment and replenished from a source of respirable air, are open circuit models. However, respirators are available in which the air is exhaled through a filter which scrubs out the carbon dioxide. The depleted oxygen is then replaced from a bottle of compressed oxygen, which renders the air respirable once again. These closed-circuit devices are often used inside containment suits in which the respirator does not communicate with the outside environment. In addition, they are used by fire fighters because of their extended duration. The drawbacks of this technology include the presence of highly reactive oxygen in the device and the fact that it is more difficult to regulate the facepiece pressure.

Fit

The distinction made in the foregoing discussion between positive and negative pressure respirators has mentioned the possibility of leaks in the face to facepiece seal, and the resulting inward leakage that can occur if the pressure inside the mask is less than that outside the mask. Accordingly, it is critically important that users of negative pressure respirators be fit tested to demonstrate that the size and model of respirator to be used fits them. The factors which can compromise the seal include facial hair, scars or other facial deformities, or dentures.

Respirator fit can be assessed using either quantitative or qualitative methods. Either will satisfy regulatory requirements, but the results of qualitative fit tests are more subject to error resulting from operator technique or lack of wearer cooperation.

Quantitative fit tests involve the simultaneous (or virtually simultaneous) measurement of a aerosol inside and outside the respirator. The aerosol is often an oil aerosol which is introduced into a chamber in which the subject sits or stands. As the subject performs various exercise designed to test the reliability of the face to facepiece seal, analytical tests are carried out to measure the relative concentration of the test agent inside and outside the mask. The resulting ratio of concentrations is then compared to the assigned protection factor for that model of respirator. If the measured fit factor exceeds the APF, the mask is said to fit the wearer. Often, respirator program administrators will increase the APF by a factor of 10 to provide a safety margin prior to making this comparison.

Qualitative fit tests involve use of an agent which elicits a sensory response from the wearer. Most often, isoamyl acetate("banana oil") is used as the test agent since it can be sensed at very low concentrations and is not unpleasant for the test subject, although irritant smoke may be used if the test subject is unable to smell isoamyl acetate or where there is some question about the subjects cooperativeness.

The fit test is conducted using a mask that is equipped with the proper cartridge for the test agent (i.e., organic vapor for isoamyl acetate, HEPA for irritant smoke). After assuring that the test subject is capable of detection of the challenge agent, the subject is asked to don the mask and to wear it until the subject is comfortable and relaxed. The test agent is introduced into the area around the mask using a method appropriate to the particular agent. If the subject detects the presence of the agent inside the mask, the mask is deemed to not fit well. In that event, a different size or manufacturer's mask should be selected, donned, and subjected until the fit test is successfully completed.

When the fit test is complete, and the masks which fit the individual have been identified, it is necessary to enable the wearer reproduce the fit in the field prior to entry into a contaminated atmosphere. The method by which this is accomplished are termed fit *checks* and should be performed after fit testing and prior to use.

Two fit checks should be used. The positive fit check is conducted by placing one's hands over the exhalation valve cover and exhaling. A well-fitting mask will rise gently off the face as the interior pressure increases. The negative pressure check is conducted by placing one's hands over the inhalation opening(s) and breathing in. As the pressure inside the mask decreases, the mask will collapse slowly in, indicating a good fit. It should be emphasized that the fit checks serve a different purpose than the fit tests, and must be used in conjunction with, and not instead of, the fit test. The purpose of the fit check is only to determine whether the original fit, which was verified via the fit test, has been reproduced in the field.

Medical Qualifications

The use of respiratory protection imposes an incremental physiological burden on the wearer; some potential users may have health conditions which would place them at elevated risk of illness or injury if they were to use a respirator. For this reason, it is essential that all respirator wearers be subjected to a medical examination to determine their fitness to wear this protective equipment.

There are a wide variety of medical conditions which may disqualify an individual from using a respirator. Among the most common are pulmonary insufficiency or cardiac problems that could be exacerbated by having to breathe against increased resistance. In addition, the use of SCBA, which may weigh in excess of thirty pounds, may be difficult for people with back problems or of particularly small stature.

Other, less common medical conditions may also present particular problems if respirators are to be used. People who are claustrophobic often find wearing a facepiece to be uncomfortably confining. Persons with a perforated eardrum should be disqualified from respirator use since the perforation may serve as a route of entry for toxic substances even when using the proper respirator.

The medical examination by which respirator users are qualified should be designed and reviewed, if not actually conducted, by an licensed and qualified physician. It should include a number of elements, including a health history, physical examination and a pulmonary function test. Additional guidance and information in this area may be found in the American National Standards Institute document which addresses medial qualifications for respirator users.

A Comprehensive Respiratory Protection Program

On hazardous waste sites, as well as other hazardous work areas, workers rely on respiratory protective devices to provide reliable and effective protection against the potential harmful agents with which they work. However, in order for the protection actually be reliable and effective, it is necessary to coordinate the different activities described in this section within the context of a comprehensive respiratory protection program.

This program should describe in careful detail how the employer will address each of the elements of respirator use discussed above. It should address, for example, how the fit and medical qualification should be done and by whom. It should outline the content and administration of respirator training. It should designate the program administrator, who should be qualified by training and experience for this responsibility. Perhaps most importantly, the program should identify the specific respirator required for each respirator use situation in the workplace, and the basis of how that selection was made.

A complete program will assure that each of the important activities associated with the use of respirators is addressed. It will also serve as a reference for employees (and, importantly, regulators) who are interested in how the program works. Most importantly, though, the written program serves as a record of the tasks and responsibilities to be undertaken by all members of the work team to assure that the protection that is intended and required is actually provided.

CHEMICAL PROTECTIVE CLOTHING

Chemical protective clothing serves two principal purposes at waste sites. First and foremost, it prevents or minimizes contact of potentially hazardous chemicals with the skin, which is the largest organ of the human body. Second, if doffed and decontaminated properly, it prevents or minimizes the transfer of potentially hazardous chemicals from the site.

As mentioned earlier, the goal is to select and use just the right amount of protective clothing to minimize negative effects on worker productivity and comfort and to control costs. The late 1980s and early 1990s have seen major advancements in chemical protective clothing. New, more chemically resistant fabrics have become available along with testing methods and test data to support claims of resistance. Attention is being given to worker productivity by means of clothing designs. Better characterization and understanding of hazards has enabled the selection of clothing that addresses workers' needs for comfort. Finally, the health and safety community is developing a better understanding of the complete cost of using clothing for protection from chemicals. This latter development is enabling more informed trade-offs with engineering controls and other approaches to protecting workers.

Most importantly these advancements are being summarized in readily available and usable documents. These include:

- *Chemical Protective Clothing*, a two-volume textbook published by the American Industrial Hygiene Association [11]
- *Guidelines for the Selection of Chemical Protective Clothing*, a two-volume field/reference manual published by the American Conference of Governmental Industrial Hygienists [5]
- *Quick Selection Guide to Chemical Protective Clothing*, a pocket-sized, paper-backed summary of chemical resistance information [12]
- The proceedings of four international conferences on protective clothing sponsored by the American Society for Testing and Materials [13, 14, 15, 16]
- *Chemical Protective Clothing Performance Index Book*, a tabulation of chemical toxicity and chemical resistance information [17]

These documents along with significantly more informative product brochures from the CPC manufacturers have greatly increased the potential for finding, selecting, and correctly using protective clothing on waste sites.

These tasks are the subject of the remainder of this chapter. The discussion begins with a brief review of the challenge represented by the various forms in which the chemical may be present.

Chemical Hazards

The proper selection and use of CPC begins with a characterization of the potential hazard, as addressed in several other chapters of this book. In summary pertinent to CPC, chemical hazards may be present in the form of solids, liquids, and vapors. Each represents one or more challenges to PPE. Solids are of special concern when particulates are involved. Respirators, of course, provide protection from the inhalation of particulates. Also important is to limit the transport of hazardous particulates from the workplace due to its accumulation in street clothing. Such particulates represent a hazard to those who associate with the worker and are not equipped with respirators. This is exemplified by the relatively higher incidence of asbestosis among the families of asbestos workers [18]. Similar concerns apply to lead and arsenic dusts, pesticide powders, and radioactive particulates. The current trend for countering such challenges is the use of porous, low air permeability fabrics which provide protection while allowing some loss of body heat generated by working.

Liquid and vapor challenges require a different level protection than that for the solids. Clothing containing a continuous (i.e., non-porous) layer of a plastic or rubber is necessary to isolate the worker from these hazards. Porous fabrics are unacceptable, although some promise is held for microporous, multilayer, breathable fabrics as splash protection.

Useful forms of the plastic or rubber (i.e., polymeric) materials for liquid and vapor protective clothing are thin, flexible films, sheets, laminates, and coatings. Many of these materials are inexpensive and in many cases can be reused multiple times. Furthermore a wide variety of candidate polymeric materials are available from which one or a select few may be applied to specific requirements. Items ranging from gloves to full-body ensembles can be made virtually air-tight and waterproof. Because of this, such items are often referred to as "impervious" clothing; however, with regard to chemical challenges, as opposed to air and water, such items may be far from impervious. Chemicals and chemical mixtures can absorb into and permeate clothing fabricated from polymers [19, 20, 21]. In the extreme, the chemicals may actually dissolve the clothing. Because of this, the chemical resistance of the clothing material to the chemicals of concern is a critical issue in the clothing/equipment selection process. This has been reviewed extensively in references 5 and 11-17, and is the subject of the next portion of this chapter.

PERMEATION

The resistance of a clothing material to liquids and vapors is judged largely on effectiveness of the material as a barrier to chemical permeation. Permeation of a chemical through a non-porous, polymeric film or coating is a three-step process involving: 1) the sorption of molecules of the chemical at the surface of the clothing exposed to the chemical, 2) the diffusion of the chemical through the material, and 3) the desorption of the molecules from the opposite or inside surface of the material. In this discussion, steps 1 and 3 will be considered fast relative to step 2; consequently, the diffusion step controls the rate of the permeation process. Classical diffusion theory (Fick's laws) states that the permeation rate (mass/time/area) is proportional to the concentration gradient of the chemical across the material [22, 23]. The proportionality becomes an equation by the introduction of the diffusion coefficient. Thus,

Eq. (1)

$$J = -D\frac{dc}{dx}$$

where
J = mass flux, $\mu g/cm^2/min$
D = diffusion coefficient, cm^2/sec
c = the chemical concentration in the material, g/cm^3
x = distance from the contacted surface, cm

The minus sign in Eq. (1) accounts for the decrease in c as x increases.

The diffusion coefficient is an intrinsic property of the chemical/material pair. It is a function of temperature and in some cases is dependent on the chemical concentration within the material. With the knowledge of D, one can estimate permeation rates for a range of material thicknesses and concentration gradients. Thus, it is worthwhile to determine diffusion coefficients for permanent/barrier pairs.

Diffusion coefficients are readily determined from the results of permeation testing. ASTM Method F739 is the recognized and practiced standard for conducting such testing, and is described in detail later in this chapter [24, 25]. The test is conducted using a two-chambered cell in which the material of interest forms the partition between the two chambers. The challenge chemical or chemical mixture is charged into one chamber (i.e., the challenge or upstream chamber) and the other chamber (i.e., the collection or downstream chamber) is monitored for the presence and concentration of the chemical that permeates the material. Initially, no chemical is detected. At some time, however, the chemical becomes evident; this is called the breakthrough time. Thereafter, the chemical appears at an increasing rate until the so-called steady-state is reached. This process is graphically depicted in Figure 9-1.

Two diffusion coefficients can be estimated from the data: the steady-state D_s and the time-lag D_L. The steady-state D_s is calculated using the steady-state permeation rate, J, and an integrated form of Eq. (1) and the assumption that the chemical concentration in the collection medium is maintained at essentially zero.

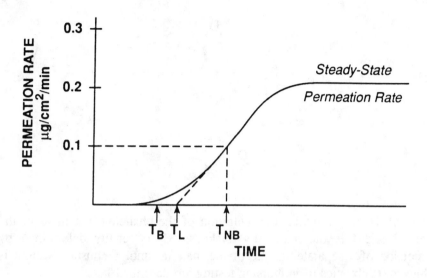

Figure 9-1. Ideal permeation through
a polymeric membrane.

Eq. (2)

$$J = \frac{D_s C_2}{\ell}$$

or

Eq. (3)

$$D_s = \frac{J\ell}{C_2}$$

where C_2 is the saturation concentration of the challenge chemical in the material and ℓ is the material's thickness. C_2 is readily determined by immersion of a separate sample of the material until a constant weight is achieved. (Subtleties of immersion testing are described later.)

The time-lag D_L is calculated according to Eq. (4).

Eq. (4)

$$D_L = \frac{\ell^2}{6T_L}$$

where T_L is the time at the intercept of the extension of the steady-state line to the time axis.

Upon rearranging Eqs. (2) and (3), one notes that the steady-state permeation rate, J, is inversely proportional to thickness while the time-lag time, T_L, is proportional to the square of the thickness. Researchers have further shown empirically that measured breakthrough times are approximately proportional to the square of the thickness [26]. Thus, doubling the thickness of the polymer layer of an item of protective clothing will theoretically quadruple the measured breakthrough time. This finding has significant implications relative to the selection and specification of chemical protective clothing. An extensive discussion of the interpretation and use of the permeation test results are in Reference 27.

Ideal permeation, as described above, involves a diffusion process in which the breakthrough time is followed by a period of smooth transition to a steady-state situation in which the permeation rate does not change with time. Ideal diffusion is most likely to occur when there is little or no other interaction between the material and the chemical. It should be recognized, however, that deviations (i.e., anomalies) from the ideal may occur in many cases [19, 22]. As the name implies, anomalous permeation is not predictable. There are, however, several conditions under which the probability for non-ideal permeation is increased:

- where there may be a reaction of the chemical with the plastic/elastomer of the CPC or some other component of the material. In some cases, the reaction will lengthen the breakthrough time and reduce permeation rate by consuming chemical. In other cases the reaction will reduce the barrier effectiveness of the CPC by degrading its properties.

- where the chemical, merely by its being absorbed, changes the properties of the CPC. Many organic liquids are known to craze (produce surface cracks) in the hard, clear plastics used for lenses and face shields. Many of these same chemicals will soften or plasticize the clothing materials.

- where the chemical extracts components from the CPC materials. For example, leaching of plasticizer from PVC clothing will significantly affect its barrier as well as functional properties.

Permeation theory can provide significant insight to clothing performance when data from testing are available. It is often necessary, however, to estimate CPC performance without the benefit of test data. This may be especially true where multi-component solutions are involved. At present, there are no established theories that provide a mechanism for this activity although several investigators have approached this problem from a basis of solubility parameter theory [28, 29]. Furthermore, experience has led to the formulation of some guiding principles relative to the probable chemical resistance of clothing materials. The first is that, in general, chemicals from the same family (e.g., the simple alcohols, the primary amines, the alkanes, the aldehydes, etc.) will tend to permeate a given CPC material at similar rates and with similar breakthrough times. There are, of course, exceptions. Other generalizations are:

- higher molecular weight members of a homologous series of chemicals permeate at slower rates than lower molecular weight members.
- pendant groups (which increase the size of a molecule) tend to slow permeation relative to that of the simple molecule.
- polar chemicals tend to permeate polar materials more rapidly than non-polar chemicals, and the converse is true.

Test Methods

The barrier effectiveness of a particular item of clothing to a particular chemical/mixture is dependent on the specific interactions between the clothing material and the chemical/mixture. This, in turn, is determined by the formulation of the clothing material, its method of manufacture, and its thickness. Temperature and other conditions of use also influence clothing barrier properties. Finally, the composition of the chemical/mixture is of major importance since relatively small percentages of a second, third, etc., component can drastically alter the way in which a chemical interacts with a material. Thus, protective clothing selection decisions should be based on the results of testing of the chemical/clothing material pair whenever possible.

Immersion Test

Immersion of a clothing material in a chemical/mixture followed by inspection for changes in appearance, strength, dimensions, and weight is the easiest and perhaps most telling test of a clothing material. Weight change information is of particular interest since in general chemicals which are absorbed at levels of 10% or more are likely to rapidly permeate the material. There appears to be a correlation between weight change and breakthrough time [30]. Furthermore, C_2 of Eq. (2) is directly estimated from the weight change of the material once it has reached a steady level.

ASTM Method D471-79 and ISO Method 2025 (International Organization for Standards) are standard methods for immersion testing. An important consideration when conducting such tests with multilayer clothing materials is that usually only the outside layer of the clothing should be exposed to the chemical/mixture. The edges of such materials should not be exposed. Absorption of the chemical layers by sublayers or supporting fabrics that would not normally "see" the chemical would confuse interpretation of the results. The calculation of C_2 for a multilayer fabric may not be practical since it is likely to be difficult to determine the amount of chemical in each layer.

Finally, it should be noted that lack of change in an immersion test does not necessarily indicate that the material is a chemical barrier. This can only be determined by permeation testing as described in the following paragraph.

Permeation Testing

Breakthrough time and permeation rate are determined by means of a permeation test. ASTM Method F739 was specifically developed for the evaluation of protective clothing materials. The method uses a test cell which is divided into two chambers at the midline by the clothing material to be tested. The challenge chemical is placed in one chamber and the other chamber (i.e., the collection chamber) is monitored for the chemical of interest. Of interest are the time the chemical is first detected (T_B), the normalized breakthrough time (T_{NB}), the rate of permeation, and the cumulative amount of chemical permeating the clothing. *The collecting medium must not interact with the clothing material; air, nitrogen, helium, or water are preferred collection media.*

The detection of breakthrough is dependent on the sensitivity of the test system, including the analytical method, the surface area of the clothing material, the volume or flowrate of the collection medium, and other experimental parameters. Because the sensitivity can vary from test-to-test and laboratory-to-laboratory, ASTM Committee F23 which is responsible for the procedure has recently defined normalized breakthrough as the time at which the permeation rate equals 0.1 µg/cm^2/min. Thus, there is now a common basis for comparison of clothing products. With reference to Figure 1 (page 12), T_{NB} is shown to occur after T_L, but this is not necessarily always the case. The sequence of events is dependent on the chemical/material pair.

Typical, preferred analytical methods for measuring permeation, include gas, liquid and ion chromatography, analysis for total combustible organics, ultraviolet and infrared spectrophotometry and radioanalysis. The properties of the chemical, the sensitivity requirements for the test, and cost are the principal factors considered in selecting an analytical method. For relatively volatile chemicals, gas chromatography and infrared spectrophotometry are the preferred methods. Liquid chromatography is used for relatively nonvolatile organic compounds. Ion chromatography is particularly useful for inorganic acids and salts. Finally, radiolabeled compounds may be preferred where high sensitivity and specificity is required. Furthermore, if the compound of interest is readily available in radiolabeled form, radiochemical methods may be significantly less costly than the development and use of the other techniques.

Permeation testing of protective clothing materials has increased significantly during the past decade. The Journal of the American Industrial Hygiene Association, and the product catalogues of the CPC vendors have become the principal vehicles for dissemination of test findings. As mentioned earlier, most of these test data have been compiled in comprehensive publications that are readily available. Furthermore, computered databases of the information are commercially available [31, 32].

ASTM F739 involves the continuous contact of the challenge chemical with the clothing material. To guide testing under conditions that may be more representative of actual exposure conditions, ASTM Method F1383 was developed. ASTM F1383 involves intermittent contact of the liquid or gas with the clothing material. The duration of and number of contacts, as well as the time between contacts, are determined by the tester. The same apparatus and analytical procedures are used.

ASTM Methods F739 and F1383 are laboratory tests. To address the frequent need for assessing chemical resistance in the field, the U.S. Environmental Protection Agency (EPA) developed the permeation cup test [33]. This test, which has been standardized as ASTM Method F1407, involves a swallow, lightweight cup and a balance. A small amount of liquid chemical is placed into the cup. A swatch of protective clothing material is secured over the mouth of the cup and the cup weighed. The cup is then inverted so that the liquid is in contact with the clothing material. Periodically, the cup is reweighed. Loss in weight indicates chemical permeation. In order to detect such permeation the chemical must be volatile. The test procedure also enables inspection of the clothing material for swelling, softening, or other signs of poor chemical resistance.

To further facilitate product comparisons, ASTM Guide F1001 defines a battery of 15 liquid and gaseous chemicals with which to challenge clothing materials. The battery includes chemicals representative of several chemical families: ketone, aldehyde, amine, linear hydrocarbon, aromatic hydrocarbon, acid, base, chlorinated hydrocarbon, and so forth.

Penetration, Including Biologically-Active Substances

In contrast to permeation, ASTM defines penetration as the movement of solids, liquids, or gases through pores, or other openings in the clothing material, seams, or closures. ASTM Method 903 describes the test, which involves pressurizing a liquid on one side of the clothing material and visually observing the other side for the appearance of liquid. Late in 1992, this method was adapted to two bio-hazard applications. ASTM Method ES21 uses a liquid that simulates the surface tension of blood as the challenge. Method ES22 uses the same liquid but with the addition of a bacteriophage ($\emptyset$X 174). Rather than visual observation of penetration, the tester swabs the outside of the clothing material and then cultures the swab. Growth of bacteriophage indicates that the material was penetrated.

Vision

Faceshields and lenses, in addition to being chemical barriers, must provide clear, undistorted vision to the wearer. Hard, inflexible faceshields and lenses fabricated from polymeric material may be subject to crazing (i.e., surface cracking) upon contact with certain chemicals. Crazing renders the surface foggy and can drastically reduce vision. Since chemical contact with the faceshield or lens is more likely to occur in uncontrolled or emergency situations when reduced vision would be an additional severe hazard, shields and lens materials should be tested for resistance to chemical attack. Crazing can also reduce the impact strength of the material.

ANSI/ASTM Method F484-77 describes a procedure for determining stress crazing by chemicals. A second method for determining the effect of chemicals on clear plastics is by measuring the transparency of the plastic before and after exposure to the chemical; ASTM D1746 describes one such method.

Other Factors

Although the focus of this discussion is chemical resistance of clothing materials, the selection and use of protective clothing involves other factors of equal or greater importance. For example, gloves must provide the wearer some minimum level of dexterity, and fabrics must have some level of tear resistance. The relative importance of the performance factors is largely dependent on the work tasks to be carried out.

At present, there is no standard, overall protocol for evaluating protective clothing or clothing materials for all the performance parameters of importance to workers on hazardous waste sites. Reference 34 is a compilation of some of the more pertinent test methods; a subset of these is presented in Table 9-3. For completeness, the chemical resistance methods mentioned above are included in the table.

TABLE 9-3. Test Methods for Chemical Protective Clothing	
Characteristic	**Test**
A. CHEMICAL RESISTANCE	
1. Permeation Resistance	ASTM F739-91: Resistance of Protective Clothing Materials to Permeation by Liquids and Gases under Conditions of Continuous Contact ASTM F1383-92: Resistance of Protective Clothing Materials to Permeation by Liquids and Gases under Conditions of Intermittent Contact ASTM F1407-92: Resistance of Chemical Protective Clothing Materials to Liquid Permeation - Permeation Cup Method
2. Penetration Resistance	ASTM F903: Resistance of Protective Clothing Materials to Penetration by Liquids
3. Swelling and Solubility	ASTM D471-79: Rubber Property--Effect of Liquids
4. Strength Degradation	ASTM D543: Resistance of Plastics to Chemical Reagents
5. Crazing	ASTM F484-77: Stress Crazing of Acrylic Plastics in Contact with Liquid or Semi-Liquid Compounds
6. Transparency	ASTM 1746-70: Transparency of Plastic Sheeting
B. BIOLOGICAL RESISTANCE	
1. Synthetic Blood	ASTM ES21: Resistance of Protective Clothing Materials to Synthetic Blood
2. Viral Penetration	ASTM ES22: Resistance of Protective Clothing Materials to Penetration by Blood-Borne Pathogens Using Viral Penetration as a Test System

TABLE 9-3. Test Methods for Chemical Protective Clothing	
Characteristic	**Test**
C. **STRENGTH**	
1. Tear Resistance/ Strength	ASTM D751-73: Testing of Coated Fabrics ASTM D412-75: Rubber Properties in Tension Fed. 191A-5102 (ASTM D1682): Strength and Elongation, Breaking of Woven Cloth: Cut Strip Method Fed. 191A-5134 (ASTM D2261): Tearing Strength of Woven Fabrics by the Tongue Method
2. Puncture Resistance	ASTM F1342-91: Protective Clothing Material Resistance to Puncture
3. Abrasion Resistance	ASTM D1175: Abrasion Resistance of Textile Fabrics
D. **DEXTERITY/FLEXIBILITY**	
1. Dexterity (gloves only)	See Reference 28
2. Flexibility	ASTM D1388: Stiffness of, Cantilever Test Methods
E. **AGING RESISTANCE**	
1. Ozone Resistance	ASTM D3041-72: Coated Fabrics--Ozone Cracking in a Chamber ASTM D1149-64: Rubber Deterioration-- Dynamic Ozone Cracking in a Chamber
2. UV Resistance	ASTM G27: Operating Xenon-Arc Type Apparatus for Light Exposure of Non-Metallic Materials--Method A--Continuous Exposure to Light

TABLE 9-3. Test Methods for Chemical Protective Clothing	
Characteristic	**Test**
F. WHOLE ITEMS	
1. Gas Tightness	ASTM F1052-87: Pressure Testing of Gas-Tight, Totally Encapsulating Chemical Protective Suits
2. Comfort & Fit	ASTM F1154-88: Qualitative Evaluation of Comfort, Fit, Function, and Integrity of Chemical Protective Suit Ensembles
3. Liquid Tightness	ASTM F135-91: Light-Tight Integrity of Chemical Protective Suits or Ensembles Under Static Conditions
4. Labelling	ASTM F1301: Labelling Chemical Protective Clothing

There are four specifications for clothing as used by first responders (typically, firefighters) to emergencies involving chemicals or injured persons. These are national Fire Protection Association (NFPA) standards 1991, 1992, 1993, and 1999 [35]. These specifications are based principally on ASTM test methods and prescribed minimum levels of performance.

Literature Provided by Vendors

The most widely available sources of information on CPC are the product catalogues of the CPC manufacturers and vendors. Much of this information has been summarized in volume two of References 5 and 11. These booklets contain descriptions of the types, sizes, and varieties of CPC produced by each manufacturer. In most cases, the basic materials of construction of the CPC are also included in the product descriptions. Many manufacturers also include information pertinent to the chemical resistance of their products or of the materials from which the products are fabricated. This information is generally in the form of tables of quantitative permeation data or qualitative recommendations for the products/materials and particular chemicals. A few vendors also provide information pertinent to abrasion, tear, etc., resistance but, in general, most catalogues do not address such application-related issues. The exception is for items which are certified to meet NFPA specifications. For those items details, specific test results and use guidance are available upon request.

The amount, level of detail, and quality of information available from the major manufacturers of chemical protective clothing has increased dramatically during the past five years. Furthermore, vendors are more knowledgeable and anxious to answer questions as to the use, maintenance, decontamination, and disposal of their products.

Performance and Purchase Considerations

The performance of CPC as a barrier to chemicals is determined by the materials and the design and quality of the clothing construction. Each application places particular demands on the clothing and, therefore, the performance requirements. For example, a less durable piece of clothing may be more than adequate for a moderate duration, mild activity (e.g., sampling), whereas it would not endure more than five minutes of a vigorous, waste site cleanup activity. Garment strength, durability, and fit, as well as worker comfort, must be addressed. Depending on the application, chemical barrier effectiveness may be more or less important than the physical attributes of the clothing.

When considering chemical resistance, three underlying factors must be taken into account:

- in general, there is no such thing as "impermeable" plastic or rubber clothing.
- no one clothing material will be a barrier to all chemicals.
- for certain chemicals or combinations of chemicals there is no commercially-available glove or clothing that will provide more than an hour's protection following contact.

Other considerations are:

- stitched seams of clothing may be highly penetrable by chemicals if not overlaid with tape or sealed with a coating. Zippers, other closure, and interfaces (e.g., sleeve-to-glove) are also pathways for chemical ingress.
- pinholes and areas where the polymer coverage is relatively thin can compromise barrier effectiveness.
- Although the generic names of the clothing material may be the same, there can be significant differences between the performance of the products of several vendors. This may be due to formulation or fabrication differences [36].

SELECTION OF PPE

When any piece or ensemble of PPE is to be utilized on a hazardous waste site, the advantages and limitations of the equipment should be carefully considered with regard to the potential exposures to chemical and physical hazards, worker productivity, worker comfort, and cost. Consequently, selection of the equipment should be performed by an individual who is familiar with both the equipment and the likely use conditions under which the PPE will be used.

Frequently, on hazardous waste sites, the solutions and mixtures of chemicals are unknown; often, the visible, physical characteristic of the chemicals (solid, gas, liquid) or the odor are the only available information. Thus, it is difficult to assess the degree of hazard to which workers may be exposed. The state-of-the-art approach for selecting PPE in such cases is to initially assume the worst exposure condition and use the highest level of PPE. Then, as the chemical and physical agents on site are characterized, the PPE can be selected to match specific hazards. A good example of this approach is demonstrated by an EPA advisory protocol for hazardous waste site entry, shown in Table 9-4.

As illustrated on the left side of Table 9-4, if any of the selection criteria listed under Level A were present on site, then Level A protective equipment must be used. As the concentration of contaminants, hazardous substances, potential for splash, and organic vapor levels are reduced, the level of protective equipment is lowered to Level C. It should be noted that Level D PPE is primarily a work uniform and should not be worn where there is potential for contamination of body parts through boots or when inhalation of gases or vapor is possible.

TABLE 9-4

Environmental Protection Agency Site Entry Protocol *

Level/Selection Criteria **	Eye/Face	Head	Hands	Feet	Full Body	Respirator
LEVEL A						
• Chemical concentration known--ABOVE SAFE LEVEL • Extremely hazardous substance (dioxin, cyanide) • Skin destructive substance • Confined spaces	See full-body SCBA	Hard hat	2 pairs gloves	Chem-resistant steel toe, shank, disposable booties	Fully-encapsulated chem-resistant suit w/disposable outer suit, gloves, boots	SCBA (pressure-demand)
LEVEL B						
• IDLH and concentrations above PF provided by full mask, air purifying • <19.5% O_2 • Skin contact unlikely to head and neck • Unidentified vapor suspected	See SCBA	Hard hat	2 pairs gloves	Chem-resistant steel-toe, shank, disposable booties	2-piece suit w/hood or disposable suit	SCBA (pressure-demand)
LEVEL C						
• Known air concentration that PF will control in air-purifying mask • No IDLH possible • No skin destruction • No unidentified vapor	See respirator	Hard hat	2 pairs gloves	Steel-toe, w/shank, disposable booties	2-piece suit or disposable suit	Full-face air-purifying mask
LEVEL D						
• No measurable concentration • No exposure to splashes or inhalation	Safety glasses	Hard hat	1 pair gloves	Steel-toe, shank	Coveralls	None

* "Occupational Safety and Health Guidance Manual for Hazardous Waste Site Activities," US DHHS (NIOSH) No. 85-115 (1986).

** Meeting any of listed criteria requires that level of protection.

The selection of the most appropriate respirators has been discussed earlier. The selection of clothing requires decisions relative to the areas of the body which must be covered and the materials of construction of clothing. The extent of body coverage is a function of the hazard to be faced. Common practice is to use the minimum amount of PPE as necessary to provide protection to the worker. PPE can be burdensome and restrictive; minimizing PPE increases the likelihood that it will be worn and minimizes the loss in worker efficiency that typically accompanies PPE utilization. In addition, PPE can be expensive. Furthermore, each time PPE is used, it must be either disposed of or decontaminated and properly maintained; therefore, it is desirable to minimize time and costs directed to these activities. The determination of the amount of clothing which is appropriate for any given job is the purview of the industrial hygienist or safety engineers. These professionals must consider in their decision all aspects of the job to be done, the conditions under which it will be done, and the capabilities of the workers.

PPE USE

In order to obtain maximum performance from any item of PPE, it must be free of defects and in good operating condition and the wearer must understand the purpose of the item and how to use and care for it. PPE should be unpacked and inspected immediately upon its reception. This initial inspection is to check that the desired items were actually received and that the items are defect-free and operational. This inspection prevents the surprise of finding non-functional or inappropriate PPE in emergency situations or losing time while replacement PPE is ordered.

Following inspection, PPE should be stored in a cool, dry place with clear and definitive labels in order to prevent mix-ups that could result in the utilization of the wrong PPE for a given application. For example, gloves made from neoprene, butyl rubber, PVC, and nitrile rubber, can be similar in appearance, yet, there can be significant differences in the barrier performances of these materials.

At the time of use, each wearer should inspect the clothing prior to donning it. Again, the objective is to identify tears, punctures, fabrication flaws or functional problems that could compromise the protection anticipated from the PPE. A post-donning inspection is essential for full-body encapsulating suits. This may be best carried out with the assistance of a second individual who is able to check closures and interconnections between, for example, gloves and sleeves, boots and pants, etc. Further reinspections should be performed throughout the work period, especially if the wearer has experienced significant contact with a chemical or suspects the integrity of the PPE has been breached.

Following completion of the work assignment or the work period, PPE is removed (doffed). A primary consideration in doffing is to avoid transfer of chemical that may be on the outside of the PPE to clean areas, skin, and underclothing. It is common practice at waste sites to doff PPE at designated areas, in many cases following a preliminary decontamination of the PPE with soap and water. The EPA has developed comprehensive doffing procedures which address doffing, decontamination, and disposal of contaminated PPE [37].

Decontamination and re-use of PPE is a matter of considerable interest and concern. (See Chapter 11, Contamination Reduction/Removal Methods.) At issue is any chemical that may have been absorbed by the PPE material. Is the chemical removed by the decontamination process? If not, what happens to this chemical during storage? Does the chemical continue to permeate the clothing such that the next time the PPE is donned, chemical is present on the inside surface? Researchers are only now beginning to address these problems; however, practitioners, must deal with the issue every day. Some have opted for the use of inexpensive, single-use disposable clothing whenever possible. Such clothing is not universally applicable, however, and the use of more expensive PPE may be required. Some full ensembles can cost $4,000 or more versus $300-500 for some limited-use garments, while the most expensive gloves are in the range of $40-50/pair versus less than a dollar a pair for the less expensive gloves. Obviously, there is an economic incentive to re-using the more expensive items; the challenge is to ensure that these items are effective and have no intrinsic hazard the second time they are worn.

SUMMARY

Since engineering controls are not readily implemented at hazardous waste sites, PPE combined with good work practices are the primary means for minimizing the exposure of workers to hazardous chemicals. PPE ranges from respirators, to supplied air systems, to gloves, to full-body encapsulating ensembles. Proper selection of PPE requires careful assessment of the risk hazard. This assessment includes the chemicals involved, the skills of the workers, the tasks, and the duration of potential exposures. PPE must then be selected on the basis of its demonstrated performance under such conditions. With regard to clothing, chemical resistance is a key concern and it must be recognized that there is no universal barrier material. Once PPE has been selected and purchased, it should be inspected for construction flaws and function. Workers must be instructed as to the use and limitations of PPE. Re-use requires special attention to decontamination and storage.

REFERENCES

1. "Environmental News Superfund Status Report," Office of Public Affairs, Environmental Protection Agency, Washington, D.C., (January 10, 1984).
2. Clayton, G.D., F.E. Clayton. *Patty's Industrial Hygiene and Toxicology*, 3rd Revised Ed., (Vols. 1-3, Wiley-Interscience).
3. Mackison, F.W., R.S. Stricoff, L.J. Partridge. "NIOSH/OSHA Occupational Health Guidelines for Chemical Hazards," DHHS (NIOSH) Publication No. 81-123 (1981).
4. *Accident Prevention Manual for Industrial Operations*, 7th Ed. (National Safety Council, 1974).
5. Schwope, A.D., P.P. Costas, J.O. Jackson, and D.J. Weitzman. *Guidelines for the Selection of Chemical Protective Clothing*. 3rd Edition. Am. Conf. of Govt. Ind. Hygienists, Cincinnati, OH, 1987). Also, National Technical Information Service (NTIS) No. AD-A179164 and No. AD-A179516.
6. Pritchard, John A. *A Guide to Industrial Respiratory Protection*, U.S. Energy Research and Development Administration (1977).
7. *General Industry OSHA Safety and Health Standards (29 CFR 1910.134: Respiratory Protection*, U.S. Department of Labor, Occupational Safety and Health Administration (OSHA 2206, June 1981).
8. J.B. Olishifski, P.E. McElroy and F.E. McElroy. *Fundamentals of Industrial Hygiene*, National Safety Council (1977).
9. Colton, C.E., L.R. Birkner, and L.M. Buosseau, Editors. *Respirator Protection: A Manual and Guidelines*, 2nd Edition. American Industrial Hygiene Association, Akron, Ohio, 1991.
10. Bolinger, N.J., and R.H. Schutz. *A NIOSH Technical Guide... NIOSH Guide to Industrial Respiratory Protection*, U.S. Dept. of Health and Human Services, NIOSH Publication No. 87-116, 1987.
11. Johnson, J.S. and K.J. Anderson, Editors. *Chemical Protective Clothing*. American Industrial Hygiene Association, Akron, Ohio, 1990.
12. Forsberg, K., and S.Z. Mansdorf. *Quick Selection Guide to Chemical Protective Clothing*. Van Nostrand Reinhold, New York, 1993.
13. Barker, R.L., and G.C. Colletta, Editors. *ASTM STP 900*, American Society for Testing and Materials, Philadelphia, Pennsylvania, 1986.
14. Mansdorf, S.Z., R. Sager, and A.P. Nielsen, Eds. ASTM STP 989. American Society for Testing and Materials, Philadelphia, Pennsylvania, 1988.

15.   Perkins, J.L., and J.O. Stull, Eds. ASTM STP 1037. American Society for Testing and Materials, Philadelphia, Pennsylvania, 1989.

16.   McBriarty, J.P., and N.W. Henry, Eds. ASTM STP 1133. American Society for Testing and Materials, Philadelphia, Pennsylvania, 1992.

17.   Forsberg, K., and L.H. Keith. *Chemical Protective Clothing Performance Index Book*, John Wiley & Sons, New York, 1989.

18.   Peters, G.A. and B.J. Peters. *Sourcebook on Asbestos Diseases* (Garland STPM Press, NY, 1980), P. B-7.

19.   Nelson, G.O., B. Lum, G. Carlson, C. Wong, and J. Johnson. "Glove Permeation by Organic Solvents," Am Ind. Hyg. Assoc. J. 42(3): 217-225 (1981).

20.   Sansone, E.B., and Y.B. Tewari. "The Permeability of Protective Clothing Materials to Benzene Vapor," Am. Ind. Hyg. Assoc. J. 41(3): 170-174 (1980).

21.   Williams, J.R. "Chemical Permeation of Protective Clothing," Am. Ind. Hyg. Assoc. J., 41(12): 884-887 (1980).

22.   Crank, J. and G. Park. *Diffusion in Polymers*, (Academic Press, NY, 1968).

23.   Crank, J. *Mathematics of Diffusion*, 2nd ed., (Claredon Press, Oxford, 1975).

24.   ASTM Standards are available from American Society for Testing and Materials, 1916 Race Street, Philadelphia, Pennsylvania 19107-1187.

25.   Henry, H.W. and C.N. Schlatter. "The Development of a Standard Method for Evaluating Chemical Protective Clothing for Permeation by Liquids," Am. Ind. Hyg. Assoc. J., 42(3): 202-207 (1981).

26.   Todd, W.F., A.D. Schwope, and G.C. Coletta. "Benzene Permeation Through Protective Clothing Materials," paper presented to the 72nd AICHE Annual Meeting, San Francisco, November, 1979.

27.   Schwope, A.D., R Goydan, R.C. Reid, and S. Krishnamurthy. "State-of-the-Art Review of Permeation Testing and Interpretation of Its Results." Am. Ind. Hyg. Assoc. j., 41(10), pp. 722-725, 1981.

28.   Zellers, E.T., and G.Z. Zhang. Three-Dimensional Solubility Parameters and Chemical Protective Clothing Permeation II. Modelling Diffusion Coefficient, Breakthrough Time, and Steady State Permeation Rate of Viton Gloves, J. App. Pol. Sci. in press, 1993.

29.   Goydan, R., A. Schwope, T.R. Carroll, H. Tseng, and R.C. Reid. Development and Assessment of Methods for Estimating Protective Clothing Permeation. EPA/600/2-87/104. U.S. Environmental Protection Agency, Cincinnati, Ohio, 1987.

30. Stampfer, J.F., M.J. McLeod, M.R. Betts, and S.P. Berardinelli. "The Permeation of Eleven Protective Garment Materials by Four Organic Solvents," submitted to Am. Ind. Hyg. Assoc. J. (1984).

31. CPCbase®, Arthur D. Little, Inc., Cambridge, Massachusetts.

32. Forsberg, K. Permeation and Degradation Database, Lewis Publisher, CRC Press, Inc., Boca Raton, Florida.

33. Schwope, A.D., T.R. Carroll, R. Huang, and M.D. Royer. "Test Kit for Field Evaluation of the Chemical Resistance of Protective Clothing." ASTM STP 989. Mansdorf, Sager, and Nielsen, Editors. American Society for Testing and Materials, Philadelphia, Pennsylvania, 1988.

34. *ASTM Standards on Protective Clothing*, American Society for Testing and Materials, Philadelphia, Pennsylvania, 1990.

35. Specification available from National Fire Protection Association, Quincy, Massachusetts.

36. Michelson, R.L. and R. Hall. A Breakthrough Time Comparison of Nitrile and Neoprene Glove Materials Produced by Different Glove Manufacturers." Am. Ind. Hyg. Assoc. J., 48(11), pp. 941-947, 1987.

37. See Appendix G of Reference 5.

38. Ross, J., and C. Ervin. Chemical Defense Flight Glove Ensemble Evaluation. AARML-TR-87-047, Armstrong Aerospace Medical Research Laboratory, Wright-Patterson Air Force Base, Ohio, 1987.

10

HEAT STRESS IN INDUSTRIAL PROTECTIVE ENCAPSULATING GARMENTS

Ralph F. Goldman, Ph.D.

There are a great many aspects to work: physical, physiological, psychological, sociological, financial, etc. Our concern for hazardous waste site workers is with the first two, and how imbalances between the physical and physiological *Demands* imposed by their tasks, and the *Capacity* of the workers to meet those demands, affect their health and performance. The ratio of the task demand to the worker's capacity is the critical element in whether a task is "comfortable." Usually, tasks demanding ≤ 20% of capacity will be "comfortable." For demand/capacity ratios from 20 to 40%, the "mild discomfort" may not seem to degrade performance; indeed this range may be best for task performance if individuals focus on the work and are less apt to relax or doze. When demands are 40 to 60% of capacity, performance of complex tasks requiring mental or manual dexterity skills may be noticeably degraded; performance of routine physical work (e.g., digging) may not appear to be altered but the work rate will probably be decreased (i.e., self-paced) to adjust the demand to 45% of a worker's capacity. Performance will become tolerance time limited as the ratio increases from 60% (tolerable for about a one hour) to 85% (tolerable for about 15 minutes). Accident rates appear to increase as demand to capacity ratios exceed 60%. At ratios above 80%, probability of illness or injury (heat exhaustion, physical exhaustion) increases. Ratios above 100% (i.e., D>C) exhaust the body's physical and physiological reserves in minutes.

Heat stress represents an imbalance between the heat produced by an individual and the heat loss allowed to the environment. The latter is as frequently controlled by the clothing worn as by any combination of environmental conditions; there is no single temperature or combination of temperature and humidity at which heat stress can be said to begin. Heat stress has occurred in men working very hard in the snow, although it is usually not recognized as such but thought to be some mysterious ailment. Typical heavy, outdoor winter clothing ensembles, e.g., clothing insulation of 4 clo, may only allow heat loss of 2.5 kcal/hr per °C difference between the skin of the wearer and the ambient environment. Even at -40°C, the maximum heat exchange by radiation and convection (H_{R+C}) through such clothing would be less than 200 kcal/hr; i.e., 2.5 kcal/hr.°C times the 75°C difference between a warm 35°C skin temperature and the ambient of -40°C. While some additional heat would be lost by respiration, since heat production for sustainable high activity is about 500 Watts (425 kcal/hr) about half of the total heat production would require sweat evaporative cooling (E_{req}) for it to be eliminated, but such clothing stringently limits the wearer's maximum evaporative cooling (E_{max}).

Using an average value of 58 kcal increase in body heat storage for each 1°C increase in mean body temperature [t_b = 1/3 skin temperature (t_{sk}) + 2/3 deep-body temperature (t_{re})] for a 70 kg man (i.e., specific heat of body = 0.83 kcal/kg. °C), it seems clear that accumulation of heat storage (ΔS,) which would lead to body temperatures above 39°C could occur within a few hours, even at -40°C.

The question of human heat balance can be analyzed by a well-defined heat balance equation. A major factor that must be considered is the metabolic energy production (M); the heat production required for a given task is a function of the total weight (body plus any load) moved, the efficiency with which this total weight is moved, and the rate of movement. The nature of the terrain over which the weight is moved is also involved. Walking on soft sand may double the energy cost for given speed and weight compared to walking on a smooth surface. Climbing stairs, or any lift (grade) work, is also very demanding in energy cost increases.

Another major factor, the non-evaporative heat exchange (H_{R+C}), is a linear function of the difference between the wearer's skin temperature (t_{sk}) and the ambient air temperature (t_a). Similarly, the maximum possible sweat evaporative cooling (E_{max}) is a linear function of the difference between the vapor pressure of sweat on the skin (P_s) and the ambient vapor pressure ($\phi_a P_a$); the latter is the relative humidity (ϕ_a) times the saturated vapor pressure of air (P_a) at ambient temperature (t_a). The heat exchange with the environment depends not only on the skin and ambient environmental conditions but also on the clothing, and the extent to which it limits the heat exchange between the skin and the ambient environment. Chemical protective clothing tends to be quite limiting both because of its insulation (clo) and its reduced moisture vapor permeability (i_m). Air motion (WV) also plays a key role in controlling these non-evaporative and evaporative exchanges, primarily by the extent to which it reduces the insulating still air layer (I_a) at the interface between the clothing surface and the ambient environment, although the intrinsic insulation of the clothing *per se* (I_{clo}) can also be reduced by wind penetration. A fourth environmental factor (in addition to t_a, $\phi_a P_a$, and WV) which frequently must be considered is the radiant heat load (H_R) produced by the sun, by such high temperature (shortwave, infrared) heat sources as blast furnaces or arc lights, or by such lower temperature "black body" sources as radiators, warm pipes, walls or ceilings. The mean radiant temperature (MRT) is an integrated expression of the average radiant temperature.

THE HEAT BALANCE EQUATION

The factors introduced so far, form the key elements in the following heat balance equation for the human body:

Eq. 1 $$(M - W_{ex}) + (H_{R+C}) - E_{req} - \Delta S = O$$

where: M = energy production (measured by oxygen consumption)
- W_{ex} = external work
- H_{R+C} = the net exchanges by radiation and convection between the body and the environment
- E_{req} = the required evaporative heat loss established by $[(M-W_{ex}) + (H_{R+C})]$
- ΔS = any change in body heat content.

Additional terms are sometimes included such as the heat exchanges by respiration, involving both humidification and heating of the inspired air, and diffusional evaporative heat losses from the skin; these respiratory and diffusional losses generally amount to about 25% of metabolic heat production at rest, and are most often ignored during work in the heat.

The amount of evaporative cooling (E_{req}) in the heat balance equation would ideally be much less than the maximum evaporative cooling that can be obtained through the clothing (E_{max}); i.e.: $E_{req} = [(M-W_{ex}) + (H_{R+C})] \ll E_{max}$.

As long as the heat losses are less than ($M-W_{ex}$), and all the evaporative cooling required can be obtained, no change in body heat storage (ΔS) is required. If heat loss by radiation and convection is greater than ($M-W_{ex}$) a heat debt will be incurred [34]. Changes of ±25 kcal in body heat content are probably not detectable by an individual, but an accumulation of body heat storage approaching 60-80 kcal generally results in the individual being unwilling to continue. Thus, satisfaction of the heat balance equation with minimal heat storage is a necessary condition for comfort and continued work. It is not, however, a sufficient condition; discomfort in the heat is largely generated by the sense of skin wettedness or dampness. The sensation of wettedness at the skin can be directly calculated as the ratio E_{req}/E_{max} [16]; i.e., the body will produce enough sweat to meet its evaporative requirements so that the relative humidity at the skin (alternatively defined as the "percent skin wettedness") can be calculated simply as the ratio E_{req}/E_{max}. If E_{req} is 50 Watts (i.e., $M-W_{ex} + H_{R+C} = 50$). and $E_{max} = 100$ Watts, then the skin need be only 50% sweat-wetted, or skin relative humidity will be 50%; expressed more precisely, the average skin vapor pressure (P_s) will be 50% of the saturated vapor pressure of water (= sweat) at t_{sk}.

As the maximum evaporative cooling (E_{max}) approaches or is less than the required evaporative cooling (E_{req}), the body cannot obtain the required evaporative cooling. The maximum evaporative cooling may be limited by the clothing, or by a high ambient vapor pressure, or even by very low ambient air motion. A necessary condition for comfort is that the relative humidity at the skin (i.e., % sweat wettedness) be less than about 20%. Note that, as discussed later, this ratio has been used as a heat stress index [HSI; [6]]. Increasing levels of sweat wettedness are associated with increasing heat discomfort. One must carefully screen and select workers for physical fitness at conditions requiring 60% sweat wettedness; at about that level, sweat will begin dripping off the skin. In general, a 60% sweat wettedness (i.e., skin relative humidity of 60% as defined by the ratio E_{req}/E_{max}) will be about the highest acceptable level for even a well-motivated, very fit and well-acclimatized workforce.

So far, the heat balance equation has been presented and its importance identified in determining whether or not a given combination of factors results in heat stress. While the reader may be concerned at the rather casual treatment of respiratory and diffusional heat losses, it must be recognized that the heat balance equation itself represents an approximation. Considering the variability in individual size, in physical and physiological states between workers, in the clothing worn and in its fit on a given individual, it is obvious that any human heat balance equation is inherently not a precision statement. Thus, this approach clearly falls within a GEGU—good enough for general use—category. This GEGU acronym will be used to emphasize adequacy, albeit imprecision, at a number of points in the subsequent discussion.

The six key parameters involved in the calculation of the heat balance equation have now been identified. Four are environmental factors: the air temperature (t_a), the ambient air motion (WV), the ambient vapor pressure ($\phi_a P_a$), and the mean radiant heat temperature (MRT). The other two factors, which are subject to behavioral temperature regulation, are the task workload (and the associated heat production of the worker) and the clothing worn by the worker. Each of these factors will be addressed in turn.

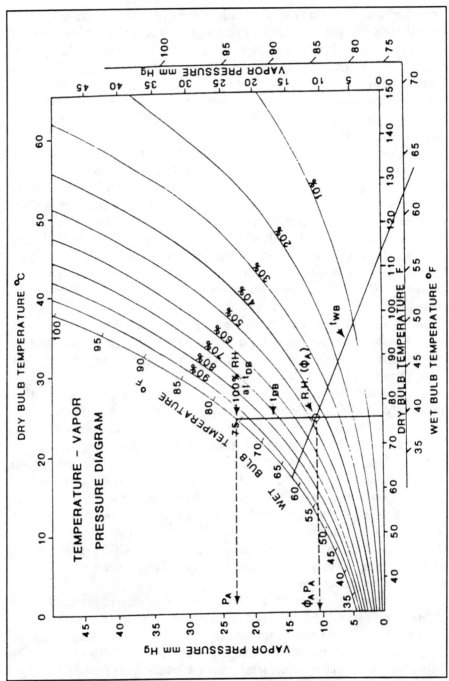

Figure 10-1. Psychrometric chart for
air at sea level showing relationships

THE SIX KEY FACTORS

1.   Ambient Air Temperature (t_a)

Surrounding every physical object is a surface film of trapped air. This "surface still air layer" contributes a very significant part of the insulation surrounding a human body (usually over 50% when dressed for indoors). This insulating air film is altered by air movement and this accounts for the perceived difference between the ambient air temperature as sensed by a still hand, and the ambient air temperature sensed when the hand is in motion. If one simply hangs a thermometer in ambient air, any radiant heat in the environment will be absorbed by the thermometer and effectively trapped there by the surface film layer around the thermometer. Accordingly, in order to measure the true psychrometric properties of air the thermometer must be ventilated, to minimize any surface still air film. This is done either by having the thermometer swung on the end of a chain (a sling psychrometer) or by having air pulled across it by a fan (an aspirated psychrometer). If the work site is close to an intense radiant heat source (smelter, glass furnace, etc.) special shielding for the thermometer bulb, or a specially shielded sensor, may also be required.

2.   Ambient Vapor Pressure ($\phi_a P_a$)

The ambient vapor pressure is usually determined from the measurement of a "wet bulb" thermometer temperature. Most psychrometers, sling or ventilating, simply pair two identical thermometers, with one bulb mounted a few centimeters below the other, and equip the lower bulb with a wettable cotton wick; hence the terminology dry bulb ($t_{db} = t_a$) and wet bulb (t_{wb}) temperature. The wick is saturated with water prior to aspirating or slinging the psychrometer. Because of both the omnipresent potential for convective heat gain from the air by the evaporatively cooled wet bulb thermometer and the potential radiant heat regain, ventilating the wet bulb thermometer to the appropriate air motion [air movement ≥ 4.5m/s (900 fpm) past the wet bulb wick] is of critical importance.

Some environmental physiologists have argued, correctly, that use of a psychrometric wet bulb to represent the potential evaporative cooling available to a worker is unreasonable—unless the worker is somehow to be ventilated or slung by the heels to produce a high air velocity across his 100% sweat-wetted skin. Accordingly, some of the environmental indices, to be discussed subsequently, incorporate a "natural"—or non-psychrometric—wet bulb (t_{nwb}). Figure 10-1 presents a standard temperature-vapor pressure (Moliere) diagram for air at sea level, which can be used to convert the measured dry bulb and wet bulb temperatures to a relative humidity; in turn, this can be converted to the ambient vapor pressure which is the key environmental parameter required for calculation of the maximum evaporative cooling capacity. Alternatively, tables of wet bulb depression at a given dry bulb temperature, or a "psychrometric slide rule," can be used to obtain the percent of relative humidity. Note that, because evaporation is a function of the difference between the skin and the ambient vapor pressures, evaporation of sweat from the skin can occur at 100% relative humidity as long as the air temperature is less than the temperature of the skin; thus ambient relative humidity *per se* is of little interest for heat balance.

The point of intersection of the wet bulb and dry bulb temperature lines on the psychrometric chart (cf. Fig.10-1) identifies the relative humidity; the uppermost curve on the graph represents the 100% relative humidity line. At 100% relative humidity, the ambient air is saturated (i.e., cannot take up any more moisture), so the wet bulb and dry bulb temperatures will, of course, be equal; no evaporation can occur unless air temperature increases. Observation of the psychrometric chart also indicates that the vapor pressure can be determined from this point of intersection of the dry bulb and wet bulb lines; it is simply read from the Y axis in either kilopascals (the SI unit) or, the more familiar, mmHg units. In the example drawn on the psychrometric chart (Figure 1) the ambient vapor pressure is one kilopascal or 7.5 mmHg. Note that at the indicated dry bulb temperature of 25.5°C, the ambient vapor pressure at 100% relative humidity would be about 25 mmHg; i.e., P_a, the saturated vapor pressure would be 25 mmHg. Multiplying this P_a by the 30 percent relative humidity indicated on Figure 1 (by the intercept of the dry bulb and wet bulb lines, ϕa) yields 7.5 mmHg, the ambient vapor pressure; simply stated, the air is holding 30% of the total moisture that it could hold when saturated at t_{db}.

Under conditions where there is little or no requirement for sweat evaporative cooling (i.e., low work with light clothing at comfortably cool to colder temperatures), ambient vapor pressure is of little concern since there is no requirement for evaporative cooling.

3.   Air Motion (WV)

The importance of the surface still air film as insulation has already been noted. For a cylinder the size of the human body, with low air motion the still-air layer film at the surface becomes a very significant contributor to the total insulation of a human. Indeed, wearing a long-sleeved shirt and trousers under still-air conditions, the contribution of the external air film (I_a; = 0.8 clo) equals or exceeds the intrinsic insulation (I_{cl}; = 0.6 clo) of the shirt and trousers. Air movement then is a major factor in heat transfer from the body to the ambient environment, with or without clothing. Even with an impermeable, encapsulating chemical protective clothing system, the external surface-air film (I_a) is still important unless reduced by wind.

Measurement of air movement requires sophisticated instrumentation, or sufficiently high but non-turbulent air motion that simpler field devices can be used. Thus, the usual approach for determining air motion indoors and outdoors, is to estimate it. One frequently sees air movement specified as 50 feet per minute (fpm), or as a seemingly more exact 44 fpm which is simply one-half mile per hour. Such values are simply GEGU estimates. With ambient air motion at about 0.13m/s (25 fpm), the natural convective air motion which results from the temperature difference between skin and air temperature becomes the primary factor; thus, lower ambient air motion is meaningless. The insulation of the surface still air layer at that low air motion is about 0.8 clo units for a human body.

In addition, if the worker is moving, body motion generates an "effective" air velocity [10]. Newburgh suggested that the effective wind velocity (V_e) generated during activity could be estimated from the heat production of the worker, using the MET unit of metabolism (one MET equals an average, "resting" heat production of 50 kcal/m²hr) he suggested the relationship:

Eq. 2 $$V_e = .07 (MET-0.85)$$

where: V_e =   effective wind motion generated (in m/s) and 0.85 = a "sedentary" MET level

Fanger suggested that the effective air velocity could be calculated as 0.1 + 0.4 $(MET-1)^{0.5}$, which gave a heat transfer coefficient (h_c) for average indoor clothing of 12.1 $(V_e)^{0.5}$ (V_e in m/s; hc in watts/m²°C). Such refinements are unnecessary for most practical work but should be kept in mind under conditions of very low ambient air movement. The effective air velocity is more important with light clothing and is particularly important with air permeable, chemical protective clothing as will be addressed further in the section on clothing.

4.   Mean Radiant Temperature (MRT)

Indoors, the temperature of the wall, windows, floor and ceiling are usually considered equivalent to the temperature of the air; however, thermal radiation can be a major contributor to discomfort and heat stress when an individual works near a large window or on the top floor of a building with an uninsulated roof. Thermal radiation is a major concern in industrial settings with such large, high-temperature heat sources as ovens, arc furnaces, etc.

The mean radiant temperature of an environment is an integrated value, representing the uniform surface temperature of a radiantly black enclosure in which an individual would exchange the same amount of radiant heat as he does in the actual, non-uniform, radiant environment. The usual mean radiant temperature measuring device is a hollow, thin-shelled, 15 cm (6-inch) copper sphere, painted flat black; the globe temperature (t_g) is measured at the center of the inside of the sphere. The mean radiant temperature (MRT) is calculated from the globe temperature [3], as a function of the ambient wind velocity (WV), by the equation:

Eq. 3 $$MRT = t_g + k \, (WV)^{0.5} \, (t_g - t_a)$$

where: k = 2.2 for t(°C) and WV (m/s)
or   k = 0.157 for t(°F) and WV (fpm)

5.   Metabolic Heat Production

As indicated above, the metabolic heat production of an individual is frequently expressed as so many Watts (= 1.163 kcal/hr) per square meter of surface area. A typical "standard" male will weigh 70 kg (154 lb), stand 174 cm (5 foot 8-1/2") tall, and therefore have 1.8 square meters (19.5 ft²) of body surface area. A "standard" female will weigh about 57 kg (125 lb), stand 164 cm (5 foot 4-1/2") tall and have a body surface area of 1.6m². The resting heat production of a standard adult male will be about 105 watts, which can be calculated quite nicely using either 1.5 watts/kg of body weight (1.3 kcal/hr kg) times 70kg, or 58 Watts/m (=1 MET=50kcal/hr m²) times 1.8m². Because of the larger amount of body fat (which is relatively inactive) in females, their resting heat production (about 85 Watts, or 80% that of the standard male) cannot be approximated by using the standard, surface area based MET unit; it can, however, be approximated using the 1.5 Watts/kg of body weight relationship. The heat production requirement for almost all physical work is a function of the weight moved (e.g., kg of body weight) and workers must move the weight of their fat, the weight-based equation presented below for estimation of energy cost (i.e., heat production) applies equally well for men and women. Since a "standard" female has about 28% body fat compared to 18% for a "standard" male, a greater thickness of the subcutaneous fat layer in females provides more insulation between the skin and the heat produced in the body. Under cool conditions, females may have cooler skin temperatures; studies suggest that women prefer about 1° C (1.8° F) higher air temperatures for comfort than men. However, under warm or hotter conditions, the circulation effectively moves heat from the core to the skin past the subcutaneous fat; thus this difference in fat, and cold tolerance, does not affect heat tolerance.

Workers seldom work at anywhere near their maximum work capacity levels during normal work. The metabolic heat production (M) at rest is, like heat loss, a linear function of body surface area. Typical office work ranges from 125 kcal/hr for "light" work to 150 kcal/hr for heavier tasks. However heavier tasks are rarely performed continuously so the energy cost (i.e., heat production) of hard work tasks must be time weight averaged with the intervening periods of resting heat production; e.g., while football players must have the capacity for very high, peak, heat production, their average heat production from the start of a game to the end of the 4th quarter is much lower. Workers performing tasks requiring heavy physical work that is machine paced, or for which overly high production quotas have been set, and marches with heavy loads, have far higher, time weighted average (TWA), heat productions. Table 10-1 presents a useful technique for estimating the energy cost of work.

Table 10-1. ESTIMATING ENERGY COST by TASK ANALYSIS		
	Typical kcal/minute	Average Range
Factor 1. Basic metabolism	1.0	0.8 to 1.2
Factor 2. Body position & movement		
Sitting	0.3	
Standing	0.6	
Walking	by formula*	2.0 to 3.0
Walk uphill	by formula* or add	0.8/meter rise
Factor 3. Type of work		
Hand work -light	0.4	0.2 to 1.2
-heavy	0.9	
One arm -light	1.0	0.7 to 1.2
-heavy	1.8	
Both arms -light	1.5	1.0 to 3.5
-heavy	2.5	
Whole body -light	3.5	2.5 to 9.0
-moderate	5.0	
-heavy	7.0	
-very heavy	9.0	

SAMPLE CALCULATION   **Average kcal/minute**
(for "standard worker")

Assembly work with heavy hand tools:

1. Basic Metabolism   1.0
2. Standing   0.6
3. Both Arms - heavy work   3.5
       Estimated TOTAL =   5.1 kcal/min

Metabolic heat production can also be estimated from a worker's heart rate. Heart rate, standing at rest, in a healthy adult male averages about 70 beats per minute, although more fit individuals may average 50 bpm; females, on average, have 10 bpm higher heart rates than males. An individual's maximum heart rate can be estimated as 220 bpm minus age in years. Heart rate during work is one of the most easily measured physiological responses (a count, for a minimum of 20 seconds, of the pulse rate, usually at the wrist). In the absence of heat stress, the rise in heart rate is linear with the rise in the metabolic cost of the work. For a fit, young, male worker, in the absence of heat stress, a simple measurement of heart rate can serve as an indicator of the difficulty of physical work, its energy cost (M), probable deep body (rectal T_{re}) temperature, and the respiration volume (in L/min) since respiratory volume usually increases linearly with M as oxygen extraction rises only slightly during moderate work, as shown in Table 10-2.

Table 10-2. Estimation of Work From Heart Rate					
Heart Rate beats/min	**Work Level**	**M kcal/min**	**Usual T_{re} °C**	**Respiration**	
				1/min	**1/min O_2**
<75	Very light	<2.5	≤37.5°	10	0.5
75-100	Light	2.5- 5.0	≤37.5°	10-20	0.5-1.0
100-120	Moderate	5.0- 7.5	37.5-38.0	20-35	1.0-1.5
120-140	Hard/heavy	7.5-10.0	38.0-38.5	35-50	1.5-2.0
140-160	Very heavy	10.0-12.5	38.5-38.8	50-65	2.0-2.5
160-180	Unduly heavy	12.5-15.0	38.8-39.0	65-85	2.5-3.0
>180	Exhausting	>15.0	>39.0	>85	>3.0

Linear interpolation can be used to fine-tune such estimation. Note that at higher heart rates, work time becomes limited (see below).

Thus, in the absence of heat stress, heart rate per se is a reasonable indicator of metabolic cost for an average, reasonably healthy worker. Work requiring heart rate to increase by < 30 bpm above the resting level is considered "comfortable;" work requiring a steady state heart rate of ≥ 120 bpm is not. Work at 140 bpm should be limited to 4 hours or less for fit, young men, while that requiring 160 bpm has a suggested time limit of about 2 hours. Heart rates ≥ 180 bpm should not be allowed for more than 15 minutes, and even then only for fit, young men. Assume that it requires an additional 35 bpm to deliver enough oxygen to meet the needs of a specific task. Given that [220 - 20] = the maximum heart rate of an average 20 year old, and assuming a resting heart rate of 70 bpm, the 20 year old has a "maximum heart rate increase" of 140 b/m (i.e., [200 - 70] b/m). The assumed task requirement of a 35 bpm heart rate increase represents 25% of the 20 year old's maximum heart rate increase. Returning to the D/C ratio concept introduced earlier, this task would be just a bit above the comfortable level for the 20 year old. It would represent about 40% of the capacity of a 60 year old (i.e., [220 - 60] - 70 = 90 bpm of maximum heart rate rise for a 60 year old) and fall just at the 40% threshold, thus changing this demand from "uncomfortable" to "performance degrading."

Alternatively, if the primary element involved in the activity is walking, the following equation has been developed [21] (and validated across a wide range of studies) to predict the heat production:

Eq. 4 $M = 1.5(W) + 2(W+L)(L/W)^2 + (\mu)(W+L)(1.5V^2 + 0.35\ VG)$

where: $W\ =$ body weight (kg); L = load carried (kg);
          $V\ =$ walking velocity (m/s); G = grade (%); and
          $\mu\ =$ a non-dimensional "terrain coefficient" ranging between a value of one, for a hard surfaced floor, to a value of two for soft sand.

The first term in the above equation simply expresses the resting energy cost of 1.5 Watts/kg of body weight, which works GEGU for males and females. The second term simply represents the energy cost of standing with a load on the back. If some portion of the load carried is not borne on the torso, adjustment should be made for the inefficiency of loading; each pound carried by hand costs roughly the equivalent of two pounds on the back, and each pound of footwear worn while walking is equivalent to five pounds carried on the back [56]. The importance of keeping the weight of protective footwear at a minimum can be seen from this relationship.; e.g., chemical protective boot covers which weight two pounds have the equivalent effect of an added ten pounds of backpack weight during walking. The weight of headgear should, in theory, be incremented by about 30% to equate it to a back-carried load, but generally this is too small an adjustment to require consideration. However, it should be recognized that the frequent complaints of the weight of protective headwear are apt to stem from too high a center of gravity, and the accompanying torque and momentum changes with body motion which result in a higher perceived weight, rather than from the actual weight of protective headgear *per se*.

The next term in the equation indicates that energy cost goes up as a function of the square of the walking speed and introduces a coefficient (μ) to adjust for the nature of the terrain being traversed [33]. Any smooth, hard surface, be it a treadmill, floor or blacktop road requires essentially the same energy cost and for these is assigned a multiplier of 1. Terrain coefficients (i.e., relative multipliers) to adjust for the energy costs of walking at a given speed across other terrain surfaces are: 1.1 for a gravel road; 1.2 for light brush; 1.3 for packed snow or ice; 1.5 for heavy brush; 1.8 for swampy terrain; and 2.1 for soft sand.

Sample Calculation: for a 70kg man, marching at 1.2 m/s with a 30kg pack in level, light brush

$$M = 1.5(70) + 2(100)(30/70) + 1.3(100)[1.5(1.2 \times 1.2)]$$

Calculated Heat Production = 456 Watts or 393 kcal/hr

    A task requiring heat production below 5 kcal/min would be considered average work, and would require a heart rate between 75 and 100 beats/min. to deliver sufficient oxygen to the working muscles. Moderate to hard work tasks would require up to 7.5 kcal/min (or 523 Watts) of metabolic energy cost; these would require heart rates in the range of 100-125 bpm. Heavy work, sustainable for about one hour by an individual of average fitness, would correspond to an energy cost of about 10 kcal/min. (700 Watts) and require heart rates between 120 to 140 bpm. Finally, physical work which corresponds to a physiological energy cost of about 15 kcal/min. (or 1,050 Watts), would present a work level that might be sustained by an average, young individual for only about 10 minutes, and would push heart rates up to 160 to 180 bpm. If the same physical work were done under hot conditions, the metabolic energy costs would be slightly, if at all, increased initially, but the heart rates would increase rapidly and dramatically as the burden of transferring heat from the working muscles to the skin increased. Eventually the heat production would also increase dramatically, as the worker became increasingly uncoordinated, dizzy and, eventually, unsteady and staggering if work continued.

    Note that these work rate-time limitations refer to reasonably fit young adult males; they really represent given percentages of such individuals' maximum oxygen uptake (VO_{2max}) or "maximum work capacity." Industrial tasks seldom demand more than 5 kcal/min, or roughly one-third of an average young adult male's (VO_{2max}). A number of studies suggest that the voluntary hard work level adopted by individuals who must sustain such work for at least three to five hours corresponds to about 45% of their capacities [~7 kcal/min for fit young men [36]]. About 33% of VO_{2max} was sustained for 8 hrs/day in one, 5 day, military field study. Although sustained, high physical work demands are rare in industrial work, individuals can sustain work demanding 60% of their individual VO_{2max} capacity for about one hour, 75% of their capacity for about 30 minutes, 85% of capacity for about 15 minutes and will be exhausted in about six minutes working at their maximum oxygen uptake, by definition of VO_{2max}. Table 10-3 is the expected VO_2max (in watts) for men (wgt=70 kg), and women (60 kg), as a function of age and fitness rating.

Table 10-3. Maximum Work Capacity (Watts) by Age and Fitness					
Age	**Poor**	**Fair**	**Average**	**Good**	**Excellent**
MEN					
17-19	<924	948-1042	1066-1161	1185-1256	>1279
20-24	<829	853- 924	948-1066	1090-1232	>1256
25-29	<805	829- 900	924-1042	1066-1184	>1208
30-34	<782	805- 877	900-1019	1042-1137	>1161
35-39	<758	782- 829	853- 971	995-1090	>1113
40-44	<711	734- 805	829- 900	924-1042	>1066
45-49	<663	687- 758	782- 829	853-1019	>1042
54-59	<616	640- 711	734- 782	805- 995	>1019
WOMEN					
17-19	<670	690-771	792-853	873-954	>975
20-24	<649	670-731	752-813	832-914	>934
25-29	<609	629-690	711-792	792-873	>893
30-34	<568	589-648	670-752	711-832	>852
35-39	<528	548-609	629-711	731-792	>813
40-44	<495	507-568	589-670	690-752	>771
45-49	<447	467-528	549-629	650-711	>731
54-59	<406	426-488	507-589	609-670	>690

To convert these values from watts to kcal/hr multiply by 0.86; convert for other body weights by ratio (e.g., wgt/70 * table).

A 1000 watt level for maximum, short term, 6 minute "peak" work by fit, young men, as shown in the above Table, can be used as the capacity term for estimating the effects of work using the D/C format; work requiring ≤ 200 watts should be comfortable, from 200 to 400 watts probably is the most productive range for physical work performance, 400 to 600 watts should produce some performance decrements, and work demanding more than 600 watts should be tolerance time limited for a 25 year old male in "good" physical condition. The values in this Table can be substituted for the generalized 1000 watts as the capacity (C) term to tailor the D/C ratio for age, sex or weight, and to estimate the effects of a physical fitness training program assuming that the improvement in work capacity will be 15% at most. The preceding relationships can be tailored for fitness level, age or sex, by using 45% of the tabulated value in place of the 500 watts which represents 45% of VO_{2max} for an average, fit, soldier.

There is little need to initiate new energy cost measurements; extensive tabulations exist for the heat production associated with almost all forms of human activity [50].

6. Clothing

The unit used to express clothing insulation (18) is of relatively recent origin; it was first proposed in 1941 by Dr. A. P. Gagge that the insulation of a typical business man's wool suit of the late 1930s be taken as one clo value of insulation. The mathematical value assigned to one clo was derived by calculating the potential difference for non-evaporative heat transfer from the human body to the ambient environment, and dividing it by the desired heat flow to calculate the resistance of the clothing worn which, it was assumed, allowed heat balance to be established for the wearer. This desired heat flow was assumed to be the resting heat production (M), one MET (58 Watt/m² or 50kcal/m²hr), less the 25% of the resting heat production lost from the body by respiration and by evaporation of body moisture, diffusing through the semipermeable skin and evaporating to the air. Using 33°C as a comfortable skin temperature and 21°C as a standard room temperature (in the early 1940s) produced a 12°C driving force for non-evaporative heat transfer. Dividing by the desired heat flow of 38kcal/m²hr (i.e., 75%M) provided a total conductance for the clothing plus the external air film at the clothing surface of 0.32°Cm²hr/kcal. In subsequent studies on nude men in still air, the still-air surface film conductance was evaluated at 0.14°Cm²hr/kcal, which left the intrinsic conductance of the heavy business suit of the early 1940s as 0.18°Cm²hr/kcal. Taking the reciprocal of this conductance established the value for one clo unit of insulation (I) as 5.55 kcal/m²hr°C (or 6.45 watt/m²°C). Under these conditions, the air temperature and mean radiant temperature were identical and the clo value is, in fact, the combined insulation against radiative and convective heat transfer. For conditions where air and mean radiant temperature are not very closely equal, one can simply substitute the adjusted dry bulb temperature (t_{adjb} = (MRT + t_a)/2). For ease in calculation, one may use the insulation per man rather than per m^2; then, for the average adult male who has a surface area of 1.8m^2, one clo of insulation results in a heat loss of 10 kcal/hr°C (11.63 Watts/°C), two clo of insulation requires the transfer of 5.8 Watts (5 kcal/hr) per °C difference between skin and air temperature, etc. The insulation of a material is almost always a linear function of its thickness, with 1.57 clo of insulation provided by each cm of material thickness (4 clo per inch); in essence, a 6.5 mm (1/4") thick blanket provides one clo unit of intrinsic insulation (I_{cl}) (45). This same general approach applies to the insulation used in building construction; the clo unit of clothing insulation is equal to 1.14 of the R units used in building insulation.

　　Thus, in calculating non-evaporative heat transfer, one simply needs to know the total clo value of the clothing worn and the surface still air film (I_a) trapped at its surface. The total insulation value of an ensemble is measured with a life-sized, heated (and when desired, sweating by means of wetted cotton "skin") manikin whose heating wires are distributed throughout the skin to produce a human skin temperature pattern. Such manikins also have temperature sensors distributed throughout their surface to measure an average skin temperature and a thermostat to demand sufficient heat to maintain a constant average skin temperature. When such manikins are run in a controlled temperature environment in steady state, the amount of heat demanded to maintain a constant skin temperature is exactly equal to the amount of heat lost. This allows direct measurement of the total insulation value of any clothing ensemble so tested, using the 6.45 W/m^2°C (5.55 kcal/m^{2}hr°C) defining value of one clo of insulation [57].

　　For cold weather conditions, one simply needs to know the heat production of the individual and the clo value of his insulation, in order to calculate whether the heat loss from the body will match the 75% of heat production available for non-evaporative losses. If it does not, any excess heat loss demand will be withdrawn from the body, in which case body cooling results; if less heat is lost than is produced, heat storage by the body must ensue unless the body can lose heat by evaporative cooling.

　　When less heat is lost through the clothing insulation than required to match the heat production at rest or work, then the 25% of resting metabolic heat production lost by respiration and diffusion of moisture through the skin, and its evaporation, must be supplemented with actual sweat evaporation; i.e., the normal 6% relative humidity of the skin (or 6%

diffusion "sweat-wetted area," equivalently) must be increased by production of sweat by the body. Note that if sweat cannot be evaporated, no cooling benefit is derived; the individual simply dehydrates at a more rapid rate unless adequate drinking water is taken. This is a frequent problem with chemical protective clothing; e.g., a well heat-acclimatized individual will produce more sweat then one who is not acclimatized [19] but, if the clothing worn is a barrier to sweat evaporation, heat acclimatization is of little benefit and may simply contribute to more rapid dehydration and earlier onset of heat exhaustion [27].

An approximate value for the clo value of a typical clothing ensemble can be calculated based on the relation that 1 kg of clothing equals 0.35 clo (0.16 clo/lb). This includes a surface air layer (I_a) which provides 0.8 Clo of insulation in still air, but only 0.2 Clo with a 5 m/sec (12 mph) breeze. The value for Ia with other air motions can be calculated by the formula: $Ia = 1/(0.61 + 1.25\sqrt{WV})$ where 0.61 represents the radiation heat transfer component and WV, the wind velocity in mph, represents the convection component of the surface air layer. Note that the insulation provided by I_a is greater than the insulation provided by any single item of clothing.

Table 10-4 suggests that the total insulation of a clothing ensemble also can be estimated by taking 80% of the sum of the individual values of the items worn (to allow for compression at overlaps) and adding 0.8 clo for the still air surface air insulation layer indoors.

Table 10-4. Calculated Intrinsic Insulation (Clo) Values Based on Individual Clothing Items Worn.			
Clothing	**Men**	**Clothing**	**Women**

Underwear
    Tank top
    T-shirt
    Underpants
	
	0.06
	0.09
	0.05
		Underwear
		    Bra + panties
		    Half slip
		    Full slip
			
			0.05
			0.13
			0.19

Shirt
    Light*: short sleeved
              long sleeved
    Heavy: short sleeved
              long sleeved
    (+5% for turtleneck or tie)
	
	0.14
	0.22
	0.25
	0.29
		Blouse
		    Light
		    Heavy
		Dress
		    Light
		    Heavy
			0.20^1
			0.29^1
			
			$0.22^{1,2}$
			$0.70^{1,2}$

Vest
    Light
    Heavy
	
	0.15
	0.29
		Skirt
		    Light
		    Heavy
			
			0.10^2
			0.22^2

Trousers
    Light
    Heavy
	
	0.26
	0.32
		Slacks
		    Light
		    Heavy
			
			0.26
			0.44

Sweater
    Light
    Heavy
	
	$.020^1$
	0.37^1
		Sweater
		    Light
		    Heavy
			
			0.17^1
			0.37^1

Jacket
    Light
    Heavy
	
	0.22
	0.49
		Jacket
		    Light
		    Heavy
			
			0.17
			0.37

Sox
    Ankle length
    Knee high
	
	0.04
	0.10
		Stockings
		    Any length
		    Panty hose
			
			0.01
			0.01

Shoes
    Sandals
    Oxfords
    Boots
	
	0.02
	0.04
	0.08
		Shoes
		    Shoes
		    Pumps
		    Boots
			
			0.02
			0.04
			0.08

* Wearers cannot reliably distinguish more than "light or heavy."
TOTAL Clo value= 0.8(Σindividual items) + still air 0.8 Clo
[1] Less 10% if short sleeved or sleeveless.
[2] Plus 5% if below knee length; less 5% if above.

SAMPLE CALCULATION:

Tshirt + shorts + light, long sleeve shirt + light pants + sox + shoes:
(.09 + .05 + .22 + .26 + .04 + .04) = (.70), and 80% of (.70)=

>   0.56 clo of *intrinsic* clothing insulation
>   + .80 clo for I_a without wind
>   1.4 clo of *total* clothing insulation

Table 10-5 gives representative values for the type of chemical protective clothing ensembles that might be worn by industrial workers. Note that these values are for normally fitted clothing. An example of the inherent variability in insulation values can be obtained by considering that the long-sleeved shirt and trousers value of 1.41 clo might go as low as 1.35 clo for a tight-fitting ensemble, and up to about 1.43 for a fairly loose-fitting shirt and trousers.

Table 10-5.
Insulation (clo) and Permeability (i_m) of
Chemical Protective Clothing Ensembles

Clothing Assembly[1]	Insulation[2] (clo)	Permeability (i_m)	Index Ratio (i_m/clo)
Category I-- Everyday Clothing			
Long-Sleeved Shirt + Trousers	1.41	0.37	0.26
Supplemented with:			
a. Safety helmet	1.49	0.37	0.25
b. Safety gloves	1.48	0.36	0.24
c. Mask, hood	1.56	0.29	0.18
d. Air back pack	1.45	0.34	0.23
e. Plastic apron	1.50	0.28	0.18
f. a+b+c+d+e	1.70	0.24	0.14
Category II-- Charcoal-in-foam			
a. Worn alone, open[3]	1.65	0.40	0.24
b. Worn alone, closed[4]	1.92	0.32	0.18
c. Worn over long shirt and trousers, open	1.97	0.42	0.21
c. Worn over long shirt and trousers, closed	2.30	0.35	0.15
Category III-- Impermeable (butyl)			
a. Worn alone, open	1.58	0.12	0.08
b. Worn alone, closed	2.05	0.09	0.04
c. Worn alone, w/wetted terry coverall	2.05	0.27	0.13

[1]Includes underwear (T-shirt, shorts), socks and shoes; values *estimated* from comparable military assemblies.
[2]All values given at 0.3m/s (0.75 mph) air motion, and include I_a of 0.8 clo.
[3]Open = without mask, hood, gloves; with open collar, etc.
[4]Closed = with mask, hood, gloves; all apertures closed.

From these changes in insulation value with clothing fit, obviously any values in the table beyond the first decimal place are more indicative than precise. An average man (i.e., surface area of 1.8m²) would lose 7.1

kcal/hr.°C difference between skin and ambient air temperature with 1.4 clo of insulation, but only 5 kcal/hr. with 2 clo of insulation. A long-sleeved shirt and trousers provide intrinsic insulation of 0.6 clo and the external air layer about 0.8 clo in still air. The total of 1.4 clo results in a heat transfer, for a standard (1.8m²) man of 7.1 kcal/hr.°C. Belding [4] suggested a radiant heat transfer of 6.6 kcal/hr.°C with such clothing and a convective heat transfer of $7(WV)^{0.6}$ kcal/hr°C in still air (e.g., WV = 0.11 m/s or 0.25 mph). This convective exchange would be 1.8 kcal/hr.°C, providing a combined transfer of 8.4 kcal/hr°C (i.e., 6.6 + 1.8) by radiation and convection. With a hot skin temperature [36°C (97°F)] and environmental temperatures of concern generally in excess of 20°C (68°F), the 15-20 kcal difference in heat loss per hour resulting from even a 0.5 clo difference in the insulation of an ensemble is clearly of minor importance; however, as discussed below, the effect of insulation is much more substantial in the extent to which it can affect evaporative heat transfer.

The evaporative cooling allowed by the environment, as discussed above, is determined from a psychrometric wet bulb thermometer. Woodcock used this in defining a moisture permeability index (i_m) for materials; Goldman [7, 29] subsequently applied this concept to measuring and calculating the maximum evaporative cooling allowed by a clothing ensemble. The permeability index (i_m) is simply the dimensionless ratio of the evaporative cooling allowed by the clothing and its surface air film (i.e., through $I_{cl} + I_a$), to the maximum evaporative cooling obtainable by a psychrometric wet bulb thermometer.

Typical permeability index values for most clothing or materials average about 0.4 (at 0.3m/s air velocity) unless impermeable layers or water repellent treatments are incorporated within the clothing assemblies, but the measured value depends in part on the insulation of the material or ensemble. Increases in insulation tend to be matched by increases in measured moisture permeability. Since impermeable materials tend to be relatively thin, covering the body surface with these materials may add only slightly to the total insulation, but will directly reduce the permeability in a linear ratio to the area covered by impermeable material [23]. Adding an impermeable layer, such as a plastic hood or mask to cover an area of previously exposed bare skin [28], will produce a much more serious reduction in the overall permeability index than covering an equivalent area of the body that is already covered with clothing [15].

The permeability index is a measure of the evaporative characteristics of the clothing materials and associated trapped air layers, but it does not provide a true measure of the evaporative cooling potential from the skin to the ambient environment. The reason it i_m generally fairly constant, at about

0.4 in still air, is that i_m really represents a characteristic moisture diffusion constant through air. The actual effective evaporative cooling obtainable by the clothing wearer is a function of this diffusion constant (i_m) (as modified by unique or water-repellent treatments, very tight weaves, or specifically introduced impermeability), divided by some expression of the length or thickness of the diffusion path; the clo insulation value provides a suitable measure of this thickness. Thus, the net evaporative cooling obtainable by the wearer of a garment system is determined by the permeability index ratio i_m/clo.

Table 10-5 includes estimated values of the permeability index (i_m) and the more critical, permeability index ratio (i_m/clo) for a series of clothing assemblies that might be worn for chemical protection. Using the 2.2°C/mmHg Lewis relationship, to link the evaporative heat transfer to the convective heat transfer, it is clear that, with one clo of insulation, one should obtain 22 kcal/hr. (i.e., 10 kcal/hr °C times 2.2°C/mmHg) of heat transfer per mmHg difference between skin (P_s) and ambient air vapor pressure ($\phi_a P_a$) for a standard 1.8m² adult male, if he behaved like a psychrometric wet bulb. Multiplying this potential maximum cooling of 22 kcal/hr.mmHg by the i_m/clo ratio determines the actual potential maximum evaporative cooling allowed through a clothing assembly. Therefore, each change of 0.1 i_m/clo produces a change of 2.2 kcal/hr.mmHg difference between skin and air vapor pressures. The vapor pressure of a hot (36°C) sweaty skin is about 44 mmHg and, at 25°C (77°F), 50% relative humidity, the ambient vapor pressure is about 12 mmHg; under that environmental condition, a change of 0.1 i_m/clo represents a change of approximately 70 kcal/hr. in the maximum evaporative cooling allowed by the ensemble [i.e., 22 x (44-12) x .1]. This direct role played by increasing insulation in the evaporative cooling obtainable by the wearer of a clothing assembly explains why individuals wearing multiple layers of heavy clothing [i.e., high insulation (clo) values] in the winter can become heat casualties during heavy work despite cool-to-cold and relatively dry ambient environmental conditions; they simply cannot get enough evaporative cooling at the skin, despite the very low ambient vapor pressure, to balance their heat production. Note that although Belding appears to have been unaware of the Lewis relationship (2.2°C/mmHg), the evaporative heat transfer he suggested of 23 $(WV)^{0.6}$ per mmHg difference between skin and ambient vapor pressure for a long-sleeved shirt and trouser ensemble is 1.9 times the 12 kcal/hr.°C he used for its convective exchange.

The role played by wind speed in altering insulation has been described above, as has the role played by body motion in inducing an effective wind [44]. Body motion has a direct effect on clothing insulation and, hence, effective evaporative cooling (i_m/clo) by "pumping" (i.e., exchanging) the air trapped within the clothing fabric and between the clothing layers. This increases the evaporative and non-evaporative heat exchange with the ambient air. Belding described a reduction of almost 50% in the total insulation of a heavy Arctic ensemble as the wearers went from rest to walking at 3.5 mph on a treadmill. Givoni and Goldman [22] have developed a family of pumping coefficients to characterize the changes in various clothing ensembles with "effective wind" (WV_{eff}), where WV_{eff} was defined as the sum of the ambient air motion and 4% of the increase in M (in Watts) above the resting heat production; i.e., $WV_{eff} = WV + 0.04$ (M-105). Although, obviously, the appropriate m/s units for air velocity cannot be rationally derived from this totally empiric estimate, this treatment of effective air motion, and the use of a pumping coefficient to characterize the changes in both the clothing insulation and the permeability index ratio, has been demonstrated to be more than adequate (GEGU) to characterize the changes in insulation and permeability of clothing during wearer activity. The pumping coefficient (p) for insulation is the slope of the line connecting two measurements of insulation at different windspeeds on a logarithmic plot; since insulation decreases with increasing wind speed, the pumping coefficient for insulation has a negative exponent. Similarly, the pumping coefficient for the permeability index (i_m) is the slope of the line connecting two determinations of i_m at different effective wind velocities; since permeability increases with increasing wind speed or wearer motion, the pumping coefficient for i_m is a positive exponent. Thus, the form of the pumping coefficient for the permeability index ratio is (i_m/clo)^{2p}.

A value of 0.25 can be taken as the pumping coefficient for a long-sleeved shirt and trousers, compared with a value of 0.20 for a completely closed, but air-permeable, charcoal-in-foam, chemical-protective ensemble. The pumping coefficient (p) for a heavy butyl garment, normally worn totally closed with mask, hood and gloves, has not yet been measured but could be less than 0.10. In summary, the insulation of chemical protective clothing is largely a function of its thickness, looseness of fit and number of layers, while its permeability is a direct characteristic of the nature of the chemical protection sought.

There are four possible approaches to provide such chemical protection. First, everyday work clothing can be supplemented with specialized gloves, aprons, face shields, etc., if only partial protection is needed against spatter or skin contact. If respiratory protection is required, this can be provided with a filtered mask [55]. If full-body protection is needed, it can take three forms. Heavy, multi-layered ensembles have been impregnated with chemicals which decompose the toxic agents; e.g., chlorocarbon impregnated underwear and outerwear. Such ensembles have some ability to sweat-wet through and thus allow some evaporative cooling, but they may also produce significant skin irritation. Alternatively, charcoal-in-foam overgarments, worn alone or over normal work clothing, can be used; these garments require liquid-repellent surface finishes to minimize local, surface concentration build-up from overwhelming the adsorbent properties of the charcoal in the garment. The charcoal-in-foam systems have been adopted by the military since they appear to be the most comfortable of the available chemical protective garments, but they may fail when they are soaked through or overwhelmed by massive surface contamination; also, while they are most comfortable when worn in a high wind because they are air permeable, the rate of air movement across the charcoal could be too rapid to insure adsorption of all the toxic chemicals. The fourth, and most frequent industrial choice, is a totally impermeable clothing system. The major drawback to the totally impermeable systems is the high potential of heat stress associated with totally blocking evaporative cooling from the human body.

Fourteen clothing materials have been evaluated for approximately three hundred chemicals, and recommendations for selection among them have been published in "Guidelines for the Selection of Chemical Protective Clothing." (See references in Chapter 9, Personal Protective Equipment.) Chemical protective clothing, considered as a subcategory of personal protective clothing, has been divided into five classifications in these Guidelines:

a. Head, face and eye protection, which encompasses hoods, face shields and goggles;
b. Hand and arm protection as provided by gloves and sleeves;
c. Footwear protection includes specialized boots and shoe covers;
d. Partial torso protection, provided by an apron, jacket, pants, coat or bib overalls;
e. Complete torso protection, including simple coveralls and full-body encapsulating suits.

A number of approaches to alleviate the heat stress associated with chemical protective clothing are commercially available or under development. These include ice vests and wettable covers, both of which can be extremely effective and simple solutions for the industrial work force, and range to microclimate cooling systems where filtered ambient air, conditioned ambient air, or liquid cooling is supplied within the impermeable ensemble using Vortex tubes, prefrozen (e.g., ice) block heat exchangers, mechanical air conditioners and the like. The potential cooling provided by such systems has been extensively explored in a number of reports [31, 51, 52, 53]. Those available commercially to date appear to require trade-offs between weight carried by the user and limited cooling duration, or require external power and umbilical connections which limit mobility.

ENVIRONMENTAL HEAT STRESS INDICES

Clearly, it would be difficult to consider simultaneously the six separate factors that must be measured to assess the heat stress of individuals at rest or work in a given clothing ensemble in any environment. Accordingly, over the years a series of environmental indices have been developed to express the interaction of two or more of these six factors. It must be recognized that an environmental index is not a precision statement. Instead, it is a ranging term and, as such, falls in the GEGU category. Extensive reviews of the indices for heat and cold are available in the published literature [5, 12, 24, 32].

1.   Direct Indices

Of the four environmental factors cited above as essential to measure in order to determine comfort and/or heat stress, air movement and black globe temperature have little meaning *per se* as environmental indices. The other two, air temperature and wet bulb temperature, can serve as direct indices, the former for thermal comfort and the latter for heat stress, under a proper set of constraints as to clothing and activity level.

a.   Air Temperature and Thermal Comfort

The simplest index of cold and warm conditions in conventional clothing in a conventional work place is obtained from the air temperature (t_{db}) itself. Given conventional indoor clothing (1.4 clo), air motion [<0.2m/s (40 fpm)] and humidity 140($\pm$20)%], and air temperature equal to mean radiant temperature, the range of dry bulb temperatures from about 22°C to 25.5°C (72 to 78°F) is generally comfortable for sedentary workers (M = 120 Watts $\pm$ 10%) [14]. Note that, having specified commonly occurring values for five of the six factors, a modest range of values can be assigned to the sixth to delineate a zone of thermal comfort; this "passband" for air temperature for comfort is about 3.5°C (6°F) wide [23]. Of course, increasing heat production moves the comfort air temperature band substantially lower, with each increment of 30 Watts (25 kcal/hr) in heat production requiring a lowering of the comfort band by about 1.7°C (3°F); indeed, as pointed out earlier, heat stress can occur at air temperatures below 0°C, given a high enough metabolic heat production and sufficient insulation.

b.   Wet Bulb Temperature and Heat Stress

Tolerance times and temperature sensations can be plotted directly on a temperature vapor pressure diagram. For cold conditions, the dry bulb temperature *per se*, appears to control discomfort with little or no adjustment for wet bulb temperature (i.e., humidity). For normally clothed or unclad individuals, the wet bulb temperature *per se* can serve as a satisfactory index of heat stress. The upper limit for unimpaired performance of most cognitive tasks can be taken as a wet bulb temperature of 30°C (86°F) for both normally clothed and unclothed subjects with air movement ranging from 0.1 to 0.5 m/s (20-100 fpm). Note, however, that for individuals wearing chemical protective clothing, where the limitation on evaporative cooling is imposed by the clothing *per se* rather than by the ambient vapor pressure, wet bulb temperature is *not* an appropriate index. In such a case, the ambient dry bulb temperature (t_a) or, making a correction for radiation, the adjusted dry bulb temperature (t_{adjb}) is a better index.

2.   Rational Indices

In unusual work situations, e.g., performing under high intensity arc lights on a movie set, MRT *per se* could serve as a rational index of heat stress, but it appears not to have been used as such.

a.   Operative Temperature (t_o)

Mean radiant temperature represents the uniform *surface* temperature of an imaginary black enclosure. Operative temperature represents the uniform *overall* temperature of the same enclosure, and encompasses an exchange of heat between the man and his environment, by both radiation and convection, to the same degree as in the actual environment. Operative temperature can be derived from the heat balance equation where one defines a combined (i.e., radiation and convection) heat transfer coefficient (h) as the weighted sum of the heat transfer coefficient by radiation (hr) and the average heat transfer coefficient by convection (h_c). The operative temperature (t_o) [17] is then derived as:

Eq. 5 $$t_o = (h_r t_r + h_c t_a)/(h_r + h_c)$$

The operative temperature represents a more precise form of the adjusted dry bulb temperature $[t_{adjb} = (t_a + MRT)/2]$; the latter should not really be used when extreme radiant temperatures are involved but, in general, is GEGU. The operative temperature can be used directly in the heat balance equation to calculate the heat exchange by radiation and convection (H_{R+C}) as:

Eq. 6 $$(H_{R+C}) = h(t_o - t_{surf}) = h(t_o - t_{sk}) F_{cl}$$

where: $t_{surf} =$ mean surface temperature of the clothing
          $t_{sk} =$ mean skin temperature

and F_{cl} is an intrinsic thermal efficiency of the clothing [47]. Note that use of the F_{cl} form of expressing intrinsic clothing thermal efficiency, as used in the ASHRAE Handbook of Fundamentals requires an adjustment for the relative increase in the area of the clothed body surface over that of the unclothed body surface. It also requires the addition of an adjusted insulating surface air film. In general, it seems preferable to express the total insulation of a clothing ensemble as directly measured from a copper man [7] in clo units and substitute to for ta to account for the combined convective and radiative heat exchanges.

b. Heat Stress Index (HSI)

The Heat Stress Index is one of the most useful indices for evaluation of heat stress, in part because Belding and Hatch provided a table of the physiological and hygienic implications of eight-hour exposures at various HSI (cf. Table 10-6). The Heat Stress Index itself is simply an application of the heat balance equation. It is the ratio of the evaporative heat loss required (E_{req}) for thermal equilibrium, to the maximum evaporation (E_{max}) allowed through the clothing that can be taken up by the environment, as discussed previously. An adjustment is required for the maximum rate of sweating which, for an average man approaches 2-3 liters/hr but this sweat rate cannot be sustained. Indeed, under such maximum strain, heat exhaustion usually occurs in less than an hour. The generally accepted value for a sustainable maximum sweat rate is 1 liter/hr, which represents a potential cooling power of some 700 Watts if all the sweat can be evaporated; i.e., each ml (one ml = one gram) of sweat evaporated produces 0.58 kcal of cooling, but unevaporated sweat provides no cooling, uselessly increasing body dehydration. Figure 10-2 presents a series of nomograms for a graphic

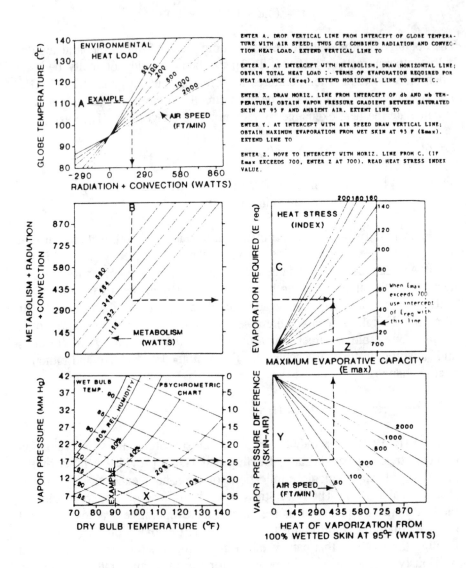

Figure 10-2. Nomograms for graphic solution of
the heat balance equation.

solution of HSI which, as developed, assumes a 35°C skin temperature, and a conventional long-sleeved shirt and trousers ($I = 1.4$ clo; $I_{cl} = 0.6$ clo + I_A = 0.8 clo) clothing ensemble; note also (cf. Block C of Fig. 2) that E_{max} is limited to 700 Watts. Although informative, it should not be used for clothing other than ordinary, indoor work clothing (i.e., long sleeved shirt and trousers).

c. Skin Wettedness (%SWA)

Percent skin-wettedness, as defined by Gagge [16], is essentially identical to HSI except that, in theory, the percent SWA uses the observed skin humidity or wettedness, rather than the required evaporative cooling as the numerator in taking the ratio to the maximum evaporative cooling power of the environment. Skin wettedness (alternatively, skin relative humidity or the percent of skin surface that is sweat-wetted) appears to be what the body uses to sense its thermal discomfort. There is little, if any, sensory input from deep-body temperature or from skin temperature, although both deep-body temperature and local skin temperature provide the control inputs for regulation of sweating. A worker will generally not continue work which results in skin-wettedness much above a 60% level [%SWA=HSI = 60 or, equivalently, a relative humidity of the skin (ϕ_s) $\geq$ 60% Ps]. At this 60% level, sweat frequently drips from the skin and begins to be wasted, except under conditions of low ambient vapor pressure, minimal clothing and/or reasonably high air movement.

Table 10-6. Physiological and Hygienic Implications of 8-hour Exposures to Various Heat Stresses	
Index of Heat Stress (HSI)	**Heat Stresses**
-20 -10	Mild cold strain. This condition frequently exists in areas where men recover from exposure to heat.
0	No thermal strain.
+10 20 30	Mild to moderate heat strain. Where a job involves higher intellectual functions, dexterity, or alertness, subtle to substantial decrements in performance may be expected. In performance of heavy physical work, little decrement expected unless ability of individuals to perform such work under no thermal stress is marginal.
40 50	Severe heat strain, involving a threat to health unless men are physically fit.
60	Break-in period required for men not previously acclimatized. Some decrement in performance of physical work is to be expected. Medical selection of personnel desirable because these conditions are unsuitable for those with cardiovascular or respiratory impairment or with chronic dermatitis. These working conditions are also unsuitable for activities requiring sustained mental effort.
70 80 90	Very severe heat strain. Only a small percentage of the population may be expected to qualify for this work. Personnel should be selected (a) by medical examination, and (b) by trial on the job (after acclimatization). Special measures are needed to assure adequate water and salt intake. Amelioration of working conditions by any feasible means is desired, and may be expected to decrease the health hazard while increasing efficiency on the job. Slight "indisposition" which in most jobs would be insufficient to affect performance may render workers unfit for this exposure.
100	The maximum strain tolerated daily by fit, acclimatized young men.

Adapted from Belding and Hatch, "Index for Evaluating Heat Stress in Terms of Resulting Physiologic Strains," *Heating, Piping, and Air Conditioning*, 27:129-136, 1955.

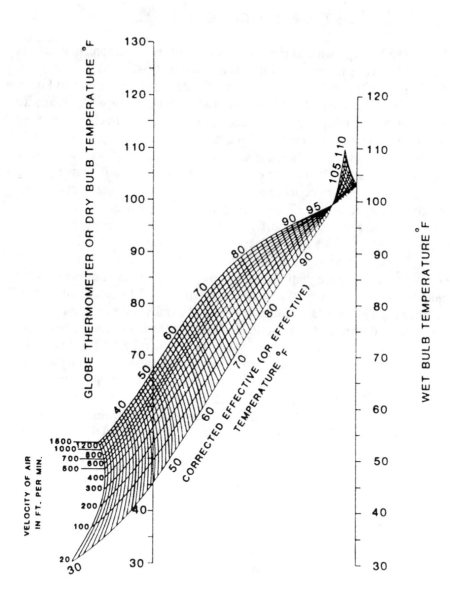

Figure 10-3. Chart showing normal scale of corrected effective temperature

3.   **Empirical Indices**

a. Effective Temperature (ET, CET and ET*):

The best known and most widely used of the environmental indices is the effective temperature (ET) index originally derived in 1923 for ASHRAE (35). It is generally calculated from the nomogram given in Figure 10-3, and combines the effects of dry bulb and wet bulb temperatures and air movement. Substituting the black globe temperature (t_g) directly in place of the air temperature produces a Corrected Effective Temperature (CET) accounting for radiation. Thus, the CET index combines all four of the key environmental factors into a single number. ET and CET were derived using subjective judgments of equivalence by a limited number of subjects. Gagge recently developed a new effective temperature, ET* which uses a 50% r.h. as the reference humidity. The ET* corresponds more closely to familiar sensations at a ta = ET* than it does to the 100 r.h. referenced ET.

Effective Temperature has been used most extensively for studies of psychological tolerance limiting conditions. It serves as the most useful guideline to the efficiency of a work-force. An ET (CET) greater than 30°C (86°F) generally is considered unacceptable and usually decreases productivity in an industrial work force. A World Health Organization scientific group has proposed tolerance limits to heat stress in terms of ET/CET [61]. The suggested limit for unacclimatized individuals doing sedentary to light work (<215 watts) was 30°C (86°F); for moderate work (to 360 watts) the suggested ET/CET limit was 28°C (82.5°F), and for heavy work (to 500 watts) a limit of 26.5°C (80°F). Fully heat-acclimated individuals (7 days of work in the heat for 2 or more hours each day) were supposed to tolerate 2°C higher ET (CET) levels for an eight-hour daily work shift. These proposed values are generally consistent with thermal environmental conditions in deep mining which resulted in stable rectal temperatures (equilibrium rectal temperatures at "safe" levels) in groups of highly acclimatized South African miners. With very large groups of workers, however, some heatstroke still occurred, probably because of the large individual variability in response to heat stress. Individuals of low maximum oxygen uptake (i.e., small body stature or poor physical condition) appear to be particularly susceptible to heat illness [59]. In addition, there was a slight reduction in productivity of these gold mine workers (5%) beginning at about ET 82°F (27.7°C), which is also the threshold reported for onset of fatal heatstroke during "hard" work.

b. Wet Bulb Globe Temperature (WBGT)

The WBGT Index (60) uses the naturally convected wet bulb as a measure of the environmental stress, rather than the psychrometric wet bulb used in all other indices presented thus far. The natural wet bulb temperature (t_{nwb}) value is taken as 70% of the WBGT; another 20% is contributed by the black globe thermometer temperature (t_g) directly, and 10% by the dry bulb temperature (t_{db}):

Eq. 7 $$WBGT = 0.7\ t_{nwb} + 0.2\ t_g + 0.1\ t_{db})$$

The WBGT index thus combines the effects of humidity and air movement (in t_{nwb}), and low temperature radiant heat and solar radiation (in t_g), and air temperature (t_{db}). WBGT instruments are commercially available from a number of manufacturers, but some misrepresent the WBGT, using a psychrometric rather than the natural wet bulb; others use smaller globes or unusual radiant heat sensors, with little validation that the adjustment (if any) made in calculating their WBGT is acceptable. Most, being battery operated and requiring calibration, can fail or be easily miscalibrated and the commercial instruments for WBGT, therefore, seem better suited for laboratory than field use. The military still use WBGT guidance for prevention of heat illness during training but it is being supplanted by a new wet globe thermometer (WGT, see below) for operational use.

As pointed out above, for individuals wearing impermeable or reduced permeability clothing, the WBGT is probably not as good an index as the adjusted dry bulb temperature alone. However, for individual workers wearing conventional clothing, WGBT remains the index of choice for expressing physiological tolerance limits at work or rest. The WBGT index was developed by Yaglou [60] to help reduce the number of heat casualties incurred during Marine training in southern U.S. military bases. Its introduction was followed by a dramatic reduction in the incidence of heat casualties when the following guidelines were mandated:

At WBGT Of:	Procedure:
82°F 85°F	Unseasoned personnel only do limited heavy exercise. Strenuous exercise such as marching at standard rate, should be suspended during the first three weeks of unacclimatized troop training; outdoor classes in the sun should be avoided.
88°F	Strenuous exercise should be curtailed for all recruits and trainees with less than twelve weeks of training in hot weather.
88-90°F	Thoroughly conditioned troops, after acclimatization each season, could carry on limited activities for up to six hours per day.

The successful reduction of heat casualties in the military community by adherence to these WBGT guidelines was not lost upon the civilian community. Brief and Confer [62] proposed WBGT limits of 32.2°C (90°F) for light work, 30°C (86°F) for moderate work, and 26.7°C (80°F) for heavy work under indoor situations in 1971.

In 1974, an Advisory Committee on Heat Stress sponsored by NIOSH developed the following table (Table 10-7) on threshold WBGT at which work should be suspended [63, 64, 65]. Note that the Committee split WBGT levels into two categories as a function of air velocity, with threshold WBGT levels at air velocities of less than 1.5 m/s (300 fpm or 3.3 mph) some 2 to 3°C below the corresponding thresholds for air velocities greater than 1.5 m/s. These WBGT threshold values are not strikingly different from those proposed by Brief and Confer for light and moderate work, if one uses the values for air velocities greater than 1.5 m/s, but are rather different for the heavy work situation. In many areas of the United States, such high WBGT's occur sufficiently often that shutting down would make the plant unprofitable, and infrequently enough that plant air conditioning was not seen as cost-effective. As a result, to date no heat stress standard has been promulgated. Perhaps the next national heat stress standard proposal [38] should follow the WBGT guidelines recommended by the American Commission of Government Industrial Hygienists for permissible heat exposure threshold limit values, given in Table 10-8 [1]. Such recommendations for work-rest cycle alteration should be much more acceptable to both management and labor. Essential work could be continued under quite severe WBGT conditions, albeit for only a limited period during each hour; e.g., at a WBGT of 30°C, heavy work could be performed for fifteen minutes of each hour, with the rest of the hour spent at rest. This would cater to those plants or regions where the occurrence of high WBGT's is infrequent, or of only a few hours duration each afternoon. No investment in major air treatment programs would be required, but there would not be a total loss of productivity, or cessation of all essential activities [25]. Industry would also have a more rational decision basis for recognizing the trade-offs between productivity losses and the economic costs of providing increased ventilation, dehumidification or frank air conditioning for indoor situations. Outdoors, fewer options are available; shading the working area is frequently the most feasible option.

Table 10-7. Threshold WBGT Values Proposed by the Standards Advisory Committee on Heat Stress, 1974 [63, 64, 65]		
Work Load	**WBGT in °C Air Velocity**	
	1.5m/s	**1.5m/s**
> 300 kcal/hr (>200 W/m²)	26.1	28.9
201 - 300 kcal/hr (135 W/m² - 200 W/m²)	27.1	30.6
200 kcal/hr (135 W/m²)	30.0	32.2

Table 10-8.
ACGIH Permissible Heat Exposure Threshold Limit
Values in °C WBGT (taken from reference 1)

Work-Rest Regimen	Work Load		
	Light	Moderate	Heavy
Continuous work	30.0	26.7	25.0
75% work-- 25% rest, each hour	30.6	28.0	25.9
50% work-- 50% rest, each hour	31.4	29.4	27.9
25% work-- 75% rest, each hour	32.2	31.1	30.0

    c.   Wet Globe Temperature (WGT)

In addition to the problem of reading and mathematically manipulating three temperatures, the WBGT apparatus tend to be set up at a fixed location, frequently quite remote from the working environment. Botsford developed a simpler device, the "Wet Globe Thermometer" (WGT or "Botsball") for use in the aluminum industry. This device is simply a three-inch globe with a black, wettable cover; a standard metallic stem thermometer is inserted into the globe through an extended neck, which contains a small water reservoir to maintain the black cover at 100% wettedness.

The device is simple, portable, and easy to read. A single number value is directly provided, rather than the three separate values provided by the WBGT. Goldman modified the WGT by color-coding the critical zones [48] to provide operational guidance during actual field operations. The WBGT is still in use. The simpler, color-coded WGT has been used in the field with remarkable success. Table 10-9 suggests Doctrine on Adjustment of Work-Rest Cycles and Increasing Water Intake. Note the guidance that the Botsball WGT's are equivalent to 2°F higher WBGT's; this 2°F offset value was obtained in several laboratory and field evaluations [31], but will not be correct in all cases. Furthermore, it may be difficult to maintain the WGT surface wet enough in a hot day environment and the offset from WBGT may be much greater than 2°F; more experience is needed. Note also that, under "GREEN" conditions (i.e., WGT between 80-83°F) water intake of between one-half and one quart per hour is recommended for 50-minute work/10-

minute break cycles. With increasing heat stress, recommended water intake is further increased and work-rest cycles are decreased.

Table 10-9. Water Intake, Work/Rest Cycles for Essential Field Operations (which cannot be curtailed) for Heat Acclimated Fit Workers			
Heat Condition	**Botsball WGT (°F)***	**Water Intake (qt/hr)**	**Work/Rest Cycles (Min)**
Green	80°-83°	0.5-1.0	50/10
Yellow	83°-86°	1.0-1.5	45/15
Red	86°-90°	1.5-2.0	30/30
Black	90° & above	2.0	20/40**

* To convert WGT to WBGT add 2°F. Below 80° drink up to 0.5 qt/hr, 50/10 work/rest cycles.
** Depending on condition of the worker.

HEAT STRESS AND PRODUCTIVITY

There have been a great many studies [2, 8, 39, 40, 41, 42] attempting to relate the productivity of a work force to the environmental heat stress. Most of these have used the effective temperature as an expression of the environmental heat stress, but very few have adequately controlled such key factors as motivation, need or expectancy. Thus, the results of studies on the effects of heat stress on productivity have varied widely. Some actually suggest improved performance under conditions of heat stress when men are in total chemical protective encapsulation. In other studies, very mild heat stress has been shown to decrement performance in men wearing normal work clothing. In response to a report by Fox et al. [11] that increasing heat stress actually improved target detection, Colquhoun and Goldman [11] evaluated the ability to detect a target as a function of increasing body heat storage. Performance in their study involved not only detection of a target, but also a judgment on the certainty with which the target was detected. The results showed that while total target detection did improve, as Fox *et al.* [11] had stated, the identification and decision-making skills of the subjects decreased. While more targets were being detected, more non-targets were erroneously identified, with increasing certainty that they were targets as body heat storage increased. One of the most massive studies on the effects of mild heat (and cold) stress on performance has just been reported by Wyon's group. Again, the interaction between environmental discomfort and performance is far from clear, with some tasks decremented and others enhanced in the various subpopulations (males and females, native and caucasian workers) studied.

To maintain physical performance:

1. Drink 1 qt. of water in the am, at each meal, and before any hard work.
2. Take frequent drinks, since they are more effective than all at once. Larger workers need more water.
3. Replace salt loss by eating 3 meals per day.
4. As the WGT increases, rest periods must be more frequent, work rate lowered, and loads reduced.
5. Use Water as a key element to maintain top efficiency by drinking each hour.

Table 10-10. Safe "Closed" Suit Times for Moderate Work (300 w; 250 kcal/hr)	
Ambient Air (Ta) Temperature (°F)	**Wearing Time (Closed)**
30° or less	8 hours
30° - 50°	5 hours
50° - 60°	3 hours
60° - 70°	2 hours
70° - 80°	90 minutes
80° - 85°	60 minutes
85° - 90°	30 minutes
90° or above	15 minutes

Decrements in performance are clearly task-dependent, as well as highly dependent on the motivation of the work force. Tasks involving decision making, judgment and complex mental functions appear to decrement at much greater rates than rote tasks such as addition. Physical task performance is relatively insensitive until the workers are affected by incipient heat exhaustion. The ability of two journeymen electricians to install duplex outlets was essentially unimpaired as Effective Temperature was increased from 21 to 27°C (70 to 80°F) across a full spectrum of relative humidities, but was reduced by 10% at 32.2°C (90°F) ET with the greatest reductions at the highest relative humidities. At 38°C (100°F) ET, productivity ranged from a low of 57% at 90% r.h., to 84% for r.h. < 40%, while at 43°C (110°F) ET, productivity was negligible above 80% RH, and ranged from 50-60% at relative humidities between 20-70%. This limited data base on a few highly trained and extremely well-motivated workers indicates that the decrements for such rote tasks can be relatively small under most heat stress conditions. In contrast, the National Association of Building Contractors suggests, as guidelines for cost estimating, that productivity for tasks involving gross motor skills will be decremented by about 30% at 27°C (80°F) ET, 40% at 32.2°C (90°F) ET, and 60% at 38°C (100°F) ET. Since these figures are used in estimating costs (and no cost estimator intends to lose money on contract bids), these estimates probably overstate the losses in productivity. Again this data base applies to normally dressed individuals, and not to individuals wearing chemical protective garments.

GUIDELINES FOR HEAT STRESS IN PROTECTIVE CLOTHING

1. Inadequacy of WBGT and WGT

Both WBGT and WGT depend primarily (>70%) on the natural evaporation allowed by the environment. This would suggest that WBGT and WGT, while perhaps the best heat stress indices for individuals wearing normal clothing (even, perhaps, with some partial, chemical protective, impermeable coverage such as aprons, masks or gloves) become increasingly inappropriate guides as one moves to the reduced permeability charcoal-in-foam overgarments, unless a very stiff breeze is blowing. WBGT and WGT values are probably quite inappropriate to use as guidance for workers encapsulated in totally impermeable chemical-protective clothing. It is important to note, however, that at upper levels of environmental heat stress [except in desert (hot-dry) environments] all these environmental indices give somewhat similar values; i.e., C.E.T., WBGT and WGT all tend to have similar values.

2.   Variability in Heat Tolerance Between Groups

Most of the well-known environmental heat stress data base was generated on physically fit, highly motivated young men in military studies, or the select population of fit young mine workers, pre-screened to eliminate individuals with lower heat tolerance, in South Africa [59]. Witherspoon and Goldman have reviewed work rate and ET interactions from large number of military and civilian data bases and produced Figure 10-4, which includes one line for significant discomfort or change in deep-body temperature for a mixed population and another line for maximum equilibrium (i.e., acceptable, steady state) values representing tolerance for at least four hours without collapse in a highly fit, young population. The data points are plotted as a function of work rate across a range of ET (or CET) values and include data from Africa, India, Germany, U.K. and U.S., and include clothed and unacclimatized populations as well as unclothed, usually acclimatized, populations. The consistency of the findings is perhaps the most remarkable thing about this diverse data base. The same authors point out the relative uniformity in heat tolerance between individuals of comparable age and fitness, as shown in Figure 10-5, where the data from seven studies between 1923 and 1967 are presented for fit, young men, wearing minimal clothing (usually shorts and boots), at work (280-350 kcal/hr) or at rest, in a range of very hot environments; the environmental heat stress is expressed as the Oxford Index WD (= $0.85\, t_{wb} + 0.15\, t_{db}$), using the psychrometric wet bulb and tolerance time is expressed in minutes. Note that even under the most severe conditions, average tolerance time is twenty minutes; as long as the pain threshold at the skin surface is not reached [a skin temperature of about 45°C (113°F)], some twenty minutes of time was provided simply by "mass damping" before body temperatures or heart rates reached critical levels [in these studies, 39.2°C (102.5°F) and 180 b/min, respectively [30, 37]]. As shown by the inset, when one compiles all the data from these seven studies on a log-log plot (adjusted to a base of 75°F for the 300 kcal/hr exercise data and to a base of 81°F at rest) the correlation coefficient is extremely high (r~0.96). This implies that about 92% (i.e., r^2) of the tolerance time can be explained simply by the environmental heat stress as expressed by this WD index. Under conditions of severe heat stress, individual variability appears to be minimal within populations of comparable fitness. In an industrial population, however, individuals vary substantially with respect to their state

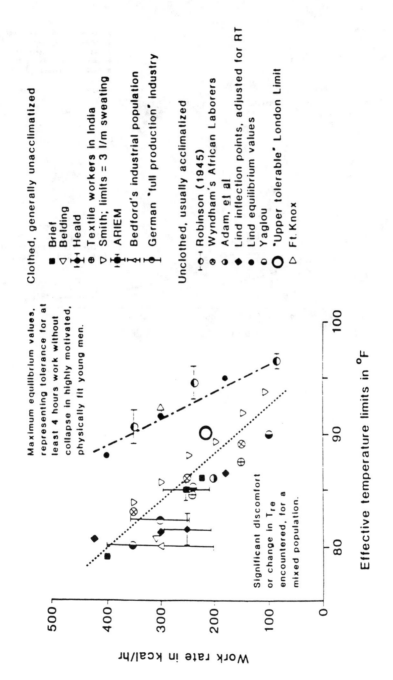

Figure 10-4. Work rate limits as a function of effective temperature.

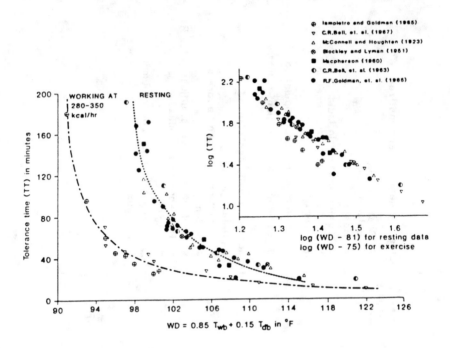

Figure 10-5. tolerance time limits (TT).

of heat acclimatization, body size and fitness, degree of hydration, congenital sweat gland distribution, etc. Thus, although Figure 4 suggests remarkable agreement in heat stress response across quite divergent populations, appropriate screening is suggested if generalized guidelines are to be used for an industrial workforce required to wear complete chemical protective clothing ensembles. Wear of totally impermeable clothing will, of course, further homogenize the responses of a population by wiping out any differences in effective sweating and differences in heat acclimatization status, other than perhaps those associated with more rapid dehydration in well heat-acclimated individuals. *Thus, given an equivalently screened population, it seems safe to conclude that conditions which are sufficiently heat stressful to produce problems for one or two workers are not far from being unreasonably stressful for the total population.*

3.   Impermeable Protective Clothing Guidelines

By now, it should be obvious that almost all the indices discussed have limited applicability to men in totally impermeable clothing [43]. The ambient vapor pressure is a meaningless measure of the environmental heat stress for individuals wearing impermeable clothing, as are all indices in which ambient wet bulb temperature (psychrometric or non-psychrometric) is a major factor. The dry bulb (air) temperature, adjusted for solar heat load by using either the adjusted dry bulb temperature, or by an increment for solar radiation of 7°C (13°F) times the percent cloud cover is probably the most appropriate index for totally impermeable garments. Custance has collated data (cf. 29) (Table 10-10) for safe "closed" impermeable suit times for moderate work (250 kcal/hr) from six U.S., Canadian and Russian studies, as a function of air temperature. As indicated below, predictive modeling has reached the stage where quite valid predictions and extrapolations can be made [27]. For specific cases, predictive modeling should provide the best guidelines for comfort, discomfort, performance or tolerance limits, and risk.

AGE, GENDER AND HEAT STRESS

The effects of age in predisposing to heat stress appear to be primarily associated with the cardiovascular system, although older individuals start to sweat later, and produce less sweat during comparable work in the heat than younger individuals. While older individuals appear to have a higher peripheral blood flow during work in the heat, their maximal work capacity (i.e., VO_{2max}) is reduced (see Table 10-3 and discussion), based on the reduction in maximum heart rate with age (220 bpm - age in years). Thus, even healthy, older individuals tend to have reduced heat tolerance to work, exhibit higher heart rates and slightly higher deep-body temperatures, and take longer to return to normal body temperatures. The effects of heat stress on individuals with specific medical problems (e.g., cardio-respiratory difficulties) can, of course, be devastating [9, 13].

The original proposed Guidelines for an OSHA Heat Standard [63] postulated differences between male and female workers with respect to their tolerance to heat. Such recommendations were based on the limited research data base available prior to 1974 [25], which suggested that females, as a group, were less tolerant than males to heat stress. Based on newer studies, however, it appears that gender-free standards can be established; brought to equivalent levels of fitness and heat acclimatization, the remaining difference between males and females of any real significance in respect to heat resistance, is body size. A smaller, less fit male is at no less or greater risk to heat stress than an equivalent-sized, less fit female while, with increasing fitness or greater opportunities for heat acclimatization, females and males appear to perform equally well in the heat.

BODY RESPONSES TO HEAT STRESS AS EXPOSURE LIMITS

By now, it should be clear that heat stress simply means: 1) heat losses by radiation and convection are less than the heat produced by metabolism so that a requirement for sweat evaporative cooling exists; and 2) the degree of heat stress is a function of the extent to which the requirement for evaporative cooling can be met. As indicated above, the ratio E_{req}/E_{max} is perhaps the best single indicator of heat stress. A chart (modified from one originally developed by Belding) delineating physiological responses to heat stress is presented as Figure 6. These responses include, as a first line of defense, an initial rise in skin temperature as a result of vasodilation. The increased blood flow to the skin raises skin temperature and thus helps increase heat loss by convection and radiation, or reduce heat gain when the operative temperature is higher than skin temperature. This first line of defense is limited however, as the available circulating heat transfer fluid of the body (i.e., the blood) becomes depleted by sweating in the absence of adequate rehydration, or becomes pooled in the periphery in the absence of continued muscle activity massaging the venous blood back, past the valves in the veins, to the heart to provide adequate venous return for continued blood flow to the brain. Inadequate blood flow to the brain leads to heat exhaustion collapse. The transition from the vertical, upright posture during work, to the horizontal, recumbent posture of heat exhaustion collapse tends to solve the problem of inadequate venous return, but at an unacceptable cost. Heat exhaustion is most likely to occur in working individuals when, upon suddenly stopping work, they incur massive peripheral pooling and inadequate venous return, and suffer the consequent blackout. It can also occur in individuals while working. Inadequate venous return to the heart leads to decreased central blood pressure and blood flow to the brain, so a signal to "beat faster" is sent to the heart. As in most pumps, sufficient filling time must be allowed between strokes and, as heart rates exceed 180/min, inadequate filling time leads to further decreases in cardiac output with a resulting transition from the vertical to the horizontal state of the worker.

Obviously, there is a general, albeit complex relationship between body temperature and heart rate [58]. In general, an increase in working heart rate of more than 30 b/min above the resting level may be considered unacceptable for an industrial work force. Performance decrements may be expected if sustained heart rates exceed 100 b/min for 8 hours, or perhaps 120 b/min for 8 hours if the workers are extremely fit and well heat-acclimatized. For very fit and acclimatized *young* workers, sustained heart rates of 140 b/min may be compatible with 4 hours of work; 160 b/min may be compatible with 2 hours of work, but heart rates above 180-190 b/min are generally considered unacceptable for any sustained period. Such values, however, are only appropriate for a relatively young work force. The maximum heart rate for individuals can be characterized as a function of age by the relationship: maximum heart rate equals 220 b/min minus age in years. A more appropriate generalization, then, would be that heart rate increases of less than 20% of the difference between an individual's age adjusted, maximum heart rate and his resting level are quite reasonable. For example, the predicted maximum heart rate for a 60-year old is 160 b/min and, if the resting rate is 70 b/min, then the working heart rate should be $\leq$ 88 b/min, i.e., [70 + 0.2 (160-70)]. As general guidelines, increases of 40% of the difference between this age adjusted maximum and the resting level probably represent an uncomfortable level of work; for the 60-year old above, this would be 106 b/min, while for a 20-year old it would be 122 b/min, given a 70 b/min resting value for both. Performance decrements may be expected at heart rates representing 40-60% of this "heart rate increase capacity," tolerance time limits will generally be associated with values between 60 and 80% of capacity, while damage may result at levels requiring more than 80% of an individual's heart rate increase capacity.

The body's second line of defense, sweating, is limited in the cooling it can provide to a sustainable rate of about 700 Watts, even if all the sweat can be evaporated efficiently at the skin surface. Sweating becomes increasingly ineffective as ambient humidities increase so that more sweat is wasted, or as sweat is absorbed into the clothing and evaporation takes place at sites more removed from the skin. Individuals wearing impregnated, but sweat permeable protective clothing frequently receive less than one-half the full cooling benefit of the sweat evaporation that takes place. Since, under conditions of work-associated environmental heat stress, the amount of sweat produced is directly titrated to the amount of sweat evaporation required and obtained, one of the best measures of the role of a clothing ensemble in stressing the wearer is the ratio of the sweat evaporated (E) during a given time period to the maximum sweat produced (P) by the individual. One simply obtains initial and final unclothed weights, adjusted for any water intake, as a measure of the total sweat production (P) and the initial and final clothed body weights as a measure of the total sweat evaporation (E). The E/P ratio with typical clothing ensembles under comfortable conditions will be close to 90%, but will decrease to about 70% with increasing humidity, decreasing air motion, or heavier than normal clothing. The E/P ratios decrease to 40% or less with most "semipermeable," encapsulating chemical protective ensembles, reaching about 20% when these are worn under hot humid conditions or during heavy work. The E/P ratio obviously approaches zero for totally impermeable, encapsulating clothing systems. Again, the relative stress can be divided into the five categories: comfortable, uncomfortable, performance decrementing, tolerance time limiting and perhaps damaging, using the 0-20%, 20-40%, etc., rubric. Thus, and E to P ratio between 80 and 100% will be quite comfortable, between 60 and 80% may be uncomfortable, between 40 and 60% will probably be performance decrementing, between 20 and 40% will be tolerance limiting, and an E/P ratio of less than 20% associated with high risk.

A common problem associated with heavy sweating is the induction of dehydration, since thirst is an inadequate stimulus for drinking enough water to prevent dehydration. Up to 2% of the total body weight may represent excess extracellular fluid that can be lost without major decrements in temperature regulation or work performance capacities, although subtle decrements in psychomotor performance may be associated with lower dehydration levels of 1 to 2%. However, individuals given unlimited access to water (albeit perhaps warm and not necessarily very palatable) have been shown [2] to incur "voluntary dehydration" levels of 8 or 9%, with associated major performance decrements and greatly increased rates of rise of deep-body temperature. Using a 10% dehydration level as a maximum, (i.e., *acute* loss of 10% of body weight by dehydration although survival has been reported at 18- 20% dehydration levels), levels of 0-2% dehydration (judged from body weight loss during a work shift) would be "comfortable," 2-4% would be uncomfortable, 4-6% would be performance decrementing, and levels above 6% would be associated with limited tolerance times, again using the 0-20, 20-40, 40-60%, etc., rubric of demand/capacity effects.

Another heat-associated syndrome which some individuals suffer is "hyperventilation," particularly in response to exposure to hot-wet environments. The overbreathing results in a reduction of the normal blood carbon dioxide concentrations. One of the first subjective sensations is a tingling around the lips and some dizziness. The phenomenon is associated with a reduction in blood flow to the brain, because of cerebral vasoconstriction, and can lead to blackout as well as to a very diagnostic cramping of the fine muscles of the hand and foot (carpo-pedal spasm). While not apt to occur in individuals performing hard work, and thus producing substantial volumes of carbon dioxide, it can cause collapse in individuals performing light work or at rest, and is probably a major contributor to the onset of heat exhaustion collapse in individuals taking a short break during periods of intensive work. In many experiments on heat stress, heat exhaustion collapse occurred during the period when the individual was asked to stop work so that his heart rate could be measured by palpation at the wrist; the resultant collapse during the one-to-two minutes subsequent to cessation of work probably is contributed to by both inadequate venous return from peripheral pooling, and reduction of the carbon dioxide levels in the blood due to hyperventilation. Hyperventilation may be more pronounced when respirators and fullface masks are worn, and the restricted visual field of a gas mask may interact with heat stress to increase dizziness and nausea. The additional dead space of such respiratory protection may not adequately compensate for potential hyperventilation.

PREDICTIVE MODELING AND HEAT STRESS GUIDELINES

As suggested previously, predictive modeling may be the most appropriate approach for establishing realistic guidelines for individuals or groups wearing chemical protective clothing. Such models are particularly well suited to simultaneously treating the possible variations in degree of protection, and the type of protective clothing worn (aprons, charcoal-in-foam, air-permeable but chemical-impermeable, or totally impermeable ensembles worn open or closed). Such models can also handle simultaneously such questions as age and gender, as well as body weight, height, air temperature, solar load, humidity and air motion, without concern as to whether an index relying on ambient vapor pressure, or on psychrometric instead of non-psychrometric wet bulb temperature needs to be used. One such model [19, 20, 22] rigorously addresses the physical heat transfers allowed by the worker's clothing between an environment and the worker, and can make adjustment for individual (or group) capacities to meet heat stress, including degree of heat acclimatization, and extent of dehydration. Model outputs include predicted subjective comfort vote (PMV, on a scale of +3 to -3, where 0 is comfortable, +3 is very hot), deep-body temperature and heart rate, Watts of required and maximum evaporative cooling, and percent sweat-wetted skin area and grams of sweat produced. This model assumes a relatively fixed skin temperature, in the 35-36°C range. The model has been programmed to provide tabulated outputs of rectal temperature and heart rate as a function of time. It can also provide values of the equilibrium rectal temperatures and heart rates that the body will attempt to achieve to establish heat balance, without recognition of whether or not these required equilibrium levels may be totally incompatible with tolerance limitations and, thus, may lead to collapse long before any equilibrium is reached. In this equilibrium state mode, the output also identifies the relative contributions of the work level [46] of any non-evaporative heat transfer limitations associated with high ambient temperatures or heavy insulation and also differentiates any problems associated with high ambient vapor pressures or inadequate permeability [26]. A sample output showing the changes associated with changing the insulation of a protective ensemble (from the 1.4 clo value of a standard long-sleeved shirt and trousers, by $\pm$ 0.2 clo increments) is presented in Table 10-11 for men, at rest or working at 250 or 500 Watts at 20°C (68°F), 25% R.H. with low air movement (0.3m/s). The output can also identify the effects of lack of (or improved) heat acclimatization and of limited (or enhanced) water ingestion programs.

   A third output format simply graphs the predicted rectal temperatures and heart rates over time as a function of any sequence of rest-work-recovery-work-recovery, etc. cycles of various durations. This allows optimum relationships between work and rest periods to be set up either to keep body heat storage below the 80 kcal/hr associated with unwillingness to continue work, or keep deep-body temperatures below the 39.2°C (102.5°F) level at which there is roughly a 25% risk of heat exhaustion collapse for individuals wearing chemical protective ensembles. For example, this could occur under conditions in which skin temperature cannot be reduced as a result of sweat evaporation with the increased effective wind velocity during work because of clothing impermeability. Such graphic outputs can be color-coded to represent acceptable heart rate and rectal temperatures for a civilian workforce under OSHA regulations in one color (i.e., T_{re} < 38.2°C; heart rate < 120 b/m). A different color can be used to reflect "safe," albeit stressful, conditions for fit young adults (i.e., T_{re} < 39.2°C; heart rate < 140, or 160, or 180 b/m depending on duration of the exposure in chemical protective garments). For older, or less fit individuals, the age adjustment in their maximum heart rate (.e., 220 bpm - age in years) should be used to modify any heart rate based limits. Transition to still another color can indicate conditions of potential heat exhaustion collapse (i.e., T_{re} between 39.2 and 41°C). Finally, another color (or symbol) can be used for temperatures above 41°C where risk of heatstroke exists.

Table 10-11. Predicted Responses to Changes in Clothing Ta=20C, RH=25%, WV=0.3m/s. Clo=a/s, Im-.43 p=.25						
REST						
Clo eff	**PMV**	**Tref**	**Ereq**	**Emax**	**% SW**	**Sweat**
.80	-1.5	36.9	-128	545	0	0
1.00	-1.2	37.0	- 82	436	0	0
1.20	-1.0	37.1	- 51	363	0	0
1.40	-0.8	37.2	- 28	311	0	0
1.60	-0.5	37.3	- 12	273	0	0
1.80	-0.3	37.3	- 1	242	1	2
2.00	+0.0	37.4	12	218	5	25
M=250 W						
.61	-0.6	37.4	- 56	934	0	0
.76	-0.3	37.5	6	747	1	7
.92	+0.1	37.6	46	622	7	61
1.07	+0.4	37.7	75	533	14	106
1.22	+0.7	37.7	97	467	21	145
1.38	+1.1	37.8	114	415	28	180
1.53	+1.4	37.9	128	373	34	211

M=500 W						
.51	+0.2	38.3	131	1365	10	120
.63	+0.6	38.4	205	1092	19	208
.76	+1.1	38.5	254	910	28	280
.88	+1.6	38.6	289	780	37	342
1.01	+2.0	38.7	315	682	46	397
1.14	+2.5	38.8	336	606	55	446
1.26	+2.9	38.9	352	546	65	490

"CONVERGENCE": THE BEST PHYSIOLOGICAL GUIDE TO HEAT LIMITS

Any tolerance limit established simply on deep-body temperature or heart rate will not address the critical problem termed "skin temperature convergence" [49]. Heat exhaustion collapse has occurred in individuals with deep-body temperatures ~38.1°C (100.6°F) with heart rates, measured only minutes before collapse ensued, on the order of 120-130 b/min after some 30 minutes of exposure to work in the heat while wearing impermeable protective garments. The critical event in such cases is that skin temperature rises, converging toward rectal temperature. A core to skin temperature difference of less than 1°C is a strong indication of inability to continue work in the heat very much longer (see Figure 10-6). As skin temperature converges toward deep-body temperature, as indicated previously, each liter of blood has a reduced capacity for moving heat from the deep-body centers to the skin from which, in normal clothing, it is eliminated. Associated with this convergence is an increased accumulation of blood in the periphery, and increased heart rates in an attempt to maintain heat balance and blood flow to the brain. In recent field trials in troops wearing chemical protective clothing ensembles, voluntary discontinuance occurred almost contemporaneously with skin temperature reaching deep-body temperature, even though deep-body temperature was well below the usual 39.5°C (103°F) used as a limiting criterion for fit, young, heat-acclimatized troops.

Except as an indicator of risk of heat stroke, deep-body temperature should not be used alone for individuals wearing chemical protective clothing since heat exhaustion collapse can occur at deep-body temperatures close to 38°C. Also, deep-body temperatures frequently continue to rise after cessation

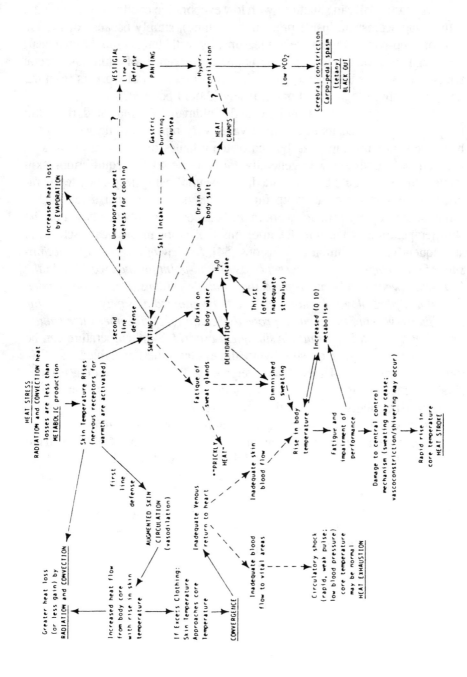

Figure 10-6.
Heat stress and its associated physiologic responses and pathologies.

of work, particularly in situations with low evaporative cooling potential (e.g., a high vapor pressure inside protective clothing), simply because of the lag time of deep-body temperature as measured by rectal temperature. Since heart rates can rise much too rapidly upon convergence of skin and rectal temperatures to be used safely as a criterion for removal of workers from the heat, what physiological end-point, if any, should be used?

Some years ago, Iampietro and Goldman [37] indicated that skin temperature achieved its equilibrium value very rapidly during work in the heat; the skin temperature at the end of ten minutes of exposure to work in a given hot condition was generally fairly close to the equilibrium skin temperature that would be established, at least until rising deep-body temperatures drove skin temperature up further. They suggested that a reasonable estimate of tolerance time for work in the heat could be obtained based on the skin temperature at ten minutes after onset of work in the heat. Schwartz, subsequently, drew similar conclusions [54]. *In view of the critical relationship of skin temperature convergence as an end-point for men working in the heat when wearing chemical protective clothing systems, it is recommended that, if any physiological end-points are to be adopted as safety criterion for individuals working in chemical protective clothing, skin temperature should be one of the most important physiological criteria.* Skin temperature can be measured at a number of sites, with three sites (chest weighted at 50%, forearm weighted at 14%, and calf weighted at 36%) usually being used to obtain a mean-weighted skin temperature. Under heat stress conditions, however, particularly when wearing complete chemical protective encapsulation systems, skin temperatures become remarkably uniform and measurement of a single skin temperature should suffice. Soule and Goldman have suggested that a lateral or medial thigh temperature is probably the most representative of average skin temperature, and a medial thigh temperature would be least apt to be influenced by direct impingement of solar or other radiant heat sources. A skin temperature at that point (or an average mean weighted skin temperature) in excess of 36°C should be considered prognostic of difficulty in maintaining an acceptable heat balance. *A skin temperature above 37°C should be cause for cessation of work in the heat.*

REFERENCES

1. ACGIH, American Conference of Governmental Industrial Hygienists, 1980, Threshold Limit Values for Chemical Substances and Physical Agents in the Workroom Environment with Intended Changes for 1980, Cincinnati.

2. Adolph, E. F., and Associates. "Physiology of Man in the Desert." NY: Interscience, 1974.

3. Bedford, T., and C. G. Warner. "The Globe Thermometer in Studies of Heating and Ventilating," *J. Hygiene (Camb.)* 34:458-473 (1934).

4. Belding, H. S. "Heat Stress," in: *Thermobiology*, A.H. Rose, Ed. (New York: Academic Press Inc., 1971).

5. Belding, H. S. "The Search for a Universal Heat Stress Index" in: *Physiological and Behavioral Temperature Regulation*, J. D. Hardy, A. P. Gagge, and J. A. J. Stolwijk, Eds., (Springfield, IL: C C Thomas, Inc., 1970).

6. Belding, H. S. and T. F. Hatch. Index for evaluating heat stress in terms of resulting physiological strain. *ASHRAE TRANSACTIONS* 62:213-236, 1956.

7. Breckenridge, J. R. and R. F. Goldman. "Effect of Clothing on Bodily Resistance Against Meteorological Stimuli," in: *Progress in Biometeorology*, S. W. Tromp, Ed. (Lesse The Netherlands: Swets and Zeitlinger, 1977), Vol. 1, Part II: 194-208.

8. Brouha, L. *Physiology in Industry*. (New York: Pergamon Press, 1960).

9. Burch, G. E., and N. P. DePasquale. *Hot Climates, Man and His Heart*, (Springfield, IL: C C Thomas Inc., 1962).

10. Colin, J., and Y. Houdas. "Experimental Determination of Coefficient of Heat Exchange by Convection of the Human Body," *J. Appl. Physiol.* 22:31-38 (1967).

11. Colquhoun, W. P., and R. F. Goldman. "Vigilance Under Induced Hyperthermia," *Ergonomics*, 15:621-632 (1972).

12. Dukes-Dobos F. N., and A. Henschel. "The Modification of the WBGT Index for Establishing Permissible Heat Exposure Limits in Occupational Work," United States Health, Education and Welfare, National Institute for Occupational Safety and Health, TR-69, (1971).

13. Ellis, F. P. "Mortality from Heat Illness and Heat Aggravated Illness in the United States," *Environmental Research*, 5:1-58 (1972).

14. Fanger, P. O. *Thermal Comfort*, (New York: McGraw-Hill, Inc., 1973).

15.   Fourt, L., and N. R. S. Hollies. *Clothing Comfort and Function*, (New York: Marcel Decker Inc., 1970).

16.   Gagge, A. P. "A New Physiological Variable Associated with Sensible and Insensible Perspiration," *Am. J. Physiol.* 120:277-287 (1937).

17.   Gagge, A. P. "Standard-Operative Temperature, a Generalized Temperature Scale, Applicable to Direct and Partitional Calorimetry," *Am. J. Physiol.* 131:93-103 (1940).

18.   Gagge, A. P., C. E. Winslow, and L. P. Herrington. "The Influence of Clothing on Physiological Reactions of the Human Body to Varying Environmental Temperatures." *Am. J. Physiol.* 124:30-50 (1938).

19.   Givoni, B. and R. F. Goldman. "Predicting Effects of Heat Acclimatization on Heart Rate and Rectal Temperature." *J. Appl. Physiol.* 35:875-979 (1973).

20.   Givoni, B. and R. F. Goldman. "Predicting Heart Rate Response to Work, Environment and Clothing," *J. Appl. Physiol.* 34:201-204 (1973).

21.   Givoni, B. and R. F. Goldman. "Predicting Metabolic Energy Cost," *J. Appl. Physiol.* 30:429-433 (1971).

22.   Givoni, B. and R. F. Goldman. "Predicting Rectal Temperature Response to Work, Environment and Clothing," *J. Appl. Physiol.* 32:812-822 (1972).

23.   Goldman, R. F. "Evaluating the effects of clothing on the wearer." Chap. 3, *Bioengineering, Thermal Physiology and Comfort*, (K. Cena, J. A. Clark, eds.) pp. 41-55, Elsevier, NY, 1981.

24.   Goldman, R. F. "Environmental Limits, Their Prescription and Proscription," *Intl. J. Environ. Sci.* 2:193-204 (1973).

25.   Goldman, R. F. "Prediction of Heat Strain Revisited 1979-1980," in: *Proceedings of the NIOSH Workshop on the Heat Stress Standard*, Cincinnati, September 1979.

26.   Goldman, R. F. "Prediction of Human Heat Tolerance," in Environmental Stress, S. J. Follinsbee et al., Eds. (New York: Academic Press, Inc. 1978), pp. 53-69.

27.   Goldman, R. F. "Tactical Implications of the Physiological Stress Imposed by Chemical Protective Clothing Systems," in: *Proceedings of the 1970 Army Science Conference*, (West Point, NY: US Military Academy, 1970).

28. Goldman, R. F. "Tolerance Time for Work in the Heat When Wearing CBR Protective Clothing," *Mil. Medicine* 128:776-786 (1963).

29. Goldman, R. F. and J. R. Breckenridge. "Current Approaches to Resolving the Physiological Heat Stress Problems Imposed by Chemical Protective Clothing Systems," in: *Proceedings of the Army Science Conference, Volume IV,* (West Point, NY: US Military Academy, June 1976) pp. 447-453.

30. Goldman, R. F., E. B. Green and P. F. Iampietro. "Tolerance of Hot, Wet Environments by Resting Men," *J. Appl. Physiol.* 20:271-277 (1965).

31. Goldman, Ralph F. and Staff. "Microclimate Cooling For Combat Vehicle Crewmen," in: *Proceedings of the 1982 Army Science Conference*, (West Point, NY: US Military Academy, June 1982).

32. Gonzalez, R. R., L. G., Berglund, and A. P. Gagge. "Indices of Thermoregulatory Strain for Moderate Exercise in the Heat," *J. Appl. Physiol.* 44:889-899 (1978).

33. Haisman, M. F. and R. F. Goldman. "Effect of Terrain on the Energy Cost of Walking with Back Loads and Handcart Loads," *J. Appl. Physiol.* 36:545-548 (1974).

34. Hardy, J. D. "Heat Transfer," in: *Physiology of Heat Regulation and Science of Clothing*, L. H. Newburgh, Ed. (London: W.D. Saunders Ltd., 1949) pp. 79-108.

35. Houghten, F. C., and C. P. Yaglou. "Determining Lines of Equal Comfort," *ASHRAE TRANSACTIONS* 29:163-176, 361-384 (1923).

36. Hughes, A. L., and R. F. Goldman. "Energy Cost of 'Hard Work'," *J. Appl. Physiol.* 29:570-572 (1970).

37. Iampietro, P. F. and R. F. Goldman. "Tolerance of Men Working in Hot Humid Environments," *J. Appl. Physiol.* 20:73-76 (1965).

38. ISO, International Organization for Standardization, 1981, Hot environments-determination of the Wet Bulb Globe Temperature (WBGT) Heat Stress Index. Draft International Standard ISO-DIS 7243.

39. Joy, R. J. T. and R. F. Goldman. "A Method of Relating Physiology and Military Performance: A Study of Some Effects of Vapor Barrier Clothing in Hot Climate," *Mil. Med.* 133:458-470 (1968).

40. Kerslake, D. M. *The Stress of Hot Environments.* (Oxford, England: Cambridge University Press 1972).

41. Leithead, C. S., and A. P. Lind. *Heat Stress and Heat Disorders.* (London: Churchill, 1964).

42. MacPherson, R. K., and F. P. Ellis. *Physiological Responses to Hot Environment.* (London: Medical Research Council, Her Majesty's Stationary Office, 1960).

43. Mihal, C. P. "Effect of Heat Stress on Physiological Factors for Industrial Workers Performing Routine Work and Wearing Impermeable Vapor-Barrier Clothing," *Am. Ind. Hyg. Assoc. J.* 42:97-103 (1981).

44. Mitchell, D. "Convective Heat Transfer in Man and Other Animals," in: *Heat Loss from Animals and Man,* J. L. Montieth and L. E. Mount, Eds. (London: Butterworth's 1974).

45. Newburgh, L. H. *Physiology of Heat Regulation and the Science of Clothing* (Philadelphia, PA: W. B. Saunders, 1949).

46. Nielsen, M. "Die Regulation der Korpertemperature bei Muskelarbeit," *Scand. Arch. Physiol.* 79:193-230 (1938).

47. Nishi, Y., and A. P. Gagge. "Moisture Permeation of Clothing: A Factor Covering Thermal Equilibrium and Comfort," *ASHRAE TRANSACTIONS* 76:1-8 (1970).

48. Onkaram B., L. A. Stroschein and R. F. Goldman. "Three Instruments for Assessment of WBGT and a Comparison with WGT (Botsball)," *Am. Ind. Hyg. Assoc. J.* 41:634-641, 1980.

49. Pandolf, K. B. and R. F. Goldman. Convergence of skin and rectal temperatures as a criterion for heat tolerance. *Aviat. Space Environ. Med.* 49:1095-1101 (1978).

50. Passmore, R., and J. V. G. A. Durnin. *Energy, Work and Leisure* (London: Heinemann Educational Books Ltd., 1967).

51. Raven, P. B., A. Dobson and T. O. Davis. "Stresses Involved in Wearing PVC Supplied-air Suits: A Review," *Am. Ind. Hyg. Assoc. J.* 40:592-599 (1979).

52. Shapiro, Y. K. B. Pandolf, M. N. Sawka, M. M. Toner, F. R. Winsmann and R. F. Goldman. "Auxiliary Cooling: Comparison of Air-Cooled Versus Water-Cooled Vest in Hot-Dry and Hot-Wet Environments," *Aviat. Space and Environ. Med.* 53:785-789 (1982).

53. Shvartz, E. "Effect of Neck Versus Chest Cooling on Responses to Work in Heat," *J. Appl. Physiol.* 40:668-672 (1976).

54. Shvartz, E., and D. Benor. Heat Strain in Hot and Humid Environments. *Aerospace Med.* 43:852-855 (1972).

55. Smith, D. J. "Protective Clothing and Thermal Stress," *Ann. Occup. Hygiene* 23:217-224 (1980).

56. Soule, R. G. and R. F. Goldman. "Energy Cost of Loads Carried on the Head, Hands or Feet," *J. Appl. Physiol.* 27:687-690 (1969).

57.   Sprague, C. H., and D. M. Munson. "A Composite Ensemble Method for Estimating Thermal Insulating Values of Clothing," *ASHRAE TRANSACTIONS* 80:120-129 (1974).

58.   Tanaka, M., G. R. Brisson and M. A. Volle. "Body Temperatures in Relation to Heart Rate for Workers Wearing Impermeable Clothing in Hot Environments," *Am. Ind. Hyg. Assoc. J.* 39:592-599 (1979).

59.   Wyndham, C. H. "The Probability of Heat Stroke at Different Levels of Heat Stress." International Symposium: Quantitative Prediction of Physiological and Psychological Effects of Thermal Environment on Man," Centre d'Etudes Bioclimatique, Strasbourg, France (1973).

60.   Yaglou, C. P., and D. Minard. "Control of Heat Casualties at Military Training Centers," *A.M.A. Archs. Ind. Hlth.* 16:302-316 (1957).

61.   World Health Organization Scientific Group. "Health Factors Involved in Working Under Conditions of Heat Stress." Who Technical Report 412, 1969.

62.   Brief, R.S. and R.G. Confer. "Companion of Heat Stress Indices." *Am. Ind. Hyg. Assoc. J.* 32:11-16, 1971.

63.   Criteria for a Recommended Standard—Occupational Exposure to Hot Environments, USDHEW (NIOSH) HSM 72-10269, 1972.

64.   Planned Update of Reference 63, scheduled for 1984.

65.   DHHS (NIOSH) Publication No. 80-132, Hot Environments, 1980.

11

DECONTAMINATION

John M. Lippitt, M.En.
Timothy G. Prothero, B.A.

The purpose of decontamination, as discussed in this chapter, is the removal or neutralization of hazardous substances on vehicles, clothing, tools, equipment and instruments. The purpose of decontamination is to prevent or minimize human exposures to hazardous substances. Decontamination is also the means to prevent the spread of contamination when workers and equipment exit contaminated sites. Controlling the spread of contamination is necessary to prevent harm to human health and the environment that can result from the spreading of contaminants to air, water, soils, plants and animals.

Decontamination is an integral part of the requirements established by the Occupational Safety and Health Administration (OSHA) for protection of workers and the U.S. Environmental Protection Agency (USEPA) for protection of human health and the environment. Although most regulatory agencies have established guidelines, it is important to note that there are no comprehensive, uniform standards for decontamination methods. This chapter discusses the principles and objectives that need to be addressed in the planning and implementation of decontamination procedures at a hazardous waste site. These discussions should be considered in the context of the related issues and requirements addressed in the other chapters of this textbook.

PRINCIPLES AND OBJECTIVES OF DECONTAMINATION

To remove a contaminant, it is necessary to consider the extent to which the contamination has permeated or penetrated the surface and the binding forces between the contaminant and the object to be decontaminated. The severity of permeation (i.e., the movement of contamination into a material at a molecular level) is related to duration of contact, the physical and chemical properties of the contaminant and the properties of the objects to be decontaminated. The severity of penetration (i.e., movement of contaminants through the structure of a materials) is a function of the physical properties of materials relative to physical properties of the contaminant. The decontamination of objects that are penetrated or permeated requires the breaking of the binding forces, and driving the contaminants to the surface for removal. The closer the contaminant is to the surface the easier it is to be removed. The nature of binding force will influence the effectiveness of the decontamination.

The basic factor of permeation is time. Simply, the longer a contaminant remains in contact with a material the more that contaminant will migrate into the material. Restricting the duration of contact is the simplest method to limit the amount of permeation. Since no material is totally impervious to all possible contaminants, appropriate time restrictions should be established for all site activities involving direct contact with contaminants. The time restrictions must be based on the suspected contaminants and the potential for permeation into the vehicles, tools, equipment and PPE used.

Permeation is related to the physical space between molecules of a material and the ability of a contaminant to move through those spaces. The density and rigidity of the molecular structure of materials will affect the ability of contaminants to permeate a material. The density, cohesive properties and mobility of the contaminants will affect its ability to permeate into another material. The greater the density and rigidity of a material the more resistant it is to permeation. This is the main reason that permeation of metals is limited, and metals are easier to decontaminate than plastics or fabrics. On the other hand, the permeability of a contaminant into another material increases as the density and cohesive properties of that material decrease and the contaminant's mobility increases. A contaminant's mobility is related to temperature and physical state as seen by the greater mobility of a liquid relative to a solid and gases relative to liquids. An increase in temperature increases the movement of contaminant molecules and provides increased energy to overcome the material's resistance to permeation.

On a larger scale, the physical restriction or filtering of contaminants will affect penetration. Penetration of personnel protective clothing and equipment (PPE) is affected by the size of the spaces between the threads of woven fabrics and the seams where sections of fabrics are joined. Penetration of structures, tools, equipment and vehicles occurs through crevices, cracks, surface irregularities, seams, hinges, and joints.

Other physical driving forces can also help to push contamination into a material. Increasing contaminant concentration increases diffusion into material to equalize the concentration gradient. Also, a contaminant propelled by as a sudden release of pressure or thrown by grinding or sandblasting can be physically pushed into a material.

Any chemical interaction between contaminants and items to be decontaminated will affect permeation and penetration. Chemical degradation of a material changes the structural integrity of the material and affects the rate of permeation. Contaminants that adhere to and coat surfaces tend to restrict permeation and penetration.

Contaminants can be bound to a material through electrostatic, chemical and physical attractive forces and mechanical entrapment. These binding forces must be broken to remove a contaminant. Methods for decontamination are discussed later in this chapter.

PLANNING AND IMPLEMENTATION OF A DECONTAMINATION PROGRAM

Decontamination procedures are established to provide four basic functions:

1. Minimizing worker contact with wastes during removal of PPE and preventing additional exposures by preventing the spread of contamination into clean areas where PPE is not worn.

2. Removing and controlling contaminants that have accumulated on PPE, tools, equipment, and vehicles used in the contaminated areas to prevent dispersal of contamination into adjacent uncontaminated areas on-site and surrounding areas off-site.

3. Preventing inadvertent mixing of wastes with other potentially incompatible wastes or compounds.

4. Removal or detoxification of wastes from equipment, vehicles, buildings, and structures to prevent further releases and/or exposures and enable future use after completing activities involving contact with contaminants.

General Design Principles

In concept, the design of a decontamination procedure is straight forward, but in practice it requires evaluation of many different variables. A general decision logic, as shown in Figure 11-1 can be used to organize decontamination procedures on a site. Within the decision logic, factors must be considered according to the site conditions, characteristics of the waste, activities being conducted, etc. The decontamination of PPE, tools, equipment, vehicles, structures, and buildings will be different because of the differences in materials and contaminants. Table 11-1 is a list of factors which impact on decontamination design requirements.

Decontamination facilities on a hazardous waste site should be located in the contamination reduction area between areas contaminated by the wastes and clean support areas, as shown in Figure 11-2. Decontamination designs and procedures must include the containment, collection, and disposal of contaminated solutions and residues generated during the process, unless the specific contaminant has been judged to be acceptable for release on the site. This must be decided on a case-by-case basis. Controls may include items such as spray booths with side walls or curtains to contain splashes and sprays, a collection tank for waste liquids, and drums for disposal of excessively contaminated materials and solid wastes from the process. Separate facilities should be provided for decontamination of large equipment to prevent cross-contamination of personnel decontamination facilities. Each stage of decontamination from gross decontamination through the repetitive wash/rinse cycles should be conducted at different stations.

Stations used should be physically separated to prevent cross-contact between stations. The stations should be arranged in order of decreasing level of contamination, preferably in a straight line. Separate flow patterns and stations should be provided when it is necessary to isolate workers from different contamination zones containing incompatible waste. Entry and exit points should be well marked and controlled. The decontamination area should be separate from the entry path to the contaminated area (exclusion zone) from the clean area (support zone). Dressing stations for entry should be separate from re-dressing areas for exit. Entry into clean areas of the decontamination facility such as the dress out locker rooms requires full decontamination.

Procedures should be established for minimum decontamination prior to use of restroom facilities. If deemed appropriate by a safety assessment, restroom facilities can be located within the contamination reduction zone preceded by the minimum decontamination procedures established.

DECONTAMINATION PROCEDURE LOGIC

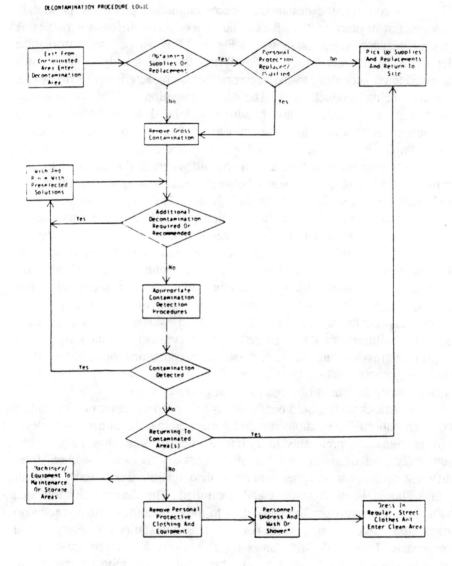

* Site clothes should be washed separately from
  non-site and other family clothing.

Figure 11-1. Decontamination procedure logic

Table 11-1. Factors Impacting Decontamination Design Requirements
1. The chemical, physical, and toxicological properties of chemical wastes.
2. The pathogenicity of infectious wastes.
3. The amount and location of contamination.
4. The potential exposures based on assigned duties, uses, activities, and functions.
5. The potential for degradation of PPE, vehicles, tools, equipment, buildings, and structures or permeation and penetration of contaminants.
6. The design and construction of PPE, vehicles, tools, equipment, buildings, and structures.
7. The proximity of incompatible wastes.
8. The reason for personnel to exit or removing equipment from the controlled contaminated area.
9. The methods available for protection of workers during decontamination procedures.
10. The impact of the decontamination process and compounds on worker safety and health

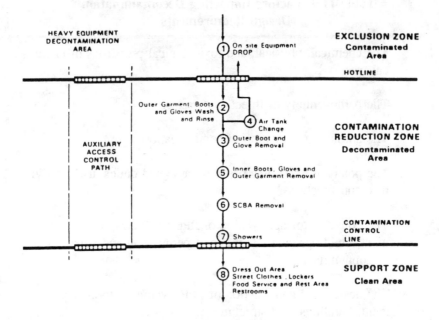

Figure 11-2. Minimum decontamination stations for
hazardous waste sites that require respiratory and skin protection

Table 11-2 is a list of recommended supplies for decontamination of personnel, clothing, and equipment. Table 11-3 is a list of recommended supplies for large equipment and vehicle decontamination. These lists are not inclusive for all needs, but should give general guidance on the types of supplies to be provided.

The actual design and setup of decontamination facilities will vary depending on:

1. The availability of utility services.
2. Mobilization time and duration of site activities.
3. Site conditions and the level of on-site activity anticipated.
4. The volume and level of decontamination required.
5. Available space in uncontaminated area contiguous with the contaminated areas of a site.
6. Potential hazards associated with the decontamination procedures and wastes generated.

The availability of utility services will determine the requirements for providing and storing portable water supplies for use in decontamination. If electrical service is necessary, portable generators could be required. Availability and access to waste water and waste water disposal systems may impact storage and handling requirements for decontamination waste waters.

Time requirements for mobilization and demobilization influence the design of decontamination facilities. Emergency response to accidents, spills, fires, or explosion do not allow sufficient time for elaborate facilities. An increasingly common practice is the use of mobile decontamination facilities that are self-contained and fully-equipped for personnel decontamination. However, in situations where mobile facilities are not available, decontamination kits should be devised. Table 11-4 is an example of a decontamination kit that could be used.

Table 11-2. Recommended Supplies for Decontamination of Personnel, Clothing, and Equipment

- Drop cloths (plastic or other suitable material) for heavily contaminated equipment and skin outer protective clothing such as overboots, second pair of gloves, monitoring equipment, drum wrenches, etc.

- Disposal collection containers (drums or suitable lined trash cans) for disposable clothing and heavily contaminated PPE.

- Storage containers for contaminated wash and rinse solutions.

- Lined box with absorbents for collection and control of wastes from scraping, wiping or rinsing off gross contamination.

- Wash tubs of sufficient size to enable workers to place booted foot in and wash off contaminants (without drains unless connected to a suitable collection tank or treatment system).

- Rinse tubs of sufficient size to enable workers to place booted foot in and hold the solution used to rinse the wash solutions and contaminants after washing (without drains unless connected to a suitable collection tank or treatment system).

- Wash solutions pretested against contaminants for effectiveness and compatibility.

- Rinse solutions (also pretested) to remove or neutralize contaminants and rinse off residues of wash solutions.

- Long-handled, soft-bristled brushes to help wash and rinse off contaminants.

- Lockers and cabinets for storage of decontaminated clothing and equipment.

- Plastic sheeting, sealed pads with drains, or other appropriate method for containing and collecting contaminated wash and rinse water spilled during decontamination.

- Shower facilities for full body wash or, at a minimum, personal wash sinks (with drains connected to collection tank or appropriate treatment system).

- Soap or wash solution, wash cloths, and towels for personnel showering.

- Clean clothing and personal item storage lockers and/or closets.

**Table 11-3. Recommended Supplies for Large Equipment
and Vehicle Decontamination**

- Containers for gross contamination involving removal of wastes and contaminated soils caught in tires, and the underside of vehicles or equipment.

- Pads for collection of contaminated wash and rinse solutions with drains or sumps connected to storage tanks or approved treatment system.

- Shovels, rods, and long handled brushes for dislodging and removing wastes and contaminated soils caught in tires, and the underside of vehicles or equipment.

- Pressurized sprayer(s) for steam cleaning or washing and rinsing (particularly hard to reach areas).

- Spray booths, curtains, or enclosures to contain splashes from pressurized sprays used to dislodge materials and clean hard to reach areas.

- Long-handled brushes for general cleaning of exterior.

- Wash solutions pretested against contaminants for effectiveness and compatibility.

- Rinse solutions (also pretested) to remove or neutralize contaminants and rinse off residues of wash solutions.

- Wash and rinse buckets for use in decontamination of operator areas inside the vehicle and equipment.

- Brooms and brushes for cleaning operator areas inside the vehicles and equipment.

- Containers for storage and/or disposal of contaminated rinse and wash solutions and damaged or heavily contaminated parts and equipment to be discarded.

Table 11-4. Example of Personnel Decontamination Kit
• Five-gallon container(s) of potable water (for decontamination only
• Soft- and stiff-bristled brushes
• Detergent (solid or liquid)
• Plastic wading pool(s)
• Buckets or sprinkler cans for rinsing
• Paper towels or other disposable cleaning cloths
• Chemical-resistant container(s) (minimum five gallons for wash/rinse solutions
• Plastic garbage bags (5 or 6 mil thick) for storage of equipment and disposal of solid/hazardous wastes.

The use of temporary facilities versus permanent facilities (such as the installation of a full-sized decontamination trailer or construction of on-site buildings and facilities) will be dependent on the type and duration of site activity anticipated. The level of on-site activity will determine, to a large extent, the potential for contamination of workers. Decontamination for investigations involving limited contact with contaminants for purposes of sampling is usually less elaborate than decontamination of workers involved in handling and packing of wastes during site cleanup. Similarly, sites on which releases of wastes have resulted in extensive contamination will require more decontamination of site workers than a site on which wastes have been contained and adequately controlled to minimize contamination.

The number and frequency of workers undergoing decontamination will impact the flow design, size, and number of stations used. Likewise, the number and frequency of vehicle and large equipment decontaminated will impact designs for those facilities.

One of the most limiting factors for decontamination facility design and setup is the availability of space in uncontaminated areas contiguous with contamination zones. Maintaining sufficient separations between stations may require use of fewer stations. Also the flow design may be arranged in rows or serpentine-fashion as opposed to the preferred straight-line design. The design of many of the mobile trailer facilities in use requires such modifications from the straight-line design to make efficient use of available space. In confined areas, it is essential that procedures and practices are implemented to minimize splashing, sprays, dusting, and aerosols that may cross-contaminate stations. In enclosed areas, such as mobile trailers, effective ventilation controls are also critical.

Concerns for cross-contamination and protection of decontamination facility workers may require special designs and controls if potential hazards during decontamination are significant. Ventilation hoods, spray booths, wet wells, chemical treatment tanks for wastes, and specialized storage containers are examples of specialized components that may be used to control dispersion of wastes during decontamination. Standard controls will prevent or minimize run-off, air diffusion/dispersion, and movement of wastes from each decontamination station.

Selection of Appropriate Decontamination Solutions

In choosing the appropriate wash and rinsing solutions for a decontamination project, one must consider the following factors:

1. *Solubility* behavior of contaminant
2. *Compatibility* of choice solutions with contaminant and object/items to be decontaminated.
3. *Accessibility and availability* of solutions
4. *Effectiveness* of solutions and methods
5. *Storage, handling, and disposal requirements* of solutions
6. *Hazards* associated with cleaning solutions (i.e., flammability and toxicity)

In general, the more common solvents and the compounds they work best on are presented below :

1. *Water*:   Dissolves low chain hydrocarbons, inorganics, salts, some organic acids and other polar compounds.

2. *Dilute Acid*:   Dissolves caustic (basic) compounds, amines, hydrazines and metal salts.

3. *Dilute Base*:   Dissolves acidic compounds, phenols, thiols, and some nitro and sulfonic compounds.

4. *Organic Solvents*: Dissolve non-polar compounds such as other organics; can also dissolve PPE fabrics and materials.

It is very important to pretest cleaning solutions for compatibility with the materials being cleaned. The choice of solvent wash and rinse solutions will depend largely on its compatibility with the material of the equipment that is being decontaminated. For example, most of the fabrics of PPE are made of polymer organics that can be dissolved or destroyed by organic solvents. The metals and gaskets of tools and equipment can be damaged by strongly acidic or caustic compounds.

Another important requirement is that the chemical waste and the cleaning solutions be compatible. Figure 11-3 diagrams the decision logic for selection of decontamination wash/rinse solutions. Incompatible reactions resulting in excessive heat, fire, or generation of toxic gases are not desired in the contamination reduction areas where decontamination crews might not be adequately protected.

The ready access to wash and rinse solutions is the most practical limitation. The availability of water has resulted in its use in most decontamination cases, despite the soluble nature of the chemical wastes. Water and detergents are easily obtained in any site's vicinity, and they are easily stored and handled.

The hazards involved with the solutions themselves must be considered during any decontamination project. Organic solvents, especially flammable and highly toxic ones, are more difficult to store, handle, and control. Besides the hazardous properties of the cleaning solutions, one must remember that even water may become hazardous after it has been used for cleaning contaminated equipment.

The disposal of cleaning solutions will depend on the type of solution (aqueous or organic), and the types and amounts of contamination it contains after use. Depending on the site and situation, cleaning solutions may be collected after use and added to waste streams at the site for disposal.

Disinfection solutions for use following removal of gross contamination will require consideration of several factors as presented in Table 11-5. A disinfection activity level based on field conditions should be established before extensive site work.

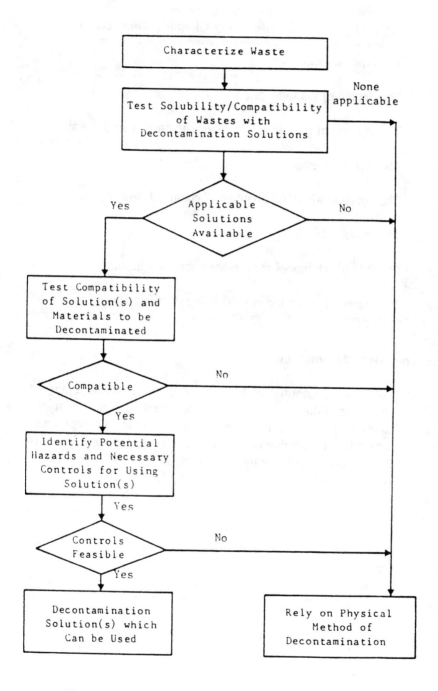

Figure 11-3. Decision logic for selecting decontamination
wash/rinse solutions

Table 11-5. Factors Influencing Chemical Disinfection
1. The types of organism
2. The degree of contamination
3. The amount of proteinaceous materials present in the waste
4. The type of chemical
5. The concentration and quantity of chemical disinfectant
6. The contact time
7. Possible interferences from other chemicals in wastes
8. The temperature of the item(s) being disinfected

Emergency Decontamination

In addition to normal decontamination procedures, emergency decontamination procedures should be established. In an emergency, decontamination may not occur at the site when immediate treatment is required to save a life. If decontamination can be provided without interfering with essential first aid and life-saving techniques, such as CPR, then it should be done. Clothing and equipment may be washed, rinsed, and/or cut-off when necessary. Otherwise, the individual should be covered with a blanket or other suitable material. Covering serves to prevent contamination of ambulance and medical personnel. Alternatively, to minimize possible heat stress to the patient, PPE may be used by the emergency response personnel (assuming appropriate training has been provided during planning stages of the project).

It is important to coordinate procedures for decontamination protection of medical personnel, and disposal of contaminated clothing and equipment. These procedures are necessary to minimize the risk of exposure to emergency medical personnel. Such procedures should be established during planning of site activities before any site work. Figure 11-4 outlines the decision logic that should be followed in an emergency.

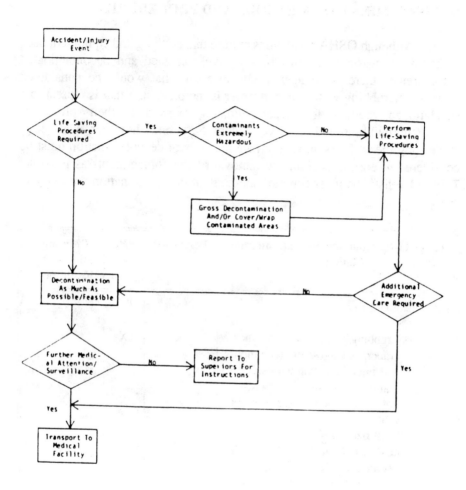

Figure 11-4. Emergency decontamination design logic

DECONTAMINATION METHODS AND PROCEDURES

Although OSHA regulations require that clothing and equipment used at hazardous waste sites must be effectively cleaned and decontaminated before reuse, there is no agency guidance on what would be considered effective. Scrubbing with soap and water is the procedure that is closest to a standardized method for decontaminating personnel, their protective equipment, buildings and heavy equipment. Scrubbing, however, is effective at cleaning the surfaces only. Alternate methods of decontamination must be considered to ensure as complete removal of the contaminants as possible. Table 11-6 lists the most common methods of decontamination presently in use.

Table 11-6. Common Decontamination Methods	Personnel	PPE	Buildings and Heavy Equipment
1. Contaminant Removal			
• Scrubbing/scraping with brushes, scrapers, sponges, etc. (commonly used in combination with solvent cleaning solutions).	X	X	X
• Water rinse (pressurized or gravity flow)	X	X	X
• Pressurized wash		X	X
• Steam jets (commonly used with solvent cleaning solutions)			X
• Evaporation/vaporization (e.g., hot air drying)		X	X
• Chemical leaching (e.g., dry cleaning or Freon cleaning)		X	
2. Detoxification			
• Oxidation/reduction (e.g., bleach)		X	X
• Neutralization		X	X
• Thermal degradation		X	X

Table 11-6. Common Decontamination Methods	Personnel	PPE	Buildings and Heavy Equipment
3. Removal of Contaminated Surfaces and Materials			
• Abrasive blasting (sand, walnut hulls, etc.)			X
• Disposal of permeated materials (e.g., seats, floor mats, clothing, coatings, disposable coveralls)		X	X
4. Disinfection/Sterilization (infectious wastes)			
• Steam sterilization		X	X
• Dry heat sterilization		X	X
• Irradiation (e.g., UV)		X	X
• Chemical disinfection	X	X	X

Personnel and Personal Protective Equipment Decontamination:

1.   *Washing with water and detergents/disinfectants.* PPE cleaning is perhaps the most frequent decontamination procedure used. Sequential wash and rinse cycles in a series of galvanized tubs are common procedures for decontamination of PPE. As contamination is reduced the layers of clothing and equipment are removed. A personnel shower is the last step of the decontamination protocol. The washing of personnel and equipment can involve the use of water, detergents or soaps, and if necessary, disinfectants. Figure 11-2 depicts a combination personnel and personal protective clothing decontamination sequence.

Washing is only effective for removal of topical contaminants. Scrubbing does not remove entrapped or permeated contaminants. Nor does scrubbing with soap and water prevent redeposition of non-polar materials that would have a greater affinity for the surfaces of non-polar materials than for the polar solution of surfactants and water. Removal of entrained, or permeated, contaminants from the fabrics of personal protective clothing requires alternate methods be used, preferably, as an addition to scrubbing with water and detergents. Alternate methods are referenced in Table 11-6 and discussed below.

2.   *Freon and dry-cleaning.* Freon cleaning has been used in some situations to remove non-polar organics from protective clothing. Removal efficiencies have been reported ranging from about 65% to 99% for removal of PCBs in firefighters' turnout gear (Ashley, 1986). Freon and dry cleaning work similarly to washing with the advantage that Freon and dry cleaning fluids are non-polar solvents able to dissolve and remove other non-polar chemicals better than water. The disadvantages of freon and dry cleaning are that the solvents can permeate the protective clothing and will then become themselves contaminants.

3.   *Hot Air Treatment.* Research has determined that permeated volatile and semi-volatile compounds may be removed from personal protective clothing by "baking" the clothing at 50°C (about 120°F) for 24 hours. The temperature is sufficiently high to drive off the organic contaminants without damaging the several types of personal protective clothing tested. At temperatures higher than 50°C, the protective clothing was damaged sometimes, either by loss of plasticizers, elastomers, or cracking of the material (Perkins, 1987).

Generally, hot air treatment is very effective at removal of organic contaminants and restores the protective clothing to very near the protective breakthrough qualities that it had when new.

4.   *Disposal of Contaminated Coverings.* Although disposal of contaminated materials is not "decontamination" per se, it is a very effective means of controlling contamination and contaminant spread. A disposable coating, for example, disposable treated paper coveralls, may be used as a barrier to contamination. Although the breakthrough times of coverings are likely to be very brief, the concentration gradients on the insides of the coverings are so low as to retard the permeation of the covered materials. Therefore, the coverings may be disposed of, and the materials that were covered will be less likely to have been seriously permeated.

5.   *Disinfectants.* Areas may be contaminated with microorganisms, such as when cleaning up abandoned medical wastes. To ensure proper decontamination in these cases, disinfectants must be used. Usually, the only decontamination that can be done by field personnel is to use topical disinfectants. Any exposures that might have occurred

from cuts or punctures should be treated by medical professionals. Factors influencing disinfectants were previously listed in Table 11-5. Table 11-7 provides disinfectant activity levels for selected classes of disinfectants.

Table 11-7. Activity Levels of Selected Classes of Liquid Disinfectants		
Class	**Use-Concentration**	**Activity Level[a]**
Glutaraldehyde, aqueous	2%	high
Formaldehyde + alcohol	8% + 70%	high
Formaldehyde, aqueous*	3% to 8%	high to intermediate
Iodine + alcohol	0.5% + 70%	intermediate
Alcohols	70% to 90%	intermediate
Chlorine compounds	500 to 5000 ppm[b]	intermediate
Phenolic compounds	1% to 3%[c]	intermediate
Iodine, aqueous	1%	intermediate
Iodophors	75 to 50 ppm[d]	intermediate to low
Quaternary ammonium compounds	1:750 to 1:500[e]	low
Hexachlorophene	1%	low
Mercurical compounds**	1:1000 to 1:500[e]	low

Courtesy of American Sterilizer Company, Erie, PA.
[a] Degree of disinfecting activity.
[b] Available chlorine.
[c] Dilution of Concentrate containing 5% to 10% phenolics.
[d] Available iodine.
[e] In appropriate diluent.

* See Section 4.7 of source reference for discussion of formaldehyde toxicity and necessary precautions for personnel protection.

** Should not be released into the environment, and therefore, is no longer used.

Source: U.S. EPA Office of Solid Waste, 1982.

Decontamination Methods for Heavy Equipment, Buildings, Structures, Vehicles, and Vessels

1.   *Steam Jetting and Pressure Washing.* Surface contaminants can be removed from heavy equipment, trucks, buildings, etc., with hot, high-pressure wash, steam jetting, at temperatures around 180°F. The higher temperatures of the water provide increased solubility for most compounds, and the high-pressures of the wash will physically "scrub" the contaminant off the surfaces being cleaned. For materials that are resistant to this method, scrubbing with brushes or brooms may help in the removal of the contaminants. These topical cleaning methods will have little effect on permeated contamination, except that the pressure differential and temperature gradients may increase permeation rates. Note that the time factors necessary for permeation are much greater than for removal of surface contaminants; therefore, pressure or steam cleaning are good methods to remove surface contamination. *Also, note that under no circumstance may any pressure or steam washing be used on a person or on a material being worn by a person, because the pressure can cause contaminants to be injected through the skin and steam will burn.*

2.   *Disinfectants.* Heavy duty disinfectants, including highly concentrated solutions, may be used on heavy equipment, buildings, or other similar materials that are contaminated with microorganisms. Tables 11-5 and 11-7 list some factors and activity levels for the use of disinfectants.

3.   *Thermal Treatment.* Structures or heavy equipment may be thermal treated through a variety of methods. Microwaves or special frequency radio waves may be used to heat up a material to drive off organic contaminants. Sufficient heat can also destroy some classes of organic contaminants.

   Thermal treatment has been used in treating a formaldehyde contaminated mobile home. The home was heated to around 90°F for several days to remove the formaldehyde from the materials of construction.

4.   *Detoxification.* In instances when the identity of the contaminant that has permeated a material is known, the contaminant may be detoxified or neutralized. For example, cyanide wastes permeated into porous media, such as bricks, may be oxidized to cyanate by using bleach. Likewise, acids or bases may be neutralized. The treatment

of penetrated or permeated contaminants in place requires careful planning and testing to ensure effective and safe treatment.

5.   *Disposal of Contaminated Coverings and Coatings*. Finally, although disposal of contaminated materials is not a method to decontaminate that material, it is a very effective method to control contamination. By prior planning, disposable coverings or coatings may be used on materials and equipment before encountering the contamination. Then the coating or covering may be removed and disposed.

Nuclear power plant containment buildings are coated inside with special permeation resistant paints that may be stripped off when contaminated (Bernaola, 1970). Sand blasting, pressure washing or stream cleaning are examples of methods used to remove protective coatings.

Measuring the Effectiveness of Decontamination Procedures

The effectiveness of decontamination procedures is often questioned because of the inability to perform real time measurements of their efficiency. Thus, it is necessary for an arbitrary decision to be made concerning the endpoint of the procedures. The state of the art in chemical analysis of surface contamination is still developing; however, several methods do exist (or can be created from available technology) for observing and measuring the decontamination procedures.

Methods available for measuring and inspecting effectiveness of decontamination includes:

1.   *Visual Inspection.*

a. *Natural Light*. Visual inspection, using natural or artificial white light, entails the search for stains, discolorations, visible dirt, or alterations in the fabric of clothing as evidence of chemical contamination. The most obvious limitation is that not all contamination will result in visible staining or other similar traces. When such visual inspections are used, it is important that the searches include problem areas such as creases, boot treads, seams, etc., of personal protective equipment. Wheel wells, tool boxes, fixtures, etc. on heavy equipment also have problem areas that are difficult to inspect visually.

b. *Ultraviolet.* Ultraviolet light is useful to detect certain contaminants that fluoresce, such as polycyclic aromatic hydrocarbons. These contaminants are common in many refined oils and solvent wastes. Ultra violet light can be used to observe skin contamination, but one must be already aware of the areas of the subject's skin that naturally fluoresces. A disadvantage of such uses of ultra violet light is the added risk of increasing carcinogenic effects on the skin and the potential of damaging the eye.

2. *Surface Analysis.* Instrumentation is currently being developed to detect, identify, and quantify contaminants on the surfaces of people, clothing, and equipment; however, at this time only large laboratory instruments are being marketed and most require the destruction of the sample. Fiberoptics is changing the technology of surface analysis and it is anticipated that as applications are identified an experienced person could fabricate field portable instruments from commercially available plans and parts.

3. *Rinse, Swab or Smear Samples.* Most available analytical methods for quantifying surface contamination are destructive of the sample. When one wishes to preserve the clothing or equipment, it is required to transfer the contaminant to another surface or solution. A smear or swab sample can be taken from selected and measured areas of the equipment or clothing. These smears or swabs can be taken using a saturated sampling swab or pad (saturated with a solution in which the contaminant is soluble) or can be used dry if the contaminant can be readily wipe off. The samples may then be analyzed by wet chemistry field tests if the contaminant is known or sent to a laboratory for further qualification or quantification. A qualified analytical chemist should choose the sampling liquids and procedure so they are compatible with the contaminant, the surface sampled, and the test(s) to be performed.

4. *Rinse Solution Testing.* Rinsing surface areas with water or other suitable solutions in which the contaminant is soluble is a common method for qualitative evaluations of surface contamination. Too much contaminant in the final rinse solution would indicate that additional cleaning and rinsing is advisable. When the type of contaminant is specifically known, a qualified chemist might devise some wet chemistry spot tests or other field tests to analyze the solutions. More complete analyses can be obtained by sending a

sample of the solutions to be tested to a laboratory; however, time constraints for laboratory analysis can limit use of this option.

5. *Disinfectant Solution Testing.* When dealing with infectious wastes, concentrations of active disinfectants can be measured in the spent solutions to determine if sufficient levels of active ingredients were available. The length of treatment with the measured level of activity can be compared to previous testing by qualified microbiologists to determine time/concentration ratios required to provide the necessary disinfection under actual or simulated conditions. As shown in Table 11-5, several factors can impact the disinfection efficiency. Therefore, it is advisable to confirm the assumed level of disinfection by laboratory culture of swab samples.

6. *Microbial Swab Samples.* Swab samples for infectious organisms taken from decontaminated surfaces or field controls (e.g., surfaces contaminated with another indicator organism, which requires similar levels of active disinfectants, length of treatment, temperatures, etc., or active cultures of the organisms of concern) should be transferred to testing laboratories for culturing under controlled temperature, atmosphere, nutrient, etc., conditions. Optimum growth and culture conditions are variable depending on the type of infectious organisms involved.

Design of appropriate sampling and laboratory testing procedures should be developed by a trained microbiologist. Every effort should be made to design and select procedures that will provide the necessary confirmation as soon as possible. Unfortunately, while some procedures require only a few hours, others can require several days.

Decisions concerning decontamination endpoints are often based on the lack of visible contamination. Unfortunately, this does not address problems of permeation, thin layers of contamination, compounds that are not readily observable with the unaided eye, or infectious organisms that can only be observed under a microscope. As a precaution, unless sufficient field experience with laboratory confirmation is available for the compounds and conditions under which decontamination is being conducted, it is advisable to assume some level of contamination may remain. If the wastes involved are extremely hazardous, repetitive decontamination may be warranted though obvious contamination has been removed. In addition, procedures for removal should be designed to prevent or minimize contact of unprotected skin surfaces with the exposed surfaces of clothing, equipment, tools, etc., which have been cleaned but may require further decontamination.

CONCLUSION

Although regulatory requirements include provisions for decontamination, no standards on effective decontamination techniques exist. The methods discussed in this chapter are in common use. The American Society of Testing and Materials (ASTM) is currently investigating effectiveness of decontamination methods to develop standards. Until then, the following guidelines are most common and effective:

- Take all reasonable precautions to prevent direct contamination.

- Limit the duration of contact with contaminated materials between decontamination and/or replacement of PPE to minimize time available for permeation and subsequent worker exposure. This can be accomplished by rotating tasks involving work in contaminated areas and work in support areas, scheduled replacement of PPE during breaks and limiting individual work shift in high risk areas.

- Establish written SOPs for worker training and monitoring of decontamination procedures. Include guidelines for replacement of reusable PPE such as respirators. Maintain records of training and field inspection to insure that decontamination is being conducted according to the SOPs.

- Remove surface contamination from PPE as soon as possible to limit the time available for permeation, especially for reusable PPE.

- At present, the most effective method for removal of permeated volatile and semi-volatile contaminants in PPE is hot air drying.

REFERENCES

1. Advisory Committee for NIOSH Carcinogen Laboratory. Protocol for the NIOSH Carcinogen Laboratory. Unpublished. National Institute for Occupational Safety and Health, Cincinnati, Oh.

2. Ashley, K.C. "Polychlorinated Biphenyl Decontamination of Fire Fighter Turnout Gear. Performance of Protective Clothing," ASTM STP 900, R.L. Barker and G.C. Coletta, Eds, American Society for Testing and Materials, Philadelphia, pages 298-307, 1986.

3. Bareis, D.L., L.R. Cook, and G.A. Parks. "Safety Plan for Construction of Remedial Actions." National Conference on Management of Uncontrolled Hazardous Waste Sites, Washington D.C., pages 280-284, 1983.

4. Barry, P.J., "Some General Considerations in Chemical Decontamination." *Health Physics*, Vol.1, No.2, pages 184-188, 1958.

5. Berardinelli, S.P., and M. Roder. "Chemical Protective Clothing Field Evaluation Methods. Performance of Protective Clothing," ASTM STP 900, R.L. Barker and G.C. Coletta, Eds, American Society for Testing and Materials, Philadelphia, pages 250-260, 1986.

6. Bernaola, O. A. and Filevich, A., "Fast Drying Strippable Protective Cover for Radioactive Decontamination." *Health Physics*, Vol. 19, No. 5, pages 685-687.

7. Brown, V.K.H., V.L. Box and B.J. Simpson. "Decontamination Procedures for Skin Exposed to Phenolic Substances." *Archives of Environmental Health*, Vol.30, pages 1-6, January 1975.

8. Department of Health, Education, and Welfare, Committee to Coordinate Toxicology and Related programs, Laboratory Chemical Carcinogen Safety Standards Subcommittee. "Guidelines for the Laboratory Use of Chemical Substances Posing a Potential Occupational Carcinogenic Risk," Revised Draft. National Institute for Occupational Safety and Health, Cincinnati, OH, 1979.

9. International Agency for Research on Cancer (IARC). "Handling Chemical Carcinogens in the Laboratory Problems of Safety." R. Montesano, H. Bartsch, E. Boyland, G. Dellaporta, L. Fischbein, R. A. Griesemer, A. B. Swan, L. Tomatis, and N. Davis, eds. IARC Scientific Publications No. 33, 1979.

10. Kominsky, J.R., and E.T. McIlvaine. "Decontamination of Fire Fighters' Protective Clothing with Trichlorotrifluoroethane." Workshop Proceedings: PCB By-Product Formation, Palo Alto, CA, December 4-6, 1984.

11. Lillie, T.H., R.E. Hampson, Y.A. Nishioka, and M.A. Hamilton. "Effectiveness of Detergent and Detergent Plus Bleach for Decontaminating Pesticide Applicator Clothing." *Bulletin of Environmental Contamination and Toxicology*, Vol.29, No.1, pages 89-94, 1982.

12. Lillie, T.H., J.M. Livingston and M.A. Hamilton. "Recommendations for Selecting and Decontaminating Pesticide Applicator Clothing." *Bulletin of Environmental Contamination and Toxicology*, Vol.27, No.5, pages 716-723, 1981.

13. Lippitt, John M., T.G. Prothero, W.F. Martin, and L.P. Wallace. "An Overview of Worker Protection Methods," in the Proceedings of 1984 Hazardous Material Spills Conference, Nashville, TN, April 9-12, 1984.

14. Mayhew, Joseph I., G. M. Sodaro, and D. W. Carroll. "A Hazardous Waste Site Management Plan." Chemical Manufacturers Assoc., Washington, D.C., 1982.

15. Mine Safety Appliances (MSA), Chemical Resistance Total-Encapsulating Suits. Data Sheet 13-00-07, Pittsburgh, PA.

16. Perkins, J.L., "Chemical Protective Clothing: II. Program Considerations." *Applied Industrial Hygiene*, Vol.3, No.1, pages 1-4, January 1988.

17. Perkins, J.L., "Decontamination of Protective Clothing." *Applied Occupational and Environmental Hygiene*, Vol.6, No.1, pages 29-35, January 1991.

18. Perkins, J.L., J.S. Johnson, P.M. Swearengen, C.P. Sackett, and S.C. Weaver. "Residual Spilled Solvents in Butyl Protective Clothing and Usefulness of Decontamination Procedures." *Applied Industrial Hygiene*, Vol.2, No.5, pages 179-182, September 1987.

19. "Permeation of Protective Garment Material by Liquid Halogenated Ethanes and a Polychlorinated Biphenyl," 81-110, National Institute for Occupational Safety and Health, January 1981.

20. Plante, D.M., and J.S. Walker. "EMS Response at a Hazardous Material Incident: Some Basic Guidelines." *Journal of Emergency Medicine*, Vol.7, No.1, pages 55-64, 1989.

21. Rosen, M. J. *Surfactants and Interfacial Phenomena*. Wiley-Interscience Publication, NY, 1978. 304 pp.

22. Rybak, Carl. "Guidelines for Operation of HERL Carcinogenic Dilution Room." Unpublished Draft. U.S. Environmental Protection Agency Health Effects Research Laboratory (HERL), Cincinnati, OH, 1981.

23. Tucker, Samuel P. "Deactivation of Hazardous Chemical Waste by Methods Other Than Conventional Incineration and Biological

Degradation." Unpublished Draft. National Institute for Occupational Safety and Health, Cincinnati, OH, 1983.

24.   U.S. Environmental Protection Agency/Hazardous Response Support Division (EPA/HRSD). Personnel Protection and Safety-Training Manual. National Training and Technology Center, U.S. Environmental Protection Agency, Cincinnati, OH, 1982.

25.   U.S. Environmental Protection Agency/Office of Emergency and Remedial Response (EPA/OERR). Interim Standard Operating Safety Guides. Edison, NJ, September 1982.

26.   U.S. Environmental Protection Agency, Office of Solid Waste and Emergency Response. Draft Manual for Infectious Waste Management. EPA-SW-957, U.S. Environmental Protection Agency, Washington, D.C., 1982. 147 pp.

27.   Vo-Dinh Tuan. "Surface Detection of Contamination: Principles, Applications, and Recent Developments." *Journal of Environmental Sciences*. January/February 1983, pp. 40-43.

28.   Vo-Dinh and Gammage. "The Use of a Fiberscope Skin Contamination Monitor in the Workplace." Chemical Hazards in the Workplace, American Chemical Society, 1981a, pp. 269-281.

29.   Vo-Dinh and Gammage. "The Lightpipe Luminoscope for Monitoring Occupational Skin Contamination." *American Industrial Hygiene Association Journal* (42), 1981b, pp. 112-120.

30.   Vogel. *Vogel's Textbook of Practical Organic Chemistry*. Longman Group Ltd., London, 1979, pp. 940-947.

31.   Vahdat, N., and R. Delany. "Decontamination of Chemical Protective Clothing." *American Industrial Hygiene Association Journal*, Vol.50, No.3, pages 152-156, March 1989.

12

TRAINING

William F. Martin, M.S., P.E.
Wm. Bryon T. Witmer, M.S., Ph.D.
Richard C. Montgomery, M.S.

Hazardous materials and hazardous waste training have long been topics of discussion among industrial personnel, emergency response teams, regulatory agencies, and allied groups. A number of successful programs have been designed to meet specific needs [1]. While it is not possible to design one single curriculum to meet all training needs, it should be equally obvious that a number of generalities and guidelines exist that are useful in developing hazardous material training programs [2].

Anyone who enters a hazardous waste site must be able to recognize and understand the potential health and safety hazards associated with the cleanup of the site. Personnel working on the site must be thoroughly familiar with work practices and procedures contained in the site health and safety plan (see Chapter 16, Site Health and Safety Plans). Site workers must be trained to work safely and use sound environmental management practices wherever there is a reasonable possibility of employee exposure to safety, health or environmental hazards.

The training program objectives for hazardous waste site activities include the following:

- to ensure that workers are aware of the potential hazards they may encounter
- to provide the knowledge and skills necessary to perform the work with minimal risk to worker health and safety, and the environment.
- to ensure that workers are aware of the use and limitations of safety equipment
- to ensure that workers can safely avoid or escape from hazardous situations that may occur

The minimum content of the training program may be found in 29 CFR 1910, 40 CFR 265 and 49 CFR 126. Workers may not participate in or supervise field activities until they have been trained to a level required by their job function and responsibility.

TRAINING REQUIREMENTS

OSHA regulation 29 CFR 1910.120 identifies the hazardous waste worker and the type of training as follows:

(e) *Training*(1) *General* (i) All employees working on site (such as but not limited to equipment operators, general laborers and others) exposed to hazardous substances, health hazards, or safety hazards and their supervisors and management responsible for the site shall receive training meeting the requirements of this paragraph before they are permitted to engage in hazardous waste operations that could expose them to hazardous substances, safety, or health hazards, and they shall receive review training as specified in this paragraph.

(ii) Employees shall not be permitted to participate in or supervise field activities until they have been trained to a level required by their job function and responsibility.

(2) *Elements to be covered.* The training shall thoroughly cover the following:

(i) Names of personnel and alternates responsible for site safety and health;

(ii) Safety, health and other hazards present on the site;

(iii) Use of personal protective equipment;

(iv) Work practices by which the employee can minimize risks from hazards;

(v) Safe use of engineering controls and equipment on the site;

(vi) Medical surveillance requirements, including recognition of symptoms and signs which might indicate overexposure to hazards.

(3) *Initial training.* (i) General site workers (such as equipment operators, general laborers and supervisory personnel) engaged in hazardous substance removal or other activities which expose or potentially expose workers to hazardous substances and health hazards shall receive a minimum of 40 hours of instruction off the site, and a minimum of three days actual field experience under the direct supervision of a trained, experienced supervisor.

(ii) Workers on site only occasionally for a specific limited task (such as, but not limited to, ground water monitoring, land surveying, or geophysical surveying) and who are unlikely to be exposed over permissible exposure limits and published exposure limits shall receive a minimum of 24 hours of instruction off the site, and the minimum of one day actual field experience under the direct supervision of a trained, experienced supervisor.

(iii) Workers regularly on site who work in areas which have been monitored and fully characterized indicating that exposures are under permissible exposure limits and published exposure limits where respirators are not necessary, and the characterization indicates that there are no health hazards or the possibility of an emergency developing, shall receive a minimum of 24 hours of instruction off the site and the minimum of one day actual field experience under the direct supervision of a trained, experienced supervisor.

(iv) Workers with 24 hours of training who are covered by paragraphs (e)(3)(ii) and (e)(3)(iii) of this section, and who become general site workers who are required to wear respirators, shall have the additional 16 hours of training necessary to total the training specified in paragraph (e)(3)(i).

(4) *Management and supervisor training.* On-site management and supervisors directly responsible for, or who supervise employees engaged in hazardous waste operations shall receive 40 hours initial training, and three days of supervised field experience (the training may be reduced to 24 hours and one day if the only area of their responsibility is employees covered by paragraphs (e)(3)(ii) and (e)(3)(iii) and at least eight additional hours of specialized training at the time of job assignment on such topics as, but not limited to, the employer's safety and health program and the associated employee training program, personal protective equipment program, spill containment program and health hazard monitoring procedure and techniques.

(5) *Qualifications for trainers.* Trainers shall be qualified to instruct employees about the subject matter that is being presented in training. Such trainers shall have satisfactorily completed a training program for teaching the subjects they are expected to teach, or they shall have the academic credentials and instructional experience necessary for teaching the subjects. Instructors shall demonstrate competent instructional skills and knowledge of the applicable subject matter.

(6) *Training certification.* Employees and supervisors that have received and successfully completed the training and field experience specified in paragraphs (e)(1) through (e)(4) of this section shall be certified by their instructor or the head instructor and trained supervisor as having successfully completed the necessary training. A written certificate shall be given to each person so certified. Any person who has not been so certified or who does not meet the requirements of paragraph (e)(9) of this section shall be prohibited from engaging in hazardous waste operations.

(7) *Emergency response.* Employees who are engaged in responding to hazardous emergency situations at hazardous waste clean-up sites that may expose them to hazardous substances shall be trained in how to respond to such expected emergencies.

(8) *Refresher training.* Employees specified in paragraph (e)(1) of this section, and managers and supervisors specified in paragraph (e)(4) of this section, shall receive eight hours of refresher training annually on the items specified in paragraph (e)(2) and/or (e)(4) of this section, any critique of incidents that have occurred in the past year that can serve as training examples of related work, and other relevant topics.

(9) *Equivalent training.* Employers who can show by documentation or certification that an employee's work experience and/or training has resulted in training equivalent to that training required in paragraphs (e)(1) through (e)(4) of this section shall not be required to provide the initial training requirements of those paragraphs to such employees. However, certified employees or employees with equivalent training new to a site shall receive appropriate, site specific training before site entry and have appropriate supervised field experience at the new site. Equivalent training includes any academic training or the training that existing employees might have already received from actual hazardous waste site work experience.

CONTENT OF TRAINING PROGRAM

The training program must contain fundamental information such as effects and risks of safety and health hazards, as well as site-specific information such as the names of site personnel in charge. Table 12-1 lists the course content proposed by OSHA for workers at hazardous waste cleanup projects and RCRA treatment storage and disposal (TSD) facilities.

Table 12-1. Proposed Content of Training Course[a]				
	40-hr	24-hr	16-hr	8-hr[b]
1 Overview of the applicable paragraphs of 29 CFR 1910.120 and the elements of an employer's effective occupational safety and health program.	X	X		
2 Effect of chemical exposures to hazardous substances (i.e., toxicity, carcinogens, irritants, sensitizers, etc.).	X	X	X	
3 Effects of biological and radiological exposures.	X	X		
4 Fire and explosion hazards (i.e., flammable and combustible liquids, reactive materials).	X	X	X	
5 General safety hazards, including electrical hazards, powered equipment hazards, walking-working surface hazards and those hazards associated with hot and cold temperature extremes.	X	X	X	
6 Confined space, tank and vault hazards and entry procedures.	X	X	X	
7 Names of personnel and alternates, where appropriate, responsible for site safety and health at the site.	X		X	
8 Specific safety, health and other hazards that are to be addressed at a site and in the site safety and health plan.	X	X		
9 Use of personal protective equipment and the implementation of the personal protective equipment program.	X	X		X
10 Work practices that will minimize employee risk from site hazards.	X	X		
11 Safe use of engineering controls and equipment and any new relevant technology or procedure.	X	X		
12 Content of the medical surveillance program and requirements, including the recognition of signs and symptoms of overexposure to hazardous substances.	X	X		
13 The contents of an effective site safety and health plan.	X	X		X
14 Use of monitoring equipment with "hands-on" experience and the implementation of the employee and site monitoring program.	X	X	X	
15 Implementation and use of the informational program.	X		X	
16 Drum and container handling procedures and the elements of a spill containment program.	X	X	X	X

Table 12-1. Proposed Content of Training Course[a]

		40-hr	24-hr	16-hr	8-hr[b]
17	Selection and use of material handling equipment.	X		X	
18	Methods for assessment of risk and handling of radioactive wastes.	X		X	
19	Methods for handling shock-sensitive wastes.	X		X	
20	Laboratory waste pack handling procedures.	X		X	
21	Container sampling procedures and safeguards.	X		X	
22	Safe preparation procedures for shipping and transport of containers.	X		X	
23	Decontamination program and procedures.	X	X	X	X
24	Emergency response plan and procedures including first-aid.	X	X		
25	Safe site illumination levels.	X		X	
26	Site sanitation procedures and equipment for employee needs.	X		X	
27	Review of the applicable appendices to 29 CFR 1910.120.	X	X	X	
28	Overview and explanation of OSHA's hazard communication standard (29 CFR 1910.1200).	X	X	X	
29	Sources of reference, additional information and efficient use of relevant manuals and hazard coding systems.	X	X	X	
30	Principles of toxicology and biological monitoring	X	X		
31	Rights and responsibilities of employees and employers under OSHA and CERCLA.	X	X		
32	"Hands-on" field exercises and demonstrations.	X	X		
33	Review of employer's training program and personnel responsible for that program.		X		
34	Final examination.	X	X	X	
35	Management of hazardous wastes and their disposal.				X
36	Federal, state and local agencies to be contacted in the event of a release of hazardous substances.				X
37	Management of emergency procedures in the event of a release of hazardous substances.				X

[a] Source: From OSHA Hazardous Waste Training 29 CFR 1910.120.
[b] Eight hour course for managers.

TYPES OF TRAINING

General Site Workers

General site workers, including equipment operators, general laborers, technicians, and other supervised personnel, should have training that provides an overview of the site, specific hazards and their risks, hazard recognition, and how to properly use the engineered controls and other means of controlling the site's hazards and risks. General site workers should receive close supervision from a trained, experienced supervisor at least during the first 24 hours following training. Some employees require additional follow-up training to develop good work practices on new tasks. Daily safety reviews just prior to commencing site work for the shift are a good way to give refresher training, make sure that everyone understands the tasks for the day, and inform workers of any new conditions on the site.

A few general site workers who may occasionally supervise others or must deal with special hazards should receive additional training in the following areas:

- site surveillance
- management of hazardous wastes and their disposal
- use and decontamination of fully encapsulating protective clothing and equipment
- federal, state and local agencies to be contacted in the event of a release of hazardous substances
- management of emergency procedures in the event of a release of hazardous substances

On-site Management and Supervisors

On-site management and supervisors, such as team leaders, who are responsible for directing others should receive the same training as the general site workers for whom they are responsible. They also need additional training to enhance their ability to provide guidance and make informed decisions. This training should include supervisory skills, planning and management of site cleanup operations, and techniques to communicate with the press and community.

Health and Safety Staff

Those with specific responsibilities for health and safety guidance on-site should be familiar with the training provided to general site workers and their supervisors and should receive advanced training in hazardous substance health and safety sampling, monitoring, surveillance, evaluation, and control procedures.

On-site Emergency Personnel

Those who have emergency roles in addition to their ordinary duties must have a thorough grounding in emergency response. Training should be directly related to their specific roles and should include subjects such as the following:

- emergency chain of command
- communication methods and signals
- how to call for help
- emergency equipment and its use
- emergency evacuation while wearing PPE
- removing injured personnel from enclosed spaces
- off-site support and how to use it

These personnel should obtain certification in first aid and CPR and practice treatment techniques regularly, with an emphasis on (1) recognizing and treating chemical and physical injuries, and (2) recognizing and treating heat and cold stress.

Off-site Emergency Personnel

Off-site emergency personnel include, for example, local fire fighters and ambulance crews, who often provide front-line response and run the risk of acute hazard exposure equal to that of any on-site worker. These personnel must be trained to recognize and deal effectively with on-site hazards. Lack of training may lead to their inadvertently worsening an emergency by improper actions (e.g., spraying water on a water-reactive chemical and causing an explosion). Inadequate knowledge of the on-site emergency chain of command may cause confusion and delays. Site management should, at a minimum, supplement off-site personnel emergency training with the following information:

- site-specific hazards
- appropriate response techniques
- site emergency procedures
- decontamination procedures

Visitors

Visitors to the site, including elected and appointed officials, reporters, and senior-level management, should receive a safety briefing. These visitors should not be permitted in the exclusion zone unless they have been trained, fit-tested, and medically approved for respirator use. An observation tower in the clean zone reduces the need for visitors to enter the contaminated area.

RECORD OF TRAINING

A record of training should be maintained to confirm that every person assigned to a task has had adequate training for that task and that every employee's training is up to date. It is very important to document the training. Performance measurements prior to site entry are good personnel management and protection against future liability.

A CONCEPTUAL FRAMEWORK FOR PROGRAM DEVELOPMENT

In order to develop a good sound hazardous waste worker training program in an orderly and systematic fashion, one must view the task in conceptual terms. Typically, program start-up involves a preparation stage, a development stage, an implementation stage, and an evaluation stage. If the program status goes beyond that of a pilot, an improvement feedback loop develops between the evaluation and implementation stages.

THE PREPARATION STAGE

During this preliminary phase, a number of considerations must be addressed, including a complete needs assessment. In assessing the needs for a hazardous material control program, questionnaires, pre-tests, and standard compilations of sociometric data can be relied upon. During this phase of operations in developing the program, staff members evaluate existing hazardous material training programs and seminars.

Audience analysis represents another often neglected part of this preparatory phase of development. The creation of a successful hazardous material control program must begin with an adequate audience analysis. Various tools may be used to compile data on potential audiences, but it remains the sole responsibility of the program development team to analyze, assimilate, and apply such data. The goals and objectives for a program on proper use and maintenance of a self-contained breathing apparatus will vary significantly depending upon whether the primary audience is composed of experienced response team members or novices. Similarly, there may be considerable gaps between the manipulative abilities of an experienced response person and those of a lab technician. Again, no single program can accommodate all of the needs of a highly diversified audience; however, in order to succeed, a program must be directed toward a specific target audience.

Before turning away from the topic of program preparation, the role of the advisory committee as a means of diagnosing needs and analyzing audiences needs to be mentioned. Well-selected advisory groups representing industry and other appropriate agencies are critical to the viability of spill and incident control training programs. One case in point is the Oil Spill Control Course Advisory Committee composed of members from the American Petroleum Institute (API) and major oil companies. Another example is the Hazardous Material Control Course Oversight Committee, chaired by the representative from a major chemical company and made up of representatives from various sectors of the chemical, transportation, and petrochemical industries.

These advisors' groups should carefully refrain from promoting any specific training program. Their purpose is not to endorse the programs, but to provide insights and information regarding how the programs might be better organized and improved in order to meet the most pressing needs of industry. Representatives from the industrial sectors offer excellent sources of information regarding basic training needs as well as valuable audience analysis data. By selecting representatives from a variety of industrial backgrounds and from different geographical locations, it is possible to avoid the parochialism that might otherwise develop in a state or regional training program.

THE DEVELOPMENT STAGE

Once the stage has been set, it is necessary to move into the developmental phase of operations. The bulk of the work to be done in this area entails the development of teaching/learning materials that will be compatible with the needs and audiences identified earlier. The use of modular training units can facilitate continuing education, flexible delivery and ease of update.

Two major areas of activity can be identified in this stage: (1) formulating objectives, and (2) selecting and organizing content [2]. As one might expect, the two areas involving objectives and content have a tendency to overlap. Therefore, it is impractical to regard them as totally separate and distinct; objectives will influence content and vice versa.

In formulating broad-based objectives for a hazardous material control program, the goals of a course should:

1. meet the general needs of those concerned with hazardous material spills including waste handling reporting regulations, control techniques, and recovery operations;

2. focus upon a variety of hazardous substances such that participants could become familiar with a wide range of hazardous materials;

3. cover lower cognitive and theoretical material in the classroom, reinforcing and expanding bases with hands-on manipulative training;

4. introduce participants to pragmatic aspects of personnel protection, toxicology, and site safety operations;

5. familiarize attendees with fire control tactics and strategies that might be relevant and applicable to hazardous material incidents;

6. offer an opportunity for participants to test and evaluate their capabilities by responding to simulated hazardous materials incidents; and

7. serve as a clearinghouse through which attendees could obtain information on the latest equipment, apparatus, and procedures for controlling hazardous material incidents [3].

By using this basic format and making modifications where necessary, it is possible to establish suitable underpinnings not only for a single program, but for a number of spin-off activities as well.

Although these objectives can certainly provide an adequate nucleus for a training program for handling hazardous materials, most instructional staff members find it useful to fine tune such broad-based objectives into more specific *behavioral objectives*. Well-defined behavioral objectives should be written clearly in a manner that incorporates: (1) a readily observable behavior; (2) the conditions or restrictions under which such behavior is to be observed; and (3) the performance level expected of the learner [4]. For example, a behavioral objective involving hazardous waste site assessment might be phrased as follows: "The learner, while wearing an encapsulated suit, will use a standard field identification kit to correctly identify an unknown waste sample taken from an overpack drum within one hour." The components of the behavioral objective are identified below:

Observable behavior -	will identify unknown waste sample
Conditions of behavior -	while wearing an encapsulated suit and using a standard field I.D. kit
Performance level -	*correctly* identify within one hour

Such behavioral objectives are useful in providing coherence and unity. Yet, if not used carefully, they may become awkward, restricting program flexibility. For instance, if such detailed objectives actually become an integral part of the course manual, then in order to remain truly accurate each time an objective is altered, the manual itself will have to be modified. For this reason, it is often helpful to include the behavioral objectives on the instructor's lesson plans where they might be altered without disrupting overall program flexibility.

The second major activity in the development stage involves selecting and organizing content. Content selection is normally thought of as a straightforward, linear process. It is commonly thought that one would be able to simply list the major topics of concern, and merely subdivide them in order to prepare a curriculum outline. Unfortunately, this approach presupposes unlimited time and a learning process that proceeds in a predictable, clockwise fashion.

Perhaps one of the greatest difficulties faced by an individual attempting to select content for a training program of this nature is in determining what to include and what not to include. As suggested earlier, a careful audience analysis and well-formulated objectives make this task easier. Still, program developers often find themselves with too much material and too little time. Content must be selected such that the material can be presented to the *target audience* within the specified time constraints. The key here lies within the ability to reach the specific target audience identified earlier. Participants on the periphery of this audience should not be ignored; nor can they expect the program to accommodate them at the expense of the target group. As a matter of fact, such peripheral participants will generally derive at least some benefit from the content selected for the target audience. Priorities must be established so that the most important information receives primary consideration.

Coincidental to content selection is content organization. Topics should generally be structured so that there is movement from the known to the unknown, from the simple to the complex, from the easy to the difficult [2]. It is often advantageous to identify certain core ideas that seem to represent the very essence of certain topics. Without fail these ideas and concepts fall within the realm of both basic and vital. Surrounding these vital kernels are myriads of information which are mostly represented in as basic. What must be done, then, is to select certain clusters of information from these areas that will selectively reinforce and expand the core ideas. This concept of organizing content with respect to core and cluster areas is not new, yet it is seldom applied in the areas of training for hazardous material and hazardous waste handling.

THE IMPLEMENTATION STAGE

The third major phase of program development, that of implementation, involves translating what has previously existed as theory into practice. Of particular interest are the subjects of selecting and organizing learning experiences, and applying teaching methodologies.

Hazardous material control training offers an excellent opportunity to apply a well-balanced mixture of classroom and field training techniques. This basic teaching-learning design was used by the Texas Engineering Extension Service's Oil Spill Control Course in 1976 as an attempt to successfully mesh traditional classroom presentations with pragmatic hands-on training. In order to achieve the necessary balance between classroom and field training for this program, it was necessary to provide traditional classroom theory as a complement to pragmatic field application. In order to subordinate formal classroom sessions to hands-on training, instructors introduced each major topic through a brief classroom presentation and relied upon field exercises for reinforcement and practical clarification. Instructors also attempted to enhance student participation through discussion groups, problem-solving exercises, and questions and answer periods. Subsequent evaluation of this early program revealed four primary benefits:

1. by encouraging participation, students benefit from *active* as opposed to *passive* learning;
2. similarly, student participation in a seminar atmosphere provides for valuable exchange of information among the students themselves;
3. introducing basics in class and reinforcing and expanding them with hands-on training tempers textbook learning with actual experience; and
4. finally, this type of arrangement allows the course to be taught effectively, by following the "spiral step" method.

The spiral step methodology is the underlying strategy inherent in this type of program. This approach exposes course participants to units of subject matter in increasing order of complexity, continuously reinforcing them with appropriate skill developing exercises. Hence, the order of moving from the simple to the complex, the known to the unknown, and the easy to the difficult is maintained. Moreover, this pedagogical approach helps to preserve the unity of the curriculum as established during the preparation and development stages by providing certain "threads" or common denominators that link basic concepts in an overall spiral configuration. One of the greatest arguments in favor of this strategy lies not in its ability to preserve order and unity, but in its tendency to promote what has been called cumulative learning. Learning involves the cumulative development of mental skills such that each succeeding idea or question requires an increasingly difficult mental operation [2]. When training in hazardous material control, however, this cumulative effect involves not only the cognitive but also the manipulative domain. Participants are thereby able to simultaneously expand both dimensions of their abilities. The schematic in Figure 12-1 depicts how one isolated area—toxicological considerations—is introduced, expanded, and reinforced in a spiral step manner. It is important to note that the curriculum is designed such that each successive upward spiral represents an increase in both the complexity of the material covered and the difficulty with which physical skills are mastered, thus helping to foster cumulative learning.

While the spiral step approach is a crucial element in curriculum design and integration, there are other teaching methodologies and precepts that also bear mentioning. One such element involves the depth with which field training is carried out. Care must be taken to avoid structuring practical

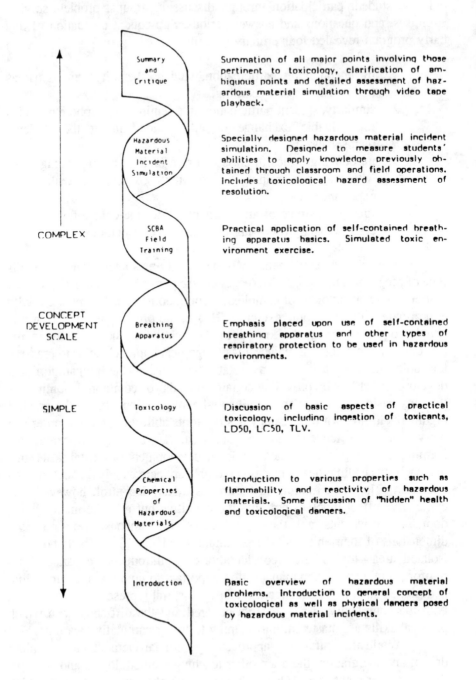

Figure 12-1. Spiral step curriculum design.

exercises as demonstrations. While certain demonstrations are useful, they simply cannot replace active student participation. In addition, field training must be carried out under realistic conditions in order to be most effective. Of course such realistic field training necessitates careful supervision by qualified instructors as well as enthusiastic participation by course attendees. Often overlooked in many programs is the need to keep such practical exercises small in order to maintain an adequate instructor-participant ratio. Depending upon the exact nature of the exercise, an adequate ratio for field training may be maintained by providing one instructor for every five to 10 participants. Going beyond a limit of 10 participants per instructor may create logistics problems as well as safety hazards under certain conditions. Likewise, it may force the instructor to rely more heavily upon strategies normally reserved for demonstrations, diminishing the desired effect of the field exercises.

In addition to the spiral step approach, techniques to help bridge the gap between theory and application need to be applied to training programs involving hazardous materials control. It has been previously noted that a well-designed spiral step curriculum can provide a sound basis for cumulative learning. Well-formulated objectives, properly selected content, and carefully chosen teaching methods all combine to form an integrated and balanced program. Basic topics are presented in classroom sessions, and expanded and specifically applied under field conditions. Thus, a student may learn a considerable amount about SCBAs in the classroom and may develop a fair amount of expertise in using them under field conditions. The same might be said for a number of other topics such as protective clothing, waste recovery, and spill control. However, there must exist a means of helping the course participants to assimilate this knowledge into a broad perspective. In other words, they must be able to take this information and apply it to a greater scenario such as a hazardous waste dump site, a train derailment, or a hazardous material spill.

One way of bridging the gap between the acquisition and the application of information is through a written problem session. Such a problem session must necessarily come after participants have covered the bulk of the course material. Inserted into the programming at this point, the problem session becomes a tool with which the instructors and participants might generate a positive attitude and response. Attempting to place the problem session too early in the programming before all basic materials have been covered would lead to confusion and probably a feeling of negativism.

Such a session usually works best if it is carefully thought out and uses accurate maps and descriptions of the problem scenario. All variables such as date, location, meteorological conditions, logistics, and available supplies and manpower are generally given by the instructor. All that remains, then, is for the participants to respond to the scenario within these guidelines. Of course some double-sided problems are included, not to trick participants, but to alert them to hidden difficulties that may not be readily apparent. As a group response this strategy works well; not only do the group members use what they have learned as a result of the training program, but they also draw upon their own experiences and those of their peers. Most importantly, they are allowed the luxury of seeing a complete scenario unfold and develop before their eyes. Quite literally, they may respond to a full-blown incident without leaving their chairs. At this point they begin to make the transition from simply acquiring the information to applying it.

Finally, some means of going beyond this armchair quarterback situation is desirable as both a measuring device and confidence builder. The full-scale field simulation provides this means. Incorporated into a program after all basic knowledge and skills have been introduced and expanded, the field simulation is designed to approximate as nearly as possible "the real thing". Because it is designed as a test of sorts, the simulation should not be used by instructors as a device to measure individual skills and competencies. Rather, it should be seen as a measure of the entire group's ability to function under the stress of an actual incident. Individuals must assess the overall situation, sort through the relevant variables, determine appropriate response measures, and initiate them accordingly. The more realistic the controlled conditions are, the more successful the simulation is likely to be. Performing under such conditions has a tendency to dispel any attitude of "it's only a game". Realistic conditions also have a way of producing stress in individuals to a point where they perform at the upper limits of their capabilities. Furthermore, such simulations often serve as confidence builders. For maximum effectiveness, it is helpful to videotape the simulated incident for prompt playback. The videotape playback serves as an informal critique of the group's overall response. Instructors must be careful to avoid playing too obvious a role in the critique. Emphasis must be placed upon constructive criticism. It is imperative that the instructor moderate this critique work skillfully to allow the participants to provide the greatest bulk of the feedback. Experience has shown in many cases that the enthusiasm from a well-designed simulation carries over so that those involved actually do a better job of evaluating their performances than the instructors.

THE EVALUATION STAGE

One of the most important aspects of any educational program involves an assessment of the success of the program as perceived by the instructor and participant. In most traditional settings the primary evaluative tool directed toward the student is the formal examination. In hazardous materials control training courses, the use of formal examinations is recommended. In addition, in these courses and other short industrial courses, it appears that the use of individualized instruction tactics might be applied effectively. Such tactics normally require that the instructors develop a rapport with course participants so that they might continuously receive and digest feedback from them. By so doing, the instructor can accommodate participants by clarifying and expanding upon course information as required. Although this tactic develops around and exists upon a relatively informal phase, it nonetheless offers a reasonable means of monitoring and improving student performance.

Another evaluative tool mentioned earlier is the hazardous material simulation. As discussed, the simulation provides the basis for a post-incident critique that may be helpful in evaluating the group's overall response; however, it rarely develops enough detail to allow for individual evaluation. Indiscriminate use of such critiques can often do more damage than good by attempting to place blame and highlight individual mistakes.

Although it is important to assess levels of student performance, it is perhaps even more important to determine the strengths and weaknesses of the program itself. This may be especially true in the case of short, continuing education courses. Course evaluations provide basic feedback essential to program improvement. Such an evaluation should be simple, easily tallied, and should allow for comments regarding each specific topic of presentation of a program. Moreover, an attempt should be made to ensure that students regard such evaluations as important tools. Accuracy and honesty must be emphasized in the name of constructive criticism. An important point here is that the actual presentation, not the instructor, should be evaluated. It is wise to prompt course participants to evaluate each session as it concludes rather than evaluating all the sessions at the end of the course. It is also important to solicit suggestions and other comments that might be helpful in improving the course. Anonymity often helps to ensure objective ratings. Figure 12-2 illustrates one typical course evaluation sheet used successfully by the Texas Engineering Extension Service.

Session Date _____

HAZARDOUS MATERIAL CONTROL COURSE
EVALUATION SHEET

This evaluation sheet will provide important feedback that will allow us to make improvements in the course. Please assist us by responding completely.

1. Circle the appropriate response. Rank only the presentation--not the instructor or topic.

Chemical Properties   1   2   3   4   5   6   7   8   9   10
of hazardous materials Poor   Average   Good

Comments: _____
_____

Toxicology   1   2   3   4   5   6   7   8   9   10
     Poor   Average   Good
Comments: _____
_____

Breathing Apparatus-   1   2   3   4   5   6   7   8   9   10
SCBA Training   Poor   Average   Good

Comments: _____
_____

Hazardous   1   2   3   4   5   6   7   8   9   10
Environment   Poor   Average   Good

Comments: _____
_____

2. What did you like least?
_____
_____

3. What additional topics or exercises would you like to see added?
_____
_____

4. Were staff members and instructors professional, well-versed and generally capable?
_____
_____

5. Were visual aids and teaching materials of a professional quality, and were they suitable?
_____
_____

Figure 12-2. Typical Course Evaluation Sheet

CULTIVATING THE IMPROVEMENT FEEDBACK LOOP

Course evaluations including written critiques and informal comments must somehow be systematically analyzed if they are to help establish a means of improving the program. Objective tallies might help to identify generic weaknesses in a program, but when used alone often fall short in offering any remedy. Hence, an instructor may receive average ratings of 2 (poor) on three of his five sessions but may receive marks of 9 (good) on the remaining two sessions. Clearly something is amiss with three sections; however, simple numerical marks offer no explanation or possible solution to the problem.

In order to move beyond the identification of generic weaknesses, one must look carefully at specific comments provided by participants. Perhaps in the earlier example a common weakness in visual aids might be suggested by student comments such as "slides were poorly developed and often out of focus" or "transparency materials were smudged and not readable." Such comments provide the functional basis for the improvement feedback loop. Such comments almost always identify what the participant perceives as a weakness. Of course, invalid criticisms are often made and must be regarded as such.

The feedback loop might also be expanded through informal discussions between instructors and course participants. In fact, the suggestion to videotape the Oil Spill Control Course simulation as a critique came about partly as a result of such an informal discussion. Advisory group suggestions often surface in this feedback loop and emerge as significant course improvements.

In summation, it is necessary to view the four-stage program development process as a dynamic one. The first stage of preparation helps to establish a basis for further development. The second stage involves formulating objectives and choosing and arranging content material in a manner to best facilitate learning. The third phase of the development process involves the actual methodologies required to translate theory into practice. The fourth stage concerns analysis of both the program and its participants. Finally, an improvement feedback loop develops as a logical outgrowth of program evaluation. It is through this link between the evaluation and implementation stages that a program may be updated and improved. The loop itself helps to ensure that the program development process remains dynamic.

ORGANIZATIONS OFFERING TRAINING PROGRAMS

A wide variety of hazardous waste training programs have been developed by other government and industrial organizations in the United States. Many of these programs are available to the public for a registration fee [1, 3, 4, 5, 6, 7, 8, 9].

A survey, sponsored by Wayne State University, was integrated into a United States Public Health Service, Bureau of Health Professions contract designed to investigate the appropriateness and adequacy of hazardous waste education in the United States. The study covers two areas; 1) hazardous waste education provided by academic institutions in the form of regular, credit course work and degrees, and 2) hazardous waste education provided through non-credit continuing education short courses, workshops, and training sessions. The results of the survey were converted into a public access electronic bulletin board. The following several pages provide an abstract of the Wayne State University Survey [1].

Data Gathering Procedure

For this part of the study, information was collected using a questionnaire. This questionnaire was designed to collect information on:

1) The type of hazardous waste education offered (undergraduate, graduate, or non-credit).
2) The colleges and/or departments participating in each type of education offered.
3) The degrees offered which contain hazardous waste education and whether that offering is required, elective or part of an option.
4) Whether the hazardous waste program is accredited.
5) The inception date of any degrees, options, certifications, individual credit courses or non-credit courses offered in hazardous waste.
6) A request for program brochures and course outlines.

It was necessary in some cases to augment the responses on the questionnaire using references such as the *1989 Peterson's Guide to Graduate Programs in Engineering and Applied Science*, the *1988 Graduate School Guide* and the *AIChE Graduate School Directory*.

Initially, the survey was mailed selectively to groups of schools which were likely to have programs. These groups included:

- National Environmental Health Association (NEHA) Educational Institution members
- Accredited U.S. Schools of Public Health
- National Institute for Occupational Safety and Health (NIOSH) funded schools
- National Institute of Environmental Health Sciences (NIEHS) funded schools
- Directors of Centers for Superfund Research
- Directors of Centers for Hazardous Waste Management
- Schools offering degrees in Industrial Safety and Health or Environmental and Occupational Health
- Members of the Association of Environmental Engineering Professors

After some replies were received and the questionnaire was refined using comments from the expert review panel, a comprehensive mailing of 1,469 was conducted. This mailing list was obtained from the *1989 HEP Higher Education Directory* which contains a listing of all accredited institutions of post-secondary education in the United States which meet the U.S. Department of Education eligibility requirements.

A telephone follow-up was used to contact institutions which did not respond to the mail survey. Sources which were used to identify institutions for the follow-up included:

- The original mailing list from the *1989 HEP Higher Education Director*
- An EPA Database on Educational Opportunities for Environmental Professionals
- The EPA National Evaluation of Training and Technical Assistance in State RCRA Programs
- An Illinois Institute of Technology list of college and university-based research centers in hazardous waste

Wayne State University Survey Results

Of the 1469 institutions contacted, 799 replied (54%). Of those 799, 591 (74%) have no hazardous waste education of any kind. Of the 208 remaining institutions, 167 offer at least one credit course as part of a degree program and 89 have non-credit training programs. Forty-one offer only non-credit continuing education courses. Of the 167 offering credit courses, about half (82) have hazardous waste courses that are required for the respective degree. The majority of degrees containing hazardous waste education are in engineering, particularly Civil, Environmental and Chemical Engineering. Offerings through Environmental Science, Public Health and Environmental Health are slightly less numerous.

Figure 12-3 provides a profile of the types of hazardous waste instruction offered at either or both (if applicable) undergraduate and graduate levels. Since courses are often offered at both levels and courses required of some students are electives for others, there is an overlap between the designated bars. While 117 universities offer at least one course at the undergraduate level and 116 at the graduate level, elimination of duplication

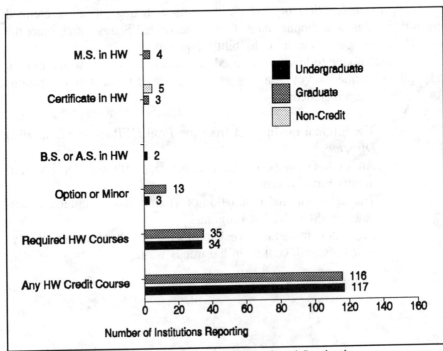

Figure 12-3. Profile of Educational Institution
Hazardous Waste Instruction Offerings [1]

yields 167 different institutions offering credit courses in hazardous waste management.

The survey identified four masters degrees, 13 graduate options, and three credit-based certificates in hazardous waste/materials management. The four masters degree programs are offered by: New Jersey Institute of Technology in Newark, Tufts University in Medford, Wayne State University in Detroit and the University of San Francisco.

A total of 675 distinct short courses were evaluated. The largest segment of the short courses deal with legal, administrative and compliance related issues. Figure 12-4 presents a breakdown of the course offerings by subject.

Courses are offered through a variety of different avenues including government, universities, professional organizations and private industry. The U.S. EPA Office of Solid Waste and Emergency Response has been identified as the largest single provider of hazardous waste related short courses, offering approximately 36 distinct short courses per quarter and 154 total courses per quarter including replications. The next three largest suppliers are Executive Enterprises, Inc., Georgia Institute of Technology, and Texas A&M University, respectively.

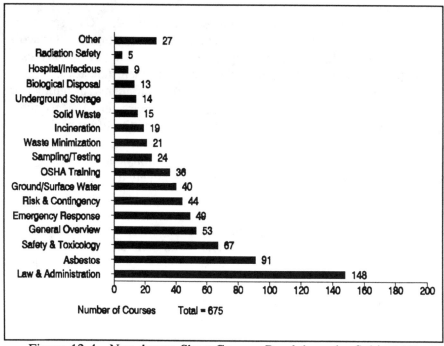

Figure 12-4. Non-degree Short Courses Breakdown by Subject [1]

Additional Sources of Training Program Information

A number of companies have developed excellent training programs, many of which began as in-house projects designed to meet specific corporate needs. One presentation developed along these lines is Texaco's videotaped hazardous materials program.

Developed in 1982, the program was targeted at the multidisciplined, broad-based spill cleanup management teams that had previously undergone Texaco's similarly developed oil spill response training program [12]. The videotape format was selected as the most viable for a number of reasons including cost and in-house availability of existing playback equipment.

The Texaco program appears to be well grounded in its topical approach to subject matter. The program is also well designed in that it makes use of a tutored videotape instruction concept that allows for student-instructor dialogue and employs strategically placed breaks to avoid taxing the attention span of the student. Texaco's premise is that if properly used, the program teaches through repetition [12]. The program appears to be a well-constructed in-house program with enough flexibility for a variety of job levels. While the program lacks significant hands-on activities, Texaco has been careful to point out that this particular program is not directed toward individuals involved in actual hands-on activities relating to hazardous materials incidents.

Other corporate developed courses are Du Pont's "RIT" series and Union Carbide's "H.E.L.P." programs. These programs, similar to Texaco's, were developed in-house for the purpose of training company employees to handle hazardous materials emergencies specific to their industries.

In addition to these types of industry programs, a number of governmental agencies offer training activities. Swiss, et al., describe a response training program developed through a cooperative effort between the Environmental Emergency Division of the Canadian Environmental Protection Service, Atlantic Region and the provincial Environment and Emergency Measures Organization. This training activity is largely directed at volunteer firefighters and is designed to be presented at various extension centers throughout each province [9].

Leading educational institutions including Iowa State University, The University of Michigan, and Louisiana State University offer various programs in hazardous material and waste control. Other training courses include those offered by cleanup contractors, consultants, and similar groups. Weiss and Leigh in their description of Texaco's in-house training program provided an interesting comparison of hazardous materials control programs offered by a number of groups [12]. Such an overview is interesting only as a topical comparison of curriculum design, methodologies, and philosophical approaches.

NIOSH developed in 1983-84, an occupational safety and health training program for superfund activities. The three-day course materials concentrate on hazard recognition and hazard control. The courses are available through educational resource centers in universities that have training grants from NIOSH, located throughout the United States [13].

The Department of Defense (DoD) has developed an entire range of training programs to prepare their employees for the environmental clean up task facing the U.S. military organizations. The Environmental Training Center, U.S. Army, Fort Sill, Oklahoma has undertaken a major portion of this task with courses specifically designed to protect the environment, personnel and the public. The Army's training courses emphasize practical hands-on training, a very good adaptation of DoD's long standing use of performance-type training. State and local employees have been given access to these courses as the DoD prepares to transfer property and facilities to local control.

The DoD has several specialized training programs that have world-wide recognition such as Explosive Ordnance Disposal (EOD) located at the Naval Ordnance Station in Indian Head, Maryland; a satellite facility at Eglin Air Force Base, Florida; and the Huntsville Corps of Engineers, Huntsville, Alabama (see Chapter 15, Ordnance, Explosive Waste, and Unexploded Ordnance for more details).

Several groups such as the states of Utah and California, and USEPA Region 7, have taken the hazardous waste training far beyond the minimum 40 hours of HAZWOPER. USEPA Region 7, Kansas City, Kansas has developed an excellent modular training program that consists of between 200 and 300 contract hours. The modular concept facilitates continuing education, ease of updates and flexibility of delivery over time. Much of the modular training content was developed by Ecology and Environmental, Inc., Overland, Kansas with direct input from EPA offices in Cincinnati, Ohio; Edison, New Jersey; and Kansas City, Kansas.

With today's emphasis on controlling hazardous materials, wastes, and by-products, a proliferation of training programs aimed at these audiences is hardly unexpected. Many diverse groups are offering programs directed at managing and controlling releases of hazardous materials. The text by Shaye, adapted from Volume II of the *EPA Directory of Hazardous Materials Response Training*, gives a regional listing of the programs being offered and their major points of emphasis [8, 11]. The *Directory* itself is approximately 190 pages long and gives detailed information about each training program.

Another similar publication, Hazardous Materials Spills Management Review, prepared for the American Petroleum Institute by the Texas Transportation Institute and the Texas Engineering Extension Service, provides statistical data about hazardous materials training programs. Of those programs documented by this review, 50 percent constitute training courses of some length while the remaining 50 percent are composed of short conferences and seminars. Hands-on training of some type appears in approximately 54 percent of the programs. Most of the programs are oriented toward public safety personnel (38 percent) with a slightly smaller percentage (34 percent) oriented toward private industry audiences. The remainder (28 percent) of the courses are directed toward governmental personnel and others [10]. These statistics suggest that high priorities are placed upon providing training to both public and private company response personnel. One might conclude that such training would emphasize emergency control and stabilization techniques as opposed to management overviews of hazardous materials. Moreover, the fact that 54 percent of the programs offer some type of hands-on training seems to indicate that programs which are both practical and applicable are favored by a majority of trainees. As in the case of the *EPA Directory*, the *Hazardous Materials - Spills Management Review* provides details including course length, topics, tuition costs, and contact person for each program catalogued.

In addition to these two major directories of hazardous material control training programs, there are several other sources of information. Federal agencies such as the Department of Transportation, the Environmental Protection Agency, the National Institute for Occupational Safety and Health, and the Occupational Safety and Health Administration may provide valuable information on program availability. Other groups such as the Chemical Manufacturers' Association, National Environmental Training Association, and the National Tank Truck Carriers Association may also be able to provide information on programs.

CONCLUSION

Today's burgeoning technology brings with it tomorrow's promise of increased production of hazardous materials and wastes. The common challenge facing industry, state and local government, and leading academic institutions is that of ensuring that such technical advances do not occur at the expense of public health and safety.

A practical part of this challenge involves hazardous material and waste control training. Those on the cutting edge of technology must endeavor to see that training should develop in conjunction with emerging technologies. Traditional approaches to training must be critically evaluated and bolstered where necessary with new and perceptive insights. Training techniques cannot remain static; for only through systematic growth and development will training help society rise to meet the challenge of the future.

REFERENCES

1. Hughes, Colleen L, R.H. Kummler, R.W. Powitz and C.A. Witt, "Hazardous Waste Management Education and Training in the United States," USEPA U.S. Public Health Service Study conducted by Wayne University, Detroit, MI, 1990.

2. Taba, Hilda. Curriculum Development: Theory and Practice (San Francisco: Harcourt, Brace and World, 1962).

3. Payne, J. L., and C. B. Strong. "Taking Technology Off the Shelf: Texas A&M's Hazardous Material Control Program," in *Proceedings of the 1980 National Conference on Hazardous Material Spills*, Louisville, KY, May 13-15, 1980.

4. Mager, Robert F. *Preparing Instructional Objectives* (Belmont, CA: Fearon Publishers, Lear Siegler, Inc., 1962).

5. "Accreditation of Training Programs for Hazardous Waste Operations." Federal Register 55, no. 18 (26 January 1990).

6. Fournier, S. *Hazardous Waste: Training Manual for Supervisors.* Business Legal Reports, 1985.

7. J.J. Keller & Associates, Inc. *Hazardous Communication Guide.* Nennah, WI: J.J. Keller & Associates, Inc., 1987.

8. Shaye, M.K. *Hazardous Waste Workers Health & Safety Training Requirements & 29 CFR 1910.120.* Detroit.

9. Swiss, J. J., W. S. Davis, and R. G. Simmons. "On-scene Response Training Program," in the *1982 Hazardous Material Spills Conference Proceedings*, Milwaukee, April 19-22, 1982.

10. *Hazardous Materials Spills - Management Review*, prepared for the American Petroleum Institute by the Texas Transportation Institute and the Texas Engineering Extension Service, (College Station, Texas: The Texas A&M University System, 1980).

11. U.S. Environmental Protection Agency, *Training Course Catalogue—EPA*. GPO Publication No. 91072969. Cincinnati: EPA, June 1990.

12. Weiss, H. J. and J. Leigh. "Development of an In-House Hazardous Materials Training Program," in the *1982 Hazardous Material Spills Conference Proceedings*, Milwaukee, April 19-22, 1982.

13. Martin, W.F., J.M. Melius, C.A. Cottrill. "Management of Hazardous Wastes and Environmental Emergencies," paper presented at National Conference and Exhibition on Hazardous Wastes and Environmental Emergencies, Houston, TX, March 12-14, 1984.

13

CONTINGENCY PLANS

Charles J. Sawyer, C.I.H., P.E.

Uncontrolled hazardous waste sites can present a broad range of potential environmental health and safety problems. Occupational exposure to hazards associated with waste site exploration, sampling, evaluation, and subsequent remediation can be controlled or avoided. The success in controlling adverse exposures depends on the detailed planning, training, scheduling, and execution of a well defined plan to remediate the hazardous wastes site. Such a plan should be drafted utilizing an interdisciplinary team of technical experts, including: analytical chemistry, geology, hydrology, environmental engineering, industrial hygiene, medicine, toxicology, safety and fire protection, civil engineering, and engineering project management.

A key element of the plan is a detailed contingency plan. Because of the range of complexities associated with various uncontrolled hazardous waste sites, site specific information must be carefully integrated to develop a satisfactory remedial action/contingency plan. A contingency plan with all its elements is necessary insurance to protect against upset conditions possibly threatening the health and safety of the workers, and/or the surrounding environment. A well developed plan should minimize the need to ever effect the call-up of a contingency plan. However, if and when an uncontrolled chain of events leads to an emergency situation, a readily adaptable contingency plan with clear responsibilities and sequenced program of activities brought into action should be effective towards prompt restoration of normal operations. Presented in this chapter are those elements that are in part essential to the remediation plan itself but by this focus are necessary to be incorporated for developing a detailed contingency plan. The key elements for discussion are divided into two categories, i.e., preventative and emergency requirements.

The impact of stricter environmental regulations in the United States has created more focus on the importance of the contingency planning process for hazardous wastes site remediation activities. In particular, the Comprehensive Environmental Response, Compensation, and Liability Act, commonly known as "CERCLA" or "Superfund" as enacted into law on December 11, 1980, was substantially amended by the Superfund Amendments and

Reauthorization Act of 1986, i.e., "SARA." On March 8, 1990, EPA promulgated a major revision to the National Contingency Plan (the original NCP was developed by EPA under Section 311 of the Clean Water Act) to serve as the blueprint for remedial response action. These revisions to the NCP serve to not only implement the statutory SARA amendments, but also to codify various procedures and requirements which have evolved during EPA's first 10 years experience with Superfund. Subpart C of the revised NCP discusses the Federal contingency plans which are to be developed, and summarizes the state and local emergency response plans which are required by SARA Title III. Subpart E (formerly Subpart F) is referred to as the National Hazardous Substances Response Plan that establishes the methods and criteria for determining the appropriate response to releases of hazardous substances.

Additionally, under the OSHA regulations entitled Hazardous Waste Operations and Emergency Response (HAZWOPER), embodied under Title 29, Part 1910, Subpart H, employee health and safety requirements and training are identified as an important resource for input to the contingency planning process. As Federal, state, and country environmental regulations changes, it is important to include such regulatory impacts on drafting contingency plans both now and in the future.

PREVENTATIVE REQUIREMENTS

The essentials of the uncontrolled hazardous wastes site contingency plan relative to preventative requirements are discussed in detail under the following individual headings.

Know the Inherent Site Characteristics

One of the key steps in the preventative aspects of a contingency plan is the need for an accurate collection and evaluation of all known and available information on the remediation waste site itself. Table 13-1 summarizes the important items needed to evaluate and understand the inherent site characteristics [1]. Information gaps should be identified and efforts made to deal with prioritizing those areas that could most influence the safe conduct of on-site activities.

Table 13-1. Site Characteristics of Uncontrolled Hazardous Wastes Sites [1]	
Site Characteristics	**Related Considerations**
Topography	Adjacent tenants
Geology	Nearby population centers
Hydrology	Hospital facilities
Climatology	Ambulance service
Wildlife (reptile, animal, insect)	Fire district
Ground cover	Utilities available/proximity
History of sampling/exploration	Industrial equipment rental
Accessibility	Law enforcement
Security	

Know the Waste Parameters at the Site

The degree of hazard in remediating the site essentially depends upon the specific waste chemical types, quantities, method of disposal, etc. Table 13-2 summarizes key information relative to assessing the waste characteristics at the site [1]. Initially (or at any time) when workers will be venturing into unknown conditions the most conservative protective requirements should be incorporated. If there are blends of wastes, controls should be set up to deal with the most toxic chemicals, or the greatest potential hazard, e.g., flammability or explosion. Extreme care is required when dealing with potential incompatibilities of various hazardous waste sources at the site.

Table 13-2. Assessment of Key Waste Characteristics at the Site
1. Sources/volume/form
2. History of waste deposits • Dates • Sources of waste • Type and quantity of wastes
3. Sources of additional information
4. Containment/confinement of waste
5. Waste containers • Types, age, condition
6. Designed confinements • Pits, lagoons, cells, trenches, cover
7. Uncontrolled practices at the site • Open dumping • Open burning • Flooding/evaporation/percolation
8. Hazardous properties of waste site chemicals • Physical and chemical properties - Flammability,   corrosivity, reactivity • Potential toxicity - Acute, chronic
9. On-site wastes compatibility considerations

Effective Project/Site Management

The conduct of cleanup activities must be under the key control of a single project manager (on scene coordinator) whose day-to-day responsibilities include:

- Monitoring and directing the site activities;
- Planning and scheduling;
- Direct resource management: manpower, materials, equipment; and
- Establishing clear communications to field staff, on-site government agency coordinators, the safety coordinator, as well as press and local government officials.

The need to maintain the highest commitment to safety and health at a site rests with one responsible party who is fully knowledgeable, experienced, and capable of acting with dispatch to monitor the day-to-day activities of personal protective procedures, industrial hygiene sampling and air monitoring, decontamination procedures, weather conditions, etc. The role of the on-site Health and Safety coordinator clearly is to provide routine advice and counsel to the project (site) manager relative to health and safety matters. Unsafe conduct or disobedience to the documented safety/health procedures serves as a clear reason for ceasing activities until corrective actions are taken.

Training

All cleanup workers must be fully trained and informed on the potential safety hazards at the site, the toxicity parameters of the waste chemicals at the site, protective equipment requirements, decontamination procedures, safe operation of remediation equipment, fire protection, emergency backup, etc. Table 13-3 presents pertinent subjects for these workers [2, 3, 4, 5]. Classroom education prior to startup is an effective means to *assure* adequate worker training. This should include instruction by various technical disciplines, e.g., industrial hygiene, toxicology, etc., as well as trial runs using requisite safety and remediation equipment for practice under controlled, no risk test environments.

The scope and length of the training program should be adjusted to fit the needs of specific worker tasks as well as the complexities and risks of the individual site. All training sessions should be attended by the official on-scene representatives of the various Federal, state, and local government agencies.

Table 13-3. Training [2, 3, 4, 5]

A. Toxicity of waste site chemicals
    1. Acute toxicity
    2. Chronic toxicity
    3. Dermatologic effects
        a. Chloracne
        b. Other
    4. Epidemiologic studies
    5. Other possible health effects
B. Material Safety Data Sheets (MSDS) for major waste site chemicals
C. Potential routes of waste chemical exposure
    1. Skin Contact
    2. Inhalation
    3. Ingestion
D. Respiratory protection
E. Protective clothing/equipment requirements
F. Industrial hygiene and safety requirements
G. Change room requirements
H. Fire fighting techniques
I. Medical monitoring requirements
    · First-aid
    · CPR
J. Trained to recognize individual medical symptoms possibly indicative of over-exposure to toxic substances:
    1. Irritation of skin, eyes, nose, throat or respiratory tract
    2. Changes in complexion or skin discoloration
    3. Headaches
    4. Difficulty in breathing
    5. Nausea
    6. Dizziness or light-headedness
    7. Excessive salivation or drooling
    8. Lack or coordination
    9. Blurred vision
    10. Cramps and/or diarrhea
    11. Changes in behavior patterns
K. Standard operating procedures
L. Equipment operation training
M. Decontamination procedures
N. Wastes handling techniques
O. Emergency response plans
P. Hazardous spill control
Q. Personal hygiene and cleanliness
R. Off-site hands-on practice
S. On-site dry runs prior to startup

Personal Protective Systems

The formulation of the preventative aspects of a contingency plan places the highest priority on the protection of the health and safety of the workers. Each phase of cleanup activities must receive a detailed review, focusing primarily on preventing possible exposures to the most toxic chemicals, and secondarily on preventing exposure to other materials of somewhat lower toxicity. Particular attention should be given to the various routes of possible exposure to workers via the respiratory tract, skin, and mucous membranes (eyes, nose, and mouth).

Typically there are four possible categories of personal protective equipment (PPE) for hazardous material workers [2, 3, 4]. Selection of specific equipment should reflect the degree of risk associated with specific remediation tasks. The four categories are summarized as follows:

Category I is the most stringent, providing both respiratory and skin/mucous membrane protection of workers engaged in work where a high potential for generation of potentially toxic levels of aerosols, dusts, mists, or organic vapors exists. This category also applies when there exists possible *unknown* risks or complexities associated with specific remedial action tasks.

Category II applies to work activities where complete skin protection is warranted, but the use of air-purifying respirators is suitable to protect against possible low level generation of aerosols, dusts, mists, or organic vapors. The Category II respirator is a combination carbon filter to remove organic chemical vapors and a HEPA-type particulate removal mechanical filter.

Category III applies to work activities where *no* generation of aerosols, dusts, mists, or organic vapors have the opportunity to impact upon the worker.

Category IV applies to providing added worker protection in the case of fire or other emergency.

All respirators must be fit-tested according to established industrial hygiene practices. Workers wearing respirators will be trained to assure proper usage, storage, and maintenance. The choice of Categories I to IV will be made after appropriate consultation with the on-site safety and health coordinator. Whenever the risk is unknown, the maximum personal protection of the workers needs to be assured so that Category I requirements are designated.

Medical Programs

All workers and supervisory personnel who are required to handle contaminated materials should be given a comprehensive preemployment physical examination. Table 13-4 summarizes the minimum medical baseline requirements for each employee [2, 3, 4]. The baseline medical tests should be modified to reflect specific health risks for certain highly toxic chemicals. (For more information, see Chapter 7, Medical Surveillance for Hazardous Waste Workers.)

Table 13-4. Health Screening Examination - Minimum Standards Requirement [2, 3, 4]

A. MEDICAL HISTORY
  Medical information questionnaire
  acquired from participant

B. PHYSIOLOGICAL TESTS
  Height
  Weight
  Blood pressure
   Systolic
   Diastolic
  Vision
   Distance visual
   Acuity
    Left eye
    Right eye
    Both eyes
   Near visual
   Acuity
    Left eye
    Right eye
    Both eyes
  Tonometry (Non-contact)
  Electrocardiogram
   12 lead
  Audiometry
  Right Ear Left Ear
   500 CPS   500 CPS
  1000 CPS 1000 CPS
  2000 CPS 2000 CPS
  4000 CPS 4000 CPS
  8000 CPS 8000 CPS
  Chest x-ray
   14" x 17" PA View
  Spirometry
   FVC
   FEV_1

C. HEMATOLOGICAL TESTS
  Hematocrit
  Hemoglobin
  Red blood count
  White blood count
  Differential (when indicated)
  MCH
  MCHC

D. BLOOD CHEMISTRY[a]
  Calcium
  Phosphorus
  BUN
  Creatinine
  BUN/Creatinine
  Uric Acid
  Glucose
  Total protein
  Albumin
  Albumin/Globulin
  Direct Bilirubin
  Total Bilirubin
  SGOT
  SGPT
  Alkaline phosphatase
  LDH
  Iron
  Cholesterol
  Sodium
  Magnesium
  Potassium
  Chloride
  GGTP
  Triglycerides

E. URINALYSIS
  Occult blood
  pH
  Protein
  Glucose

[a]SMA-24 is routine, (standard test conducted by auto-analyzer).

Among the list of the key employee medical history and physical examination parameters evaluated by a physician to establish worker preclearance are:

a. History of nervous disorders, drinking habits.
b. Evidence of preexisting chronic illnesses.
c. Skin and liver function evaluation.
d. Evaluation of suitability to wear respiratory protective equipment.

Upon completion of all remedial and closure work, the workers should be given a follow-up physical examination, and another one 6 to 12 months later. This baseline and follow-up documentation reflects appropriate tracking of hazardous waste site workers medical health information.

Site Work Zones

One method for the reduction of possible contamination or release of toxic materials is to class the uncontrolled hazardous waste site into specific delineated work zones or work areas wherein expected or known levels of contamination exist. Within these zones, prescribed operations occur utilizing appropriate personal protective equipment. Movement between areas should be controlled at specified checkpoints. The three recommended zones are:

1. *Exclusion Zone* - The contaminated area typically requiring the most stringent categories of personal protective equipment (Category I or II). Within this area protective equipment requirements may vary slightly based on different levels of contamination within the zoned area.
2. *Contamination Reduction Zone* - An intermediate buffer zone between contaminated and uncontaminated work areas. (All decontamination activities occur in this area.)
3. *Noncontaminated or Clean Zone* - The outermost area of the site where no contamination exists. Typically this area contains the bulk of the administrative and support services, and serves as the focal point for controlled access of authorized support personnel and equipment.

Figure 13-1 represents a typical layout delineating the three zones [7, 8].

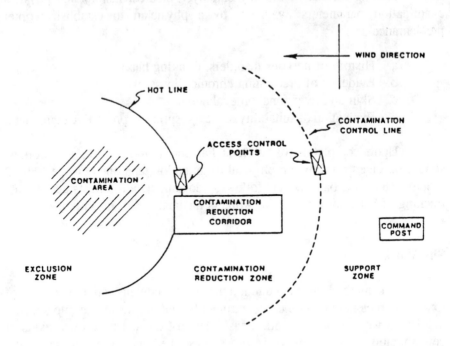

Figure 13-1. Site work area classification.

Air Monitoring Requirements

A variety of air monitoring equipment is necessary to characterize and monitor the ambient air at a hazardous waste site. Air monitoring can document that toxic materials are not being released at the perimeter boundaries (both in upwind and downwind directions) during site activities, as well as to provide information for selecting the proper respiratory equipment. In addition, continuous air monitoring is required because workers may encounter hazards such as explosive atmospheres or high levels of radiation for which their existing protective equipment would not be adequate. Such continuous monitoring then serves as a basis by which the Health and Safety Coordinator can establish the minimum level of protective equipment consistent with maintaining worker health and safety. Table 13-5 provides a detailed list of air monitoring equipment available for ambient and perimeter boundary air sampling, and personal breathing zone sampling [8].

Meteorological Monitoring

During all on-site activities, continuous analysis of the site and vicinity weather is necessary. A portable wind station should be established at a point as high as possible on the site. Continuous recording of prevailing wind speed (mph) and average wind direction (degrees) is important to establish locations of upwind and downwind perimeter boundary air sampling. In addition, wind monitoring will provide readily available documented wind condition information by which an uncontrolled release of airborne toxic materials can be tracked immediately after the incident. Because of certain instrument calibration requirements for on-site industrial hygiene monitoring equipment, it is good practice to routinely record relative humidity at all times during the site remedial activities.

Table 13-5. Ambient/Boundary and Personal Breathing Zone Air Sampling Equipment [8]		
Ambient/Boundary:		
Hazard	**Direct Reading**	**Collection System**
Explosive atmosphere[a]	Combustible gas indicator	Not used
Oxygen-deficient atmosphere[b]	Oxygen level meter	Not used
Toxic atmosphere	1. Portable photo-ionization detector (PID) 2. Portable flame ionization detector (FID) w/gas chromatograph (GC) option 3. Colorimetric tubes	Sampling pumps in conjunction with adsorption tubes, filters, and impingers (similar to personal breathing measurements)
Radioactivity[c]	1. Radiation survey (alpha, beta, gamma) 2. Passive monitors (alarms)	Dosimeters (film badges)
Personal Breathing Zone:		
Pollutant	**Collection Media[d]**	**Laboratory Analysis**
Volatile organics	Carbon tubes, Tenax tubes, XAD-2 tubes, Silica gel tubes	Gas chromatograph/Mass spectroscopy (GS/MS)
Particulate organics	Gas fiber filters	GC/MS
Pesticides (including PCBs)	Florisil tubes, Polyurethane plugs	GC/MS GC/Electron capture
PBBs	Glass fiber filters	GC/MS
Metals	Membrane filters	Atomic absorption (AA)
Volatile inorganics	Impingers/reagent solutions	Wet chemical methods
Particulate inorganics	Membrane filters, Glass fiber filters	Wet chemical methods
Cyanides	Filters/impingers	Wet chemicals

[a]At a vapor explosiveness of greater than 20%, all work activity in the site where reading taken is ceased. At 10%, an alert is made to carefully evaluate explosiveness at various levels in reference to ground level.

[b]At less than 19.5% oxygen, supplied air or SCBA is required.

[c]0.02MR is normal; at levels greater than 2.0MR, operations should cease.

[d]Any of these, depending on the specific site hazards, can be used with a sampling pump to monitor at the uncontrolled site boundaries for possible off-site release.

Security

As much as possible, the site should be fenced and isolated from the surrounding population environment. Only those people approved by the project (site) manager will be allowed access to the noncontaminated work zone. Only those workers having completed the employee medical examination will be allowed into the intermediate and/or contaminated work zones. Daily reports from the on-site manager should be made to local government representatives and/or the press to describe remedial progress and activities. A security guard service should be employed on a 24-hour basis to provide on-site security notice of potential exposure problems, e.g., fire, weather, etc. The guard should maintain a security log for all workers and visitors entering the site. The log should indicate name, organization, dates, and arrival and departure times for each worker or visitor. At least one or more access routes for emergency vehicles must be maintained throughout the site activities. Walkie-talkie communications to remote field locations are needed to communicate potential hazard conditions. If at all possible, Federal Aviation Administration (FAA) air space restrictions over the site at key activity periods should be enforced using USEPA to facilitate the requirements.

EMERGENCY REQUIREMENTS

Regardless of the care undertaken to address the major elements of a remediation plan that can protect (routinely) against an unforeseen event, there always exists the potential of an upset condition. The basic objectives for an emergency contingency plan are threefold: 1) to be prepared to minimize, control, and contain any possible release of hazardous wastes from the remediation site; 2) to provide coordination of all related emergency response groups in a safe manner; and 3) to promote safety in any necessary cleanup operation so as to prevent harm to the workers, the surrounding community, or to the environment. The heart of the documented contingency plan, as identified below, deals with specific emergencies and how each best could be handled [2, 3, 4]. Users should review the latest regulations, such as 29 CFR 1910.120 pp "q."

Fire

a. Fire extinguishers designed for solvent and electrical fires must be within easy access of various phases of site remediations. (No worker should have to move more than 75 lineal feet to obtain fire extinguishers.) Backup foam systems and emergency fire water supplies should be available as needed to protect against the spread of fire.

b. All personnel must be trained in the use of the fire extinguishers.

c. A skilled Fire Brigade must be available, and on call, should a major fire occur. Workers in close contact with the source of the fire should be in Category IV emergency equipment with at least two people participating together.

d. Telephone (or radio) contact must be made immediately with the local fire department to obtain their response, if necessary, to contain the blaze. Before remedial operations are begun, all fire department personnel should be briefed on the chemical waste hazards at the site.

e. All site activities will be immediately terminated until the threat of fire hazard is removed. If possible, evacuation from the affected areas should be in an upwind direction.

f. Electrical power to the work area must be disconnected until the hazard is removed.

g. All personnel not involved in fire fighting activities should be evacuated to a safe location.

h. The general plant fire alarm should be activated to notify all personnel of the problem. (Portable air horns will be distributed across the site area for easy access to sound an emergency alarm.)

i. All appropriate Federal, state, and local government agencies must be notified of the fire.

j. After the fire has been extinguished, the damage should be immediately assessed and any required spill control or clean-up activities initiated.

Severe Storm

a. At the imminent presence of severe weather conditions, all clean-up activities must cease.

b. Workers should be instructed in proper procedures for securing the site before leaving the work area.

c.   As soon as the work area has been secured, all personnel must evacuate the work area, decontaminate, and proceed to a safe area.

d.   All electrical power must be disconnected to the work area.

e.   As soon as the severe weather passes, the work area should be assessed for damage and any required spill control or clean-up measures initiated.

Toxic Vapor Release

a.   Although extremely unlikely, should an unsatisfactory air quality measurement be noted, all site activities must be ceased until the problem is corrected. A well designed system will have taken into consideration the occassional release of hazardous materials with adequate on-site controls.

b.   If necessary, all downwind persons should be notified and evacuated.

c.   All appropriate Federal, state, and local agencies must be notified.

d.   Personnel in appropriate protective equipment will determine the source of the release and proceed to correct the problem.

Medical Emergency

a.   Personnel from local medical facilities must be briefed on the nature of the project so they can make preparations for medical emergencies.

b.   Emergency medical transportation must be notified immediately, as well as the nearest hospital.

c.   The medical problem should be treated with emergency first aid procedures by qualified trained persons from the site crews until medical help arrives.

d.   The affected person, as soon as practicable, will be removed from the work area and protective clothing will be removed, if possible.

e.   A designated supervisory person should accompany the person to the hospital to provide the medical team with an accurate description of how the accident or emergency occurred.

Liquid or Solid Wastes Spill

a.   Adequate spill control and containment materials must be available on-site to deal with any spill which might occur.

b.   All areas subject to potential spills must be diked to prevent migration from the work area off the site boundary.

c.   All personnel should be trained in proper spill control measures and must respond immediately to contain, then clean up, the spilled material.

d.   All appropriate Federal, state, and local agencies must be notified. Any other unforeseen emergencies should be dealt with by the on-site project manager, and all appropriate agencies will be notified of any additional problems as warranted.

Evacuation

In the unlikely event that the release of toxic materials and/or flammable or explosive mixtures threaten nearby population centers, the following steps should be directed to facilitate the evacuation process:

a.   Have a preestablished means to quickly inform nearby population areas. Alternative information contacts include going door-to-door, radio/television broadcasts, or a public address system attached to a motor vehicle driven through the nearby population areas.

b.   Have pre-assigned evacuation routes to facilitate transport by private automobile to safe centers wherein temporary food and shelter is available.

c.   Secure, monitor, and decontaminate as necessary affected areas prior to any inhabitants returning to their dwellings.

d.   Have the evacuation protocol on file with local authorities, i.e., Civil Defense, National Guard, fire and police departments, EPA, and local hospitals.

e.   Have a readily available list of phone numbers and name contacts for emergency situations:

Agency	Telephone	Person to Contact
Fire		
Police		
Ambulance Service		
Hospital Emergency Room		
EPA and EPA Emergency Response Team		
Mayors of Nearby Communities		
Civil Defense		
Local National Guard Units		
Cleanup Contractor Management Officials		

f.   A local communications spokesperson must be established to assure rapid, accurate, thorough, and timely communications to the public during any threat of emergency or evacuation. This is typically the responsibility of the project (site) manager. Joint communications should be drafted and issued among the project (site) manager, USEPA, and local government authorities to assure continuity and consistent appraisal of the emergency status. The utmost care *must* be taken to prevent a public communications vacuum that can lead to possible panic and misunderstanding to the surrounding populace.

Hazard Risk Assessment

Before startup of any major activity at the uncontrolled hazardous wastes site, an attempt to address the logical consequences of various uncontrolled exposure incidents should be made. Table 13-6 lists several of the uncontrolled incident cases to which responses can be drafted in case such emergency situations arise [1]. These scenario responses should be documented as a key part of any contingency plan. The response to these issues requires probable and worst case answers by which careful analysis and study can identify beforehand important areas of uncertainty or high hazards.

**Table 13-6. Uncontrolled Hazardous Waste Site
Incident Cases [1]**

1. Fire and/or explosion of flammable or combustible solvents or pesticide mixtures.

2. Explosion of waste containers containing shock, pressure or heat sensitive materials.

3. Penetration or rupture of compressed gas cylinders (buried or at the surface) containing toxic materials.

4. Penetration of protective gear by toxic liquids, gases or vapors.

5. Penetration of protective gear by equipment movement, flying debris, or contact with sharp objects.

6. Interruption or contamination of supplied breathing air.

7. Excavation and surface cave-ins.

8. Equipment rollovers.

9. In transit leaking or rupture of sample containers.

10. Rupture or leakage of sample containers while in storage.

11. Violent reaction of waste samples with analytical reagents.

12. Medical emergency in hazardous area (e.g., heart attack).

13. Severe storms.

14. General loss of utilities.

15. Public protests and harassments.

CONCLUSION

This chapter has dealt In broad terms with the key elements of a contingency plan for remediation at uncontrolled hazardous waste sites. The focus has been to relate those elements of a contingency plan that are truly preventative in nature with those that deal with an emergency situation arising from the remediation activities at the site. No one uncontrolled hazardous waste site is exactly like any other. There is no real substitute for a definitive contingency plan in order to protect workers, the surrounding community, and the environment. Each contingency plan needs to be modified reflecting those site or wastes characteristics unique to a particular situation. However, the core elements addressed in this chapter must all be considered preparatory to fine tuning for specialized hazard situations.

REFERENCES

1. Allcott, G. A., J. V. Messick and R. Vandeewort. "Practical Considerations for the Protection of Personnel During the Gathering, Transportation, Storage, and Analysis of Samples from Hazardous Waste Sites," in *Management of Uncontrolled Hazardous Waste Sites* National Conference--October 28 to 30, 1981, Washington, D.C., (Silver Spring, Maryland: Hazardous Materials Control

2. Sawyer, C. Unpublished material (1984).

3. Sawyer, C. J. "Environmental Health and Safety Considerations for a Dioxin Detoxication Process," in *Detoxication of Hazardous Wastes*, J. H. Exner, Ed. (Ann Arbor, Michigan: Ann Arbor Science Publishers, 1982), pp. 289-297.

4. Sawyer, C. J., and K. E. Stormer. "Environmental Health, Safety, and Legal Considerations for the Successful Excavation of a Dioxin-Contaminated Hazardous Wastes Site," American Chemical Society Meeting-Dioxin Symposium, Washington, D.C., (August 1983).

5. Streng, D.R., W.F. Martin, L.P. Wallace, G. Kleiner, J. Gift, and D. Weitzman. "Hazardous Waste Sites and Hazardous Substance Emergencies," DHHS (NIOSH) Publication No. 83-100 (1982), p. 20.

6. Graciano, R., OH Materials Inc., Findlay, Ohio. Personal Communication (1983).

7. Partridge, L. J., Arthur D. Little, Inc., Cambridge, Massachusetts, Personal Communication (1983).

8. Mathamel, Martin S. "Hazardous Substance Site Ambient Air Characterization to Evaluate Entry Term Safety," in *Management of Uncontrolled Hazardous Waste Sites* National Conference-October 28 to 30, 1981, Washington, D.C., (Silver Spring, Maryland: Hazardous Materials Control Research Institute, 1981, pp. 281-184.

14

RADIATION SAFETY

Leslie W. Cole, M.S.

INTRODUCTION

The presence of radioactive materials cannot be ruled out at any location, particularly one where other hazardous materials are present. Radioactive materials have been generally well controlled but, in the past, there are radioactive materials that were either not recognized or not controlled. For instance, in oil fields there may be contamination from the naturally occurring radioactive materials (NORM). This contamination is the result of cleaning pipes and casing on which compounds containing NORM have "plated out" in the oil extraction process. The presence of the NORM contamination may not have been known to the oil firms or their employees. NORM are based on the three principal radioactive series: the uranium-radium series (U238), the uranium 235-actinium series and the thorium 232 series all of which began with the creation of the earth. The radioisotope radium is the principal constituent of the NORM associated with oil fields.

Radium may be in other places also. It was in wide use for many years in the manufacture of watch dials and aircraft instruments. Paint washes from this manufacturing in New Jersey have been the focus of landfill remediation efforts that cost over $16 million in the early 1970s. These same type wastes were the object of several Superfund site studies in Ottawa, Il where watch dials and instruments were painted at two companies beginning in the 1920s. Coal clinkers from a heating furnace in one plant became radioactive when paint wastes were burned in the furnace. The clinkers were subsequently incorporated into road materials and cement on both private and municipal properties. Radium paint washes have contaminated several disposal and landfill sites in the area.

Thorium has been in wide use for many years and some of these uses are still not fully regulated. The small mantels used in Coleman lanterns contain a thorium compound. At the consumer level, this material is not regulated at all. In recent times, the processing of thorium up to the point of distribution of the finished product has been brought under a strict regulatory system. There may be sites in several places in the country where waste from thorium process wastes are present that may be unknown to these who may be required to work at these sites.

Uranium is quite well known to most people as a radioactive material. In the early days of the nuclear industry, uranium was mined in many locations thorough the country. The residue materials from the mining and milling process are quite hazardous. It was not properly controlled and has cost a great deal to bring under control. There may be areas where this material is present that have not yet been discovered and it could be present with other hazardous materials.

Most other radioactive materials are "man made," that is, they are not present in nature. These man made radioactive materials are generally more hazardous than the materials mentioned above. In recent times, radioactive cobalt has been involved in a major problem in the steel industry. A small, but very active, bit of radioactive cobalt was apparently smelted into some steel in a Mexican steel mill. The steel was used in several applications from outdoor furniture to building construction materials.

In another highly publicized incident, some radioactive cesium was carried from a "junk yard" and left in a residential area. Some small children found the material and thought it was a wonderful toy. The result of this incident was the lose of several lives and serious injury to many others.

While the products containing the radioactive cobalt presented only a small health hazard and the radioactive cesium incident was a real tragedy for the people involved, neither of these incidents are related here as being something hazardous waste workers are likely to encounter. These two incidents point out that very dangerous radioactive materials can be in places where they are unexpected. They *could* end up in a waste site.

These examples document the necessity of including radiation surveying in a Phase I site assessment. Survey requirements may extend to cover municipal water treatment sludge, hard mining areas and other locations as the regulation of NORM becomes more widespread and the people become more aware of its potential hazards.

The purpose of this chapter is to outline some simple procedures to identify radiological hazards in a hazardous waste site and to assist in minimizing the health hazards to workers in the area. The workers in this discussion are non radiation workers, that is, the workers are not trained in all aspects of radioactive materials handling. As a prologue, it should be pointed out that the health hazards from radioactive materials that may be found in any inadvertent location are probably not nearly as great as most chemical hazards. In addition, the initial individual protective actions taken for chemical hazards are appropriate for most radiological hazards.

COMMON TERMS

ALPHA PARTICLE (alpha radiation) - A positively charged particle having a mass and charge equal in magnitude to a helium nucleus (two protons and two neutrons). They are emitted by certain radioactive materials. They will travel only a few inches through the air before being stopped by air molecules. They are most dangerous when they are inhaled or ingested.

BECQUEREL (Bq) - A unit of activity equal to one nuclear transformation per second (1 Bq = 1s^{-1}). The former special named unit of activity, the curie, is related to the becquerel according to 1 Ci = 3.7 x 10^{10} Bq.

BETA PARTICLE (beta radiation) - A charged particle emitted from the nucleus of an atom, with a mass and charge equal in magnitude to that of the electron. They are faster and lighter than an alpha particle.

CONTROLLED AREA - A defined area in which the occupational exposure of personnel to radiation or radioactive material is under the supervision of an individual in charge of radiation protection.

CURIE (Ci) - See also Becquerel. (a) Formerly, a special unit of activity. One curie equals 3.7 x 10^{10} disintegrations per second exactly or 1 Ci = 3.7 x10^{10} Bq. (b) By popular usage, the quantity of any radioactive material having an activity of one curie.

DECAY, RADIOACTIVE - A spontaneous nuclear transformation in which particles or gamma radiation is emitted, or x radiation is emitted following orbital electron capture, or the nucleus undergoes spontaneous fission.

DOSE - A general form denoting the quantity of radiation or energy absorbed. Most people receive between 150 and 200 millirems a year, and any level less than 5,000 millirems a year is considered low-level. Scientists have found that radiation doses of over 100,000 millirem will usually cause radiation sickness. Doses of over 500,000 millirems, if received in three days or less, will usually kill a person.

GAMMA RADIATION - A type of radiation that is released in waves by unstable atoms when they stabilize. They are a very strong (range of energy from 10 keV to 9 MeV) type of electromagnetic wave. Gamma waves have no weight and travel even faster than alpha and beta radiation.

GAMMA-RAY SCINTILLATION DETECTOR - A gamma-ray detector consisting of a scintillation, such as sodium iodide, thallium-activated, NaI(Tl), and a photomultiplier tube housed in a light-tight container.

HEALTH PHYSICS - The science of radiation protection.

MONITOR, RADIATION - A radiation detector the purpose of which is to measure the level of ionizing radiation (or quantity of radioactive material). It may also give quantitative information on dose or dose rate. The term is frequently prefixed with a word indicating the purpose of the monitor such as an area monitor, or air particle monitor.

MONITORING, RADIATION (RADIATION PROTECTION) - The continuing collection and assessment of the pertinent information to determine the adequacy of radiation protection practices and to indicate potentially significant changes in conditions or protection performance.

NEUTRON - A non-charged particle in the center of the atom. Together with the proton it forms the nucleus.

OCCUPATION DOSE (REGULATORY) - Dose (or dose equivalent) resulting from exposure of an individual to radiation in a restricted area or in the course of employment in which the individual's duties involve exposure to radiation (see 10 CFR 20.3)

RADIATION PROTECTION - All measures concerned with reducing deleterious effects of radiation to persons or materials (also called "radiological protection").

RADIATION HAZARD - A situation or condition that could result in deleterious effects attributable to deliberate, accidental, occupational, or natural exposure to radiation.

RAD - A former unit of absorbed dose; 1 rad = 10^{-2} Gy = 10^{-2} J/kg {see gray (Gy)}

RADIOACTIVE MATERIAL - A material of which one or more constituents exhibit radioactivity. NOTE: For special purposes such as regulation, this term may be restricted to radioactive material with an activity or a specific activity greater than a specified value.

REM - A former unit of dose equivalent. The dose equivalent in rems is numerically equal to the absorbed dose in rads multiplied by the quality factor, the distribution factor, and any other necessary modifying factors (originally derived from roentgen equivalent man).

ROENTGEN (R) - A unit of exposure; 1 R = 2.58 x 10^{-4} C/kg.

SCINTILLATION COUNTER - A counter in which the light flashes produced in a scintillation by ionizing radiation are converted into electrical pulses by a photomultiplier tube.

RESTRICTED AREA - Any area to which access is controlled for the protection of individuals from exposure to radiation and radioactive materials.

SIEVERT (Sv) - The special name of the unit of dose equivalent. It is given numerically by 1 Sv = 1 J * kg^{-1} (= 100 rem).

RADIATION HAZARDS

Radiation is classed as a carcinogen. Exposures to man made or technically enhanced radioactive materials are regulated by the U.S. Nuclear Regulatory Commission (NRC) or by the individual states through agreement with the NRC. Regulation of naturally occurring radioactive materials (NORM) is through the Environmental Protection Agency and state regulatory agencies. NORM are not fully regulated in many states. Where regulations exist there are limits on exposures for radiation workers and for members of the public. The regulatory limits on doses for radiation workers are set to provide risks as low or lower than the risks associated with "safe" industries. Since the workers in this discussion are not radiation workers, the regulatory limits appropriate for them are the same as for the general public and that is one-tenth the level for radiation workers. The level of risk is in proportional to the dose, thus the risk for radiation exposure as discussed here is much lower than the total risk in "safe" industries.

The risk that exists is directly proportional to the radiation dose. Radiation doses are measured in units of either rem or sieverts (Sv). The risk of cancer is approximately four in one hundred per sievert (four in ten-thousand per rem). The sievert is a large unit. The limit on the annual dose for a non-radiation worker is five millisieverts (500 mrem) per year and will soon be changed to one millisievert (100 mrem). A dose of five millisieverts translates to a cancer risk of two chances in ten thousand (2×10^{-4}). The risk from one year's exposure to the average background radiation level of about one millisievert (100 mrem) is 4×10^{-5}. The lifetime risk from background radiation is approximately 3×10^{-3}.

RADIATION DETECTION

Field exposures usually concentrate on detection gamma-ray emissions as a means of detecting the presence of radioactive materials. A simple hand held sodium iodide crystal detector is adequate for initial assessments. Positive indication on the survey meter will determine the presence of radioactive materials but it cannot be quantitative measure of the long-term hazard. The absence of a positive measurement with the survey meter is not sufficient to rule out the presence of radioactive materials. Some radioactive materials will not cause the sodium iodide instrument to respond and buried materials may be sufficiently shielded to be not detectable. Land contamination can be determined only through laboratory analysis. If there is any indication of the presence of radioactive materials it may be prudent to include sampling and analysis of materials from the suspected site.

Some states require the sampling and analysis of land contamination where the evidence of a land radiation survey indicates radiation levels are twice background in small areas (usually defined as 100 square meter or less) or 1.5 times background in large areas (usually defined as several hundred square meters).

MODES OF EXPOSURE

Individuals may be exposed to radiation in several ways. The exposing material may be outside the individual's body or it may be inside his body. These are the two modes of exposure.

External exposure

The radiation emissions from a radioactive substance, a source, outside an individual's body travel through the space between the source and the individual and impact on and inside his body. The materials between the source and the body absorb some of the energy. Even the individuals clothing and the outer layer of dead skin absorb some of the energy. In the case of alpha radiation the dead skin is capable of absorbing all the energy. If one were to pick up a piece of a pure alpha emitter, no harm at all would come of it since the inert layer of skin on the hand would provide adequate shielding. The same may be true of some beta emitting substances because the inert layer of skin on the hands is relatively thick. Some beta particles may penetrate into the live skin, however, and the most energetic beta particles from some radioactive materials may penetrate into the tissue below the skin. It is quite unlikely that any significant damage would result to the vital organs inside the body from beta radiation. Gamma radiation is capable of penetrating into the body and interacting with the internal organs. Some gamma radiation will be stopped by the skin if it is of "low" energy but there are many radioactive substances that emit gamma radiation of quite powerful energies.

Most of the NORM substances emit more than one type of radiation and can all be classed as potentially harmful from an external exposure viewpoint. The same is true from man made radioactive materials. One cannot assume that any radioactive material is harmless. Even the pure alpha emitter mentioned above could lead to some harm if one were to pick it up and transfer some residual material that may be left on his hand to his mouth. That would fall into the other category of exposure.

Internal Exposure

Radioactive materials inside the body can irradiate the internal organs directly. There is no intervening mater to act as a shield as with the external radiation. Even the alpha particle can cause significant damage when it decays inside a cell or in body fluids. In fact, alpha emitters are potentially the most dangerous type of radioactive substances. It is not possible to prevent some internal exposure. Part of the element potassium is radioactive. We all carry around about a microcurie of radioactive potassium. It is a gamma emitter that gives us a dose of about 0.15 millisievert (15 mrem) a year. Most of us receive the largest portion of our radiation dose internally from the radioactive gas radon. This gas is present everywhere. The average person receives about two millisieverts (200 mrem) a year from radon.

Internally deposited radioactive materials may stay in the body for long period and continue their irradiation all the time they are present. This requires the use of adequate protective measures when radioactive substances are encountered that may be either inhaled or ingested.

INDIVIDUAL PROTECTIVE MEASURES

The actions taken for individual protective action against chemical hazards are all appropriate for protection against radiation hazards. While it is true that the energetic gamma radiation can penetrate the protective clothing worn to avoid the chemical hazards, the very fact that they are so penetrating makes it easy to detect them. If the simple measure of beginning each remedial action or survey with a simple radiation survey always taken, the risk is easily quantifiable. Radiation safety specialists can quickly evaluate the hazard level to determine if the use of specially trained radiation workers are necessary. If the potential exposure level is below the regulatory level for exposure to the general public, there should be little concern for the radiation risk. The dose at that level of exposure is less than half the dose received by an x-ray examination of the back or a lower GI examination.

When the potential for the radioactive material to become airborne, it may be necessary to wear individual respiratory protection. Again the radiation safety specialist should be called on to make that evaluation. The respiratory protection requirement is no different than the one for airborne chemical hazards. There may be a different or additional filter device on the respirator but all other requirements are the same.

The one difference that may exist is the requirement to actively monitor personnel and equipment when departing a radiologically contaminated area. Each individual must be monitored as he departs an area where radioactive materials are present in an exposed or potentially exposed condition. If contamination is found on an individual, he must be decontaminated before departing from the area. Note again that sensitive but simple equipment exists to monitor individuals leaving a contaminated area and the decontamination measures are also simple.

RADIATION CONTROL MEASURES AT A HAZARDOUS WORK SITE

Restricted Areas

If radioactive materials are identified in work site, the first control measure is to restrict the area from inadvertent entry. This will require the establishment of a restricted area or controlled area. The area must be clearly delineated and posted. There are special signs required for this posting. They are generally familiar to most people. The specification for the posting is contained in CFR Title 10 Part 20. All personnel who enter the controlled area must be instructed as to the requirements inside the area, i.e. requirement for respiratory protection, personal radiation monitoring, and the requirements for exiting.

Protective Clothing

Protective outer garments are essential in working in a contaminated area. No one can ever be allowed in a controlled area who is not fully clothed. Disposable gloves and shoe covers are almost essential for working in controlled areas. These can be easily removed as the individual exits the controlled area and can provide a high level of assurance of no contamination remaining on the individual. The other outer clothing can be monitored and worn again if it is not contaminated.

Personal Radiation Monitors

Each individual working in an area where radioactive materials exist should be assigned a radiation monitor that will provide a permanent record of his radiation dose. The regulatory requirement is that an individual who may be exposed to more 10 percent of the occupational limit is required to be monitored in this way. Even though the thrust of this discussion is that the dose will be below that level, it is still recommended that all individuals be assigned a monitoring device. This will provide a permanent record that will allay any difficulties in the future regarding the level of exposure. The recommended device is a thermoluminescent detector (TLD). These devices are available from several vendors and are inexpensive, rugged and accurate.

Air Monitoring

If there is any potential for airborne radioactive contamination, air monitoring is an absolute requirement. The collection procedures are much the same as for chemical hazard sampling. Evaluation requires knowledge of the air sampling procedures for radioactive materials. The radiation specialist should be called on for assistance in this procedure.

REFERENCES

1. Code of Federal Regulations Title 10 Parts 19, 20, 60, 61 & 62.
2. Code of Federal Regulations Title 49 Parts 173-178.
3. Manual for Conducting Radiological Surveys in Support of License Termination. NUREG/CR-5849, ORAD-92/C57 (Draft for Comment) U.S. Nuclear Regulatory Commission, June 1992.
4. Methods for Evaluating the Attainment of Cleanup Standards, Volume 1: Soils and Solid Media, EPA 230/02-89-042, U.S. Environmental Protection Agency, February 1989.
5. Procedures for Sampling Radium-Contaminated Soils, GJ/TMC-13, UC-70A, U.S. Department of Energy, March 1984.
6. Regulatory Guide 4.15, Quality Assurance for Radiological Monitoring Programs - Effluent Streams and The Environment, U.S. Nuclear Regulatory Commission, February 1979.

15

ORDNANCE, EXPLOSIVE WASTE AND UNEXPLODED ORDNANCE

James P. Pastorick, B.A.

Environmental scientists and project managers working on active and former Department of Defense (DOD) facilities are frequently finding that their environmental investigation and remediation sites are potentially contaminated with ordnance and explosive waste (OEW). The U.S. Army Corps of Engineers has identified of 7,600 formerly used defense sites of which approximately 1,200 are potentially contaminated with OEW.

The ability to safely perform environmental remediation projects in an environment contaminated, or potentially contaminated, with OEW is critical to the safe and efficient performance of field activities on many current or former DOD installations. Accidents involving OEW usually result in severe consequences, including death, for those involved. An example of such an incident occurred recently at Peterborough, England [1] where explosives that were being transported accidently detonated.

The U.S. Army Corps of Engineers has been dealing with the issue of OEW for several years. Specifically, Congress established the Defense Environmental Restoration Program (DERP) in 1986 under Public Laws 99-190 and 99-499. The two subprograms established under DERP are the Installation Restoration Program (IRP), which deals with active DOD installations, and the Formerly Used Defense Sites (FUDS) Program which deals with formerly owned or used DOD sites that are no longer under DOD control.

On April 5, 1990, the Huntsville Division of the Corps of Engineers was designated as the Mandatory Center of Expertise (MCX) and Design Center for Unexploded Ordnance (UXO). As the UXO MCX, Huntsville is responsible for the investigation and remediation of OEW at active facilities and FUDS sites. The Huntsville Division MCX works in cooperation with local Corps of Engineers Districts, local officials, and interested citizens to examine and remediate OEW contamination.

OEW is defined by the Huntsville MCX [2] as "anything related to ordnance designed to cause damage to personnel or materiel through explosive force, incendiary action, or toxic effects. OEW is: Bombs and warheads; guided and ballistic missiles; artillery, mortar, and rocket ammunition; small arms ammunition; antipersonnel and antitank land mines; demolition charges; pyrotechnics; grenades; torpedoes and depth charges; containerized and uncontainerized high explosives and propellants; depleted uranium rounds; military chemical agents; and all similar and related components, explosive in nature or otherwise designed to cause damage to personnel or material (e.g., fuzes, boosters, bursters, rocket motors). Uncontainerized high explosives/propellants or soils with explosive constituents are considered explosive waste if the concentration is sufficient to be reactive and present an imminent safety hazard."

UXO, therefore, is one component of OEW and is defined by the DOD as "Explosive ordnance which has been primed, fused (sic), armed or otherwise prepared for action, and which has been fired, dropped, launched, projected or placed in such a manner as to constitute a hazard to operations, installations, personnel or material and remains unexploded either by malfunction or design or for any other cause." [3]

Personnel Qualifications for UXO Specialists

Personnel working with UXO require specialized training. All four branches of the armed forces use the designation of Explosive Ordnance Disposal (EOD) technician to describe their specialists in this field. EOD training has been standardized at the U.S. Naval School of EOD, located at the Naval Ordnance Station in Indian Head, Maryland.

This site has been the main EOD training center for all of the U.S. armed services since World War II and attendance and graduation from this school are still the basic requirements for performing UXO work by the Huntsville MCX. A satellite facility of the U.S. Naval School of EOD has recently been opened at Eglin Air Force Base, Florida, and this new facility may take on a larger role in EOD training in the future.

Civilian contractor specialists in this field are referred to as UXO specialists to differentiate them from their active duty counterparts. The skill classifications of UXO Specialist, UXO Supervisor, and Senior UXO Supervisor generally relate to the military designations of Basic EOD Technician, Senior EOD Technician, and Master EOD Technician (also known in the military as "Master Blaster") although all of the services have their own criteria for achieving these various military EOD skill levels. Although always subject to change, the current training and experience requirements, as determined by the Huntsville MCX, for UXO project personnel and their primary on-site duties are as follows [4]:

Project Title	Qualifications/Duties
Senior UXO Supervisor	A graduate of the U.S. Naval School of EOD with at least 15 years of EOD/UXO experience (3 years of contractor experience can apply, at least 12 years of active duty EOD experience is required). Serves as the leading UXO specialist on site. Has ultimate responsibility for UXO procedural and safety decisions and serves as overall field project director. The same qualifications enable this person to serve as the UXO Site Safety Officer or Quality Control Specialist.
UXO Supervisor	A graduate of the U.S. Naval School of EOD with at least 7 years of EOD/UXO experience (at least 3 years of active duty EOD experience is required). Reports to the Senior UXO Supervisor and is responsible for a specific work crew or the personnel involved with a specific project phase.
UXO Specialist	A graduate of the U.S. Naval School of EOD with 3 years of active duty EOD experience or a graduate of an EOD Assistant course with 5 years of combined military and contractor EOD/UXO experience. Reports to the Senior UXO Technician and performs all UXO field tasks, including excavation, identification, and disposal of UXO by detonation. Can serve as a supervisor of small work units such as a magnetometer survey crew.
UXO Assistant	A graduate of the EOD Assistant course at the U.S. Naval School of EOD or Redstone Arsenal, Alabama. Must be supervised in the field by a UXO Technician. Can perform most UXO field tasks with the exception of unsupervised excavation and disposal of UXO.
Skilled Laborer	No minimum experience qualifications but must be trained in the specific skill required by the assigned duties, such as magnetometer operator or surveyor assistant.

UXO Projects

UXO projects are identified by examining the past use of the project site. Any active or formerly used DOD facility has the potential to be contaminated with UXO. Most often the past use by the DOD is obvious and documented. But, some DOD operations were not widely publicized due to war-time secrecy requirements and may not be obvious to the casual observer today. Conducting thorough site historical research is necessary to completely rule out the possibility of UXO hazards on an active or formerly used DOD installation.

One recent example of this is the toxic chemical UXO discovered inside the city limits of Washington, D.C. in December 1992. Buried chemical UXO was discovered at this site, located in a subdivision of Washington, by a backhoe operator digging a utilities trench approximately twenty feet away from a newly completed home. The subdivision had been owned by the developer since the 1920's when it was purchased from a university. After the UXO was discovered the investigation determined that the university assisted the government with chemical weapons research during World War I and the UXO discovered was from a burial site used during the era of chemical weapons research.

UXO projects fall into two main categories: UXO remediation/ investigation and UXO safety support services. UXO remediation/investigation involves the location and disposal of UXO from the project site and, although other mixed waste considerations are frequently associated with these projects, the explosive hazard presented by the UXO is the overriding safety consideration.

UXO Remediation/Investigation

During a UXO remediation/investigation project, the performance of UXO operations is the main project objective. These projects are usually contracted by the Huntsville MCX or, if the project is being conducted under another program, the Huntsville MCX will often have some degree of project oversight responsibility. For example, the Huntsville MCX may review the work plan prior to approval by the contracting authority.

UXO remediation/investigation projects are often considered to be emergency removals of imminent and substantial hazards to the local population and are subject to Comprehensive Environmental Response, Compensation, and Liability Act (CERCLA) Section 104 and the Final National Contingency Plan (NCP). This interpretation has been supported by state and local agencies because it tends to streamline the remediation process in order to eliminate the extreme hazard of UXO on uncontrolled former DOD installations.

The level of effort required to complete a UXO remediation project depends on the size of the project and the conditions at the site. But generally, UXO work crews can work most efficiently when they are divided into distinct teams to accomplish specific objectives.

A field work team will generally work under the direction of a UXO Supervisor and be staffed by a group of from three to ten UXO specialists, assistants, and skilled laborers. The exact number and type of personnel chosen depends on the work objective for which the team is being selected. A large surface survey team may have several skilled laborers trained in the use of the low sensitivity magnetometers. UXO work crews performing intrusive operations, such as UXO excavation, will be comprised of UXO specialists because this higher level of training is required to safely perform that operation.

UXO Safety Support

During UXO safety support operations, in contrast to UXO remediation/investigation projects, UXO specialists are called upon to provide their specific area of knowledge and expertise to a project with different objectives. An example of this is any remedial investigation/feasibility study (RI/FS) project requiring the generation of field data from an active or formerly used DOD installation. Because the installation is or was used by the DOD, the possibility of UXO or explosives being present should at least be considered. If the site history indicates that UXO was used or disposed of in the vicinity of project sampling activities, the project management authority will probably require that the work plan and safety plan consider UXO hazards.

Examples of UXO safety support to environmental sampling efforts are the removal of UXO hazards to allow access to well drilling sites and performing downhole magnetometer checks during well drilling operations to preclude contact with UXO. UXO specialists may escort field sampling teams to locate potentially hazardous UXO and ensure that such items are avoided. The emphasis of UXO safety support is not the removal and disposal of UXO hazards, but rather the avoidance of UXO hazards by non-EOD trained site personnel. This is the main difference between UXO support and UXO investigation/remediation operations.

UXO safety support operations are usually staffed with the minimum number of UXO specialists required to ensure the safety of field sampling personnel. Generally, the level of UXO staffing required is one UXO specialist for every individual field operation being conducted simultaneously. For example, if two well drilling rigs and one soil gas sampling team are working simultaneously in areas suspected to contain UXO, a total of three UXO specialists can be used to ensure the safety of the three sampling teams. Each field team should be assigned a UXO specialist who is responsible for the detection and avoidance of UXO for the team.

The disposal of UXO hazards may not be possible during a UXO support project because sufficient UXO personnel are not likely to be available to perform these functions. Intrusive activities, such as excavation of suspected UXO items, require at least two UXO specialists, with support personnel nearby in case of the occurrence of an emergency. This level of staffing is rarely available on a UXO support project which has other field priorities and usually involves the minimum number of UXO specialists required to escort the sampling teams.

Explosives Contamination in Soil

Some hazardous materials sites may not be contaminated with UXO but may be contaminated with explosives. This is particularly true of active and former weapons production and demilitarization facilities where explosives settling lagoons were commonly used to separate residual explosives from water used in the production and demilitarization process.

Explosives settling lagoons (commonly referred to as "pink water lagoons") can possibly have accumulated enough bulk explosive to become reactive. Explosive contaminated soil exhibits reactivity to shock down to levels of 15% explosive content in the soil and reactivity to flame is retained down to 12% explosive content. In light of these reactivity characteristics the U.S. Army Environmental Center has established 10% explosive content of soil as the maximum explosive content allowable without instituting explosive safety controls during the handling of the explosively contaminated soil.

Field testing procedures to determine the percentage of TNT [5], RDX [6], and 2,4 DNT [7] explosives have been developed by the U.S. Army Cold Regions Research and Engineering Laboratory under funding by the U.S. Army Environmental Center. It should also be noted that explosive compounds are extremely toxic and are very hazardous even in quantities below reactive levels [8].

Explosive content in soil of 10% necessitates the institution of strict safety precautions when working with this potentially reactive media. Extreme measures should be taken to avoid subjecting a potentially reactive or explosive substance to the stress of heat, shock, and friction. The project work plan and safety plan should identify the specific methods for obtaining samples that do not subject the sample area to stress. Examples of methods that reduce or reduce the chances of stressing potentially reactive soil are using non-sparking (beryllium) sampling and excavating tools, wetting the sampling or excavation area to reduce friction, and using snap-top instead of screw-top sampling containers.

Also, the basic safety concept of minimizing the number of workers exposed to the hazard and minimizing the amount of time those workers are exposed should be enforced. Only the amount of personnel required to safely accomplish each work task should be allowed within the established exclusion area when working with potentially explosive or reactive soils.

If laboratory analysis of samples taken from the site indicate that the soil has an extremely high explosives content, consideration should be given to using remotely operated equipment for excavation and sampling. Remotely operated equipment is expensive and time-consuming to use but it has the advantage of not exposing any site workers to an extreme hazard.

There are alternatives to the open burning of explosive contaminated soil [9]. Some successful remediation methods are incineration [10], composting [11], and chemical treatment [12]. Soil with high levels of explosive content can be more safely handled after lowering the explosive content in the soil to below 10% by blending it with uncontaminated filler material [13].

UXO Project Plans

All field activities involving or potentially involving UXO should be performed in accordance with a work plan and a safety plan. The work plan should clearly state the project objective and provide detailed procedures governing the UXO related field operations.

If the project is being accomplished under the cognizance of the U.S. Army, the safety plan should include an accident prevention plan prepared in the format specified in the U.S. Army Corps of Engineers' Safety and Health Requirements Manual [14]. The procedures and guidance contained in the work plan and safety plan should not conflict with the specific safety procedures contained in the Huntsville MCX UXO safety criteria document [15] and this document should also be included as an appendix to the safety plan to ensure that it is available for reference at the project site.

One common exception to routine field safety practices involves the wearing of steel-toed safety shoes and hard hats by UXO specialists. UXO specialists must take precautions to avoid dropping heavy objects during normal UXO field activities in order to avoid disturbing potentially hazardous UXO. Steel-toed safety shoes also interfere with the operation of UXO detection instruments which can create a very hazardous situation by causing a UXO to be undetected during the geophysical survey. UXO specialists, therefore, are usually exempted in the project safety plan from wearing safety shoes and hats unless they are working with a drop hazard such as when using a mechanized excavator to access a deeply buried UXO.

UXO TOOLS AND TECHNIQUES

This section provides a brief overview of the tools and techniques employed to perform UXO operations. The common tools and equipment used by UXO teams are designed for UXO detection, excavation, and disposal.

Geophysical Detection Equipment

Although locating UXO by visual observation should never be discounted, most UXO is extremely difficult to locate by sight alone because it is usually in a deteriorated condition and camouflaged by soil, grasses, and leaves. Because of this, geophysical instruments are usually used to help locate potential UXO anomalies. A complete evaluation report of UXO detection methods has recently been completed by the U.S. Naval EOD Technology Center [16].

One concern unique to the UXO field is electromagnetic radiation (EMR) [17]. Some types of ordnance fuzing uses electrical firing systems that can potentially be initiated, under ideal conditions, by electromagnetic radiation. Because of this, the safest approach to UXO detection is to use a detection instrument that is completely passive or emits only low levels of EMR.

The most common types of geophysical instruments used on UXO projects are described below:

Low Sensitivity Magnetometer (LSM): The low-sensitivity magnetometer is the most commonly used instrument for UXO detection because it is cost-effective and easy to use. Instruments used are typically the dual-fluxgate type originally developed for the detection of underground utilities. They are inexpensive, readily available, and easy to use. In addition, they have the added benefit of being completely nonintrusive in that they do not emit even low levels of electromagnetic radiation, which can be a potential source of initiation for some electrically initiated UXO. A minor disadvantage of LSMs is that they detect only ferrous items, however, nonferrous UXO is fairly rare. LSMs are most frequently used to augment visual observation during surface and near-surface UXO searches and during safety escort operations.

High-Sensitivity Magnetometer (HSM): HSMs operate on the same principal as the LSM but can be calibrated and are much more sensitive. Some HSMs are designed specifically for subsurface UXO detection and are used by military EOD teams for that purpose. Some specific models have been extensively tested by the U.S. Naval EOD Technology Center and are capable of locating large UXO up to 20 feet underground. They may be equipped with a fluxgate sensor probe that can be detached from the electronics package and lowered underwater and downhole. The primary disadvantages of this instrument are cost ($17,000 compared to $650 for the LSM) and increased weight and bulk. As such, an HSM is used only when greater detection capabilities are required or as a quality control tool to check areas previously searched by less capable instruments.

Metal Detector: Metal detectors, similar to those commercially available as treasure finders, are useful if the project requires a second method of UXO location. These instruments are inexpensive and can locate nonferrous objects. However, they do emit low-frequency radiation, which has the remote possibility of initiating certain UXO under ideal conditions. Underwater versions are also available for use by divers.

UXO Detection Techniques

The following general description of UXO methodology is not intended to train the reader in UXO operations and handling, but rather to make the reader aware of standard and accepted practices. This will allow the reader to more easily recognize potentially unsafe situations.

A group of UXO specialists surveying an area for UXO will most likely begin the project by marking the boundary of the area to be surveyed with wooden stakes. The location of all stakes should be checked with a geophysical instrument to ensure that no UXO are present prior to hammering a stake in the ground. They will then divide the area into five-foot-wide search lanes by stringing surveyors line between stakes hammered in at opposite ends of the survey area. The UXO survey team will then use the low-sensitivity magnetometer, described earlier, to examine each survey lane thoroughly.

Upon detecting a possible subsurface UXO, the UXO specialist will mark the spot with a pin flag or a spot of spray paint. A team of two UXO specialists will then excavate the marked items. Consistent with the concept of exposing the minimum number of site personnel to the hazard of detonation, UXO excavation should not take place until the magnetometer survey team has advanced beyond the hazard area of a possible accidental detonation caused by the excavation team.

UXO Excavation Techniques

Anomalies suspected to be UXO can only be positively identified by a trained UXO specialist after the item is recovered by excavation. The vast majority of UXO are located within two feet of the surface and a variety of common hand tools are used to excavate these relatively shallow UXO. A backhoe can be used by a skilled UXO specialist/equipment operator for large projectiles and bombs that can be imbedded from 10 to 20 feet underground. Although the objective is to gain access to UXO, the UXO excavation process is still governed by OSHA [18] and U.S. Army [19] worker protection requirements.

Upon locating the suspected item, the members of the excavation team will attempt to identify it. First they will determine if it is UXO. If it is not UXO and is not hazardous, such as a piece of metallic scrap, the hole may be backfilled and the non-hazardous metallic item may be removed and discarded.

If the item is identified as UXO, the excavation team will attempt to positively identify it. This may or may not be possible depending on the item and its state of deterioration. The results of the excavation should be recorded in a field UXO log book.

UXO Disposal Options

The following information, describing the rationale and logic for properly handling and disposing of UXO is also illustrated in the logic diagram in Figure (1).

If the UXO item is positively identified as armed and unsafe to move, or if it cannot be positively identified, it will be blown in place (BIP). If the item is positively identified and the fuze is determined to be unarmed and safe to move, the UXO may be moved to a secure storage facility for collection and later disposal by detonation at a designated and prepared disposal site. This is most efficient on larger projects where a secure storage area is constructed and maintained for the storage of UXO and working explosives in proper and approved magazines.

UXO discovered during safety escort operations are usually reported to the military EOD team responsible for supporting the area because UXO disposal is usually not included in the statement of work for such projects. An important consideration during the planning for this kind of operation is to establish a clear understanding of who has custody of, and responsibility for, any UXO discovered during the project.

UXO DISPOSAL TECHNIQUES

Disposal of UXO during a UXO remediation project can become a major task if large amounts of UXO are discovered. The following sections discuss the accepted methods of UXO disposal and the critical factors that must be considered when designing a safe and efficient UXO disposal operation.

Unpredictability of UXO

UXO is most often discovered in a deteriorated condition that results from years of exposure. It may have been buried for long periods of time or highly stressed by being fired downrange and failing to function as designed or being kicked out of an improperly constructed disposal detonation.

UXO fuzing is usually mechanical or electric, or a combination of both, and it is frequently impossible to tell the effect on the UXO of stress, such as the heat and shock of being propelled from an improperly constructed disposal detonation, and deterioration. For these reasons, it is sometimes impossible to determine the condition of certain UXO and, therefore, those UXO should be considered unsafe to move.

Positive Identification

Before considering whether or not it is safe to move a UXO it must be positively identified. Positive identification is made more difficult by the stress to which the UXO has been subjected. Stress such as heat, shock, weather, and time, tend to obliterate the key identification features that are used to positively identify UXO.

Positive identification by UXO specialists is made more difficult by the fact that UXO specialists do not have easy access to EOD publications. These publications are produced, by the EOD Technology Center in Indian Head, Maryland, as reference documents for EOD technicians and provide them with detailed information on the identification and functioning of specific ordnance.

These publications are frequently classified and are available to UXO specialists through the Huntsville MCX only on an as-needed basis for a specific type of UXO. UXO specialists are not authorized to maintain EOD 60 Series libraries which would require that the publications be guarded with the proper security and updated when changes to the publications are promulgated by the EOD Technology Center in Indian Head, Maryland.

UXO specialists, therefore, are frequently required to identify UXO based on their experience. They must always err on the side of safety and consider a UXO not positively identified unless it is a common UXO and they are thoroughly familiar with its characteristics and operation. If a UXO cannot be positively identified, it must be considered to be not safe to move and should be disposed of by blow-in-place (BIP) or, if the area cannot withstand a high order detonation, moved only after military EOD have performed an approved render-safe procedure (RSP).

Determining if UXO is Safe to Move

It is often much more efficient to consolidate UXO for disposal in a large disposal detonation as opposed to disposing of all UXO on a project by BIP. This requires that the UXO be moved to the disposal site and safely stored until enough UXO is amassed for an efficient disposal detonation.

Before a UXO can be moved it must be positively identified as previously described. Once positive identification is made the decision to move a UXO is based on an understanding of the UXO's fuzing and condition.

The UXO specialist will determine if the UXO item's fuze has been armed. Ordnance is designed so that fuze arming occurs when the ordnance is fired or otherwise deployed. Therefore, UXO that have been fired or otherwise deployed, and have failed to function as designed, are considered to be armed. Usually, armed UXO will be disposed of by BIP but some specific UXO are safe to be moved even in an armed condition. Detailed knowledge of the specific UXO is required to safely move armed UXO.

Even if the condition of a UXO is considered to be not armed the UXO specialist may decide that it is not safe to be moved based on the appearance of the particular UXO item. UXO that has been subjected to stress such as heat and shock may be damaged internally and not safe to move. The UXO specialist should err on the side of safety and BIP any UXO that are questionable.

Disposal by Blow-In-Place

Another common method of disposal by detonation is the BIP. This method is used to dispose of ordnance, that cannot be safely moved, by detonating it where it is found and is done by detonating a small initiation charge of explosives that has been properly placed in contact with, or close to, the UXO.

The advantage of disposing of UXO by BIP is that the UXO is not moved and, therefore, the maximum degree of safety is realized. On the other hand, some sites cannot withstand a high order detonation because of their proximity to valuable or sensitive assets and disposal by BIP is not possible. BIP is also very time consuming and costly method to dispose of large quantities of UXO.

Render Safe Procedures

One option that a UXO specialist is not authorized by the Huntsville MCX to perform [20] is the RSP. These procedures require detailed knowledge of the UXO and the recommended RSP which is only available from EOD 60 Series publications. The issues involved with procuring, maintaining, and safeguarding EOD 60 Series publications have been discussed earlier.

Performing an RSP involves a detailed procedure designed to eliminate the possibility of detonation of the UXO. Most RSPs require the removal or disablement of the fuze. The act of performing an RSP is itself inherently hazardous and preparations for a high order detonation should be taken in the event that the RSP is not successful. For this reason EOD technicians will frequently perform an RSP remotely and not subject themselves to the hazard of a detonation caused by an unsuccessful RSP.

Disposal of UXO in a Prepared Disposal Area

UXO specialists usually will establish a disposal operation using standard EOD procedures [21] for disposal by detonation. An important aspect of a UXO disposal operation is the minimization of shock and fragmentation caused by the disposal operation, to lessen the impact on the surrounding area. Common methods for reducing blast and fragmentation effects are to tamp each disposal shot using earth or sandbags.

It is often preferable to dispose of UXO by detonation in a prepared disposal area as opposed to performing all disposals by BIP. UXO disposal in a prepared disposal area has the advantages of being safer and more efficient and has less of an impact on the surrounding area. The increased efficiency occurs because setting up one large disposal detonation only takes slightly longer than preparing a BIP. And large quantities of UXO can be disposed of at once at a prepared disposal area while a BIP will usually involve a single UXO or possibly a cluster of UXO found in close proximity to each other.

The selected site will have less of a lasting impact on the environment because the disposal site can be chosen instead of being dictated by the location the UXO was found in. Previously disturbed sites can be selected for the UXO disposal area thereby limiting the impact to such areas. Also, the environmental impacts are contained in the selected area and it can be completely remediated after UXO disposal operations are finished.

UXO disposal in a prepared detonation area improves the safety of the overall disposal process because the disposal site can be selected to have favorable conditions and access to it can be positively controlled. UXO disposal areas should be designed to be easily accessible by UXO and emergency personnel, and easily and positively secured when UXO disposal operations are being conducted.

Another advantage of using a prepared UXO disposal site is that it is possible to perform larger detonations while minimizing the effects of blast and fragmentation. This is usually accomplished by tamping the disposal detonation, which is accomplished by burying it. A properly tamped disposal detonation will consist of a hole, in which the UXO is placed and covered by at least three feet of earth prior to detonation. This will help to contain the detonation and reduce the amount of blast and fragmentation.

Storage and Security

The security requirements of a UXO disposal operation vary from site to site. Active military facilities may have fenced and guarded perimeters which provide adequate security without modification. On the other hand, a FUDS site that is no longer under DOD control may have no existing security and require that a considerable effort be expended to prevent the possibility of unauthorized personnel gaining access to the UXO.

Because of the extreme hazard presented by UXO, combined with the attractiveness of UXO to children as souvenirs, appropriate action must be taken to ensure the security of the disposal site. Appropriate actions to enhance site security may include the erection of fencing and implementation of security patrols. Explosives magazines, in compliance with federal regulations [22] can also be used to enhance the safety and security of stored explosives and UXO.

Detonation Size Limits

The maximum size of disposal detonations allowable will depend on the specific site exclusion area available around the disposal site. The size of the exclusion area required is determined by the size, in pounds net explosive weight (lbs. NEW), of the UXO disposal detonation, including the explosive used for initiation of the detonation. There are two governing references for determining the required exclusion area and, in order to comply with both of them, the greater exclusion area should be observed.

The Huntsville MCX governing reference to determining the detonation exclusion area [23] states that an unoccupied radius of 1250 feet is required for detonation of non-fragmenting explosive material. Fragmenting UXO requires an unoccupied radius of at least 2,500 feet for disposal detonations of UXO smaller than 5 inches, and 4,000 feet for UXO 5 inches and larger.

The EOD standard governing reference [24] provides the following formula for determining the exclusion area:

In order to comply with both governing references, a detonation exclusion area smaller that 1,250 feet cannot be used. An exclusion area of 2,500 feet can be used to detonate UXO smaller than 5 inches in size and totaling no more than 570 lbs. NEW. A 4,000 foot exclusion area is required for disposal detonations containing UXO larger than 5 inches and totaling no more than 2,350 lbs. NEW.

REFERENCES:

1.   "Peterborough Explosion: A Report of the Investigation by the Health and Safety Executive into the Explosion of a Vehicle Carrying Explosives at Fengate Industrial Estate, Peterborough on 22 March, 1989," *Health and Safety Executive*, London (England), Report No.: ISBN-0-11-885572-7.

2.   This definition of OEW has been developed by the Huntsville MCX and has been used frequently in their statements of work to contractors.

3.   "Department of Defense Dictionary of Military and Associated Terms," Joint Publication 1-02, 1 December, 1989.

4.   These training and experience requirements have been established by the Huntsville MCX and are frequently used as requirements in their statements of work to contractors.

5.   "Development of a Simplified Field Method for the Determination of TNT in Soil," Special Report 90-38, November 1990, Thomas F. Jenkins, U.S. Army Cold Regions Research and Engineering Laboratory, Hanover, New Hampshire.

6.   "Development of a Field Screening Method for RDX in Soil," Special Report 91-7, June 1991, Thomas Jenkins and Marianne Walsh, U.S. Army Cold Regions Research and Engineering Laboratory, Hanover, New Hampshire.

7.   "Field Screening Method for 2,4 DNT in Soil," Special Report 91-17, October 1991, Thomas Jenkins and Marianne Walsh, U.S. Army Cold Regions Research and Engineering Laboratory, Hanover, New Hampshire.

8.   "Determination of the Chronic Mammalian Toxicological Effects of RDX: Twenty-Four Month Chronic Toxicity/Carcinogenicity Study of Hexahydro-1,3,5-Trinitro-1,3,5-Triazine (RDX) in the Fischer 344 Rat," Final Report, November 1983, B.S Levine, E.M. Furedi, V.S. Rac, D.E. Gordon, and P.M. Lish, IIT Research Institute, Chicago, Illinois.

9.   "U.S. Army Armament, Munitions and Chemical Command Study on Demilitarization Alternatives to Open Burning/Open Detonation (OB/OD)," Project No. DEV 12-88, June 1990, the U.S. Army Defense Ammunition Center and School, Evaluation Division, Savanna, Illinois.

10.   "Incineration of Explosive Contaminated Soil as a Means of Site Remediation," Technical Report, November 1992, M.A. Major and J.C. Amos, U.S. Army Biomedical Research and Development Laboratory, Fort Detrick, Maryland.

11. "Proceedings of the Workshop on Composting of Explosives Contaminated Soils," September 1989, U.S. Army Toxic and Hazardous Materials Agency (Technical Support Division), Aberdeen Proving Ground, Maryland.

12. "Economic Feasibility Analysis for Development of Low-Cost Chemical Treatment Technology for Explosive Contaminated Soils," Final Report May 1990, M.C. Crim and C.W. Brown, Tennessee Valley Authority, Muscle Shoals, Alabama.

13. "Materials Handling of Explosive Contaminated Soil and Sediment," Installation Restoration General Environmental Technology Development Task 6, June 1985, Lawrence J. Bove, M. Ramanathan, John W. Noland, and Peter J. Marks, Roy F. Weston, Inc. West Chester, Pennsylvania.

14. "U.S. Army Corps of Engineers Safety and Health Requirements Manual," EM 385-1-1, April 1981, Revised October 1987.

15. "Safety Concepts and Basic Considerations for Unexploded Explosive Ordnance (UXO)," Revised September 1992, U.S. Army Corps of Engineers, Huntsville Division.

16. "Range Clearance Technology Assessment," Final Report, Revision 1, March 1990, U.S. Naval Explosive Ordnance Disposal Technology Center, Indian Head, Maryland.

17. "Electromagnetic Radiation (EMR) Hazards of Unexploded Explosive Ordnance (UXO)," Revised September 1992, U.S. Army Corps of Engineers, Huntsville Division.

18. U.S. Code of Federal Regulations chapter 29, Part 1926, Subpart P.

19. "U.S. Army Corps of Engineers Safety and Health Requirements Manual," EM 385-1-1, Chapter 23, Revised October 1987.

20. UXO specialists are specifically prohibited from performing render safe procedures by all statements of work issued to contractors by the Huntsville MCX.

21. "EOD Disposal Procedures," EOD Publication 60A-1-1-31, Classified "For Official Use Only, November 1983, The U.S. Naval Explosive Ordnance Disposal Technology Center, Indian Head, Maryland.

22. U.S. Code of Federal Regulations Chapter 27, Part 55, Subpart K.

23. "Safety Concepts and Basic Considerations of Unexploded Explosive Ordnance (UXO)," Revised September 1992, U.S. Army Corps of Engineers, Huntsville Division.

24. "EOD Disposal Procedures," EOD Publication 60A-1-1-31, Classified For Official Use Only, January 1982, The U.S. Naval Explosive Ordnance Disposal Technology Center, Indian Head, Maryland.

16

SITE HEALTH AND SAFETY PLANS

William F. Martin, P.E.

The hazardous waste site health and safety plan is the document that brings all the various health and safety information into an operational plan. It is a dynamic document in that it must be continually updated if and when new information is discovered.

These health and safety plans vary greatly depending on the experience of the contractor, reviewing agency, and scope of project. Health and safety plans may be only a few pages that list the operational procedures which are then followed up by hundreds of pages of background and training materials selected employees are required to study.

Most plans will identify the hazards, evaluate the risk to workers and provide methods or work practices to minimize potential exposure or accidents, thus preventing illness/injury. Lines of authority and responsibility along with communication channels are normally required by state and federal agencies. The training and/or experience required for each task is generally included.

Many health and safety plans will reference the state or federal regulation such as 29 CFR 1910.120, then leave it up to the on-site health and safety officer to interpret and enforce the appropriate regulations. It has become a more common practice to restate the key applicable regulation in the health and safety plan.

Due to the potential for high cost liabilities at hazardous waste sites, it is a good idea to train the site personnel using the indepth site specific health and safety plan. This accomplishes the mandated training requirements, assures the employers that site personnel have read the health and safety plan, and documents by employee signature that training and instructions were received.

The documentation of employee training brings us to another potential legal problem. The health and safety plan must be specific enough to give good clear instructions but broad enough to allow the work to be accomplished without violating the written instructions. No employer wants to be brought into court in violation of his/her own health and safety plan. The health and safety plan must be written with the expectation that any disputes or accidents that occur on the site will reach the courts. Thus, do not say more than you can do; do not write anything you do not know, and prepare the health and safety documents with the expectation that they will be interpreted by the *Judge*. The longer and more extensive the health and safety plan, the more likely that an opposing lawyer can find a challenging point. However, an indepth and well documented health and safety plan can be used as evidence that the employer went to great lengths in their efforts to protect the workers and the environment. Each site and subsequent health and safety plan has to be evaluated with these legal dilemmas in mind.

An example of a site health and safety plan has been provided in this chapter. This is a military base investigation and clean up with a dollar value in the range of $5 to $15 million covering a variety of activities. The hazardous waste regulations have not specified any particular format, however most regional EPA and state agencies will often identify the minimum topics that must be covered by the particular site health and safety plan. The United States Environmental Protection Agency (USEPA) has developed a generic Health and Safety Plan (HASP) available on both 3.5- and 5.25-inch disks for most computer floppy drives. This publicly available health and safety planner can be ordered from the USEPA, Response, Engineering and Analytical Contract (REAC) at 2890 Woodbridge Avenue, Edison, New Jersey, 08837-3679, or call 1-800-999-6990.

Also see EPA publication 9285-8-01, March, 1992 for guidelines on the use of the computer disk.

Early contact with the local environmental plus health and safety regulatory agencies may save a lot of time, expense and delays.

EXAMPLE

SITE HEALTH AND SAFETY PLAN

FOR

(name) HAZARDOUS WASTE SITE

_____(location)_____

CONTRACT #_____

NATIONAL PRIORITY LIST #_____

Submitted to:

_____
_____
_____

Prepared by:

_____
_____
_____

Date: _____

Revisions: _____

TABLE OF CONTENTS

SECTION 1.0 INTRODUCTION

This Site Health and Safety Plan (SHASP) has been prepared to provide specific procedures and guidelines for all tasks at _____ Site under this contract. It is a dynamic document which is subjected to revisions in response to various conditions which may be encountered.

The purpose of the SHASP is to provide general procedures for defining responsibilities, identify hazards, and designate procedures to be followed for each activity at each designated location. This Plan should be viewed as standard operating procedures for all on-site activities. The Site Safety Officer (SSO) should be thoroughly familiar with the information contained in this Plan.

Applicability of the SHASP extends to all employees, contractors, subcontractors, and visitors entering this controlled location. All personnel must review the SHASP and sign an agreement to comply with its provisions prior to commencing any on-site work.

SECTION 2.0 ORGANIZATION

The following personnel are designated to carry out the stated job function on-site (one person may occupy more than one position).

Project Manager (PM) - The PM is responsible for overall coordination of all activities.

Site Manager (SM) - The SM is responsible for the daily operation of the site.

Health and Safety Coordinator (HSC) - The HSC is responsible for the overall coordination of all safety matters and has stop work authority. The HSC is responsible for the review of health and safety of all operations and will periodically perform audits of all operations. In addition, the HSC will be responsible for the review of all site documentation relating to monitoring, protective equipment, and accident reporting. In addition, the HSC will supervise health and safety during the initiation of Level B operations and at the initiation of each new phase of the project.

Site Safety Officer (SSO) - The SSO is responsible for the daily implementation and enforcement of the SHASP. The SSO also will be responsible for:

- Daily safety meetings.
- Overseeing the safety of daily operations.

- Monitor for worker and ambient exposures.
- Evaluate daily weather and chemical hazards.
- Notify the HSC of discrepancies or violations of the SHASP.
- Maintain required on-site records.
- Maintain daily records of activity, monitoring, protective equipment employed, employee exposure roster, and accidents reported.
- Maintaining safety and monitoring equipment.

Site Health and Safety Technician (SHST) - The SHST will report to the SSO and will receive his specific duties from the SSO.

All Other Personnel - Contractor/Subcontractor/Visitors. All personnel entering this controlled site will be responsible for:

- Review and compliance with the provisions of the SHASP as minimal requirements.
- Submission of required paper work.
- Completion of site specific training as required.

SECTION 3.0 TRAINING REQUIREMENTS

Consistent with OSHA's 29 CFR 1910.120 regulations covering Hazardous Waste Operations and Emergency Response (HAZWOPER), personnel will be trained in accordance with the applicable requirements. This will require forty (40) hours of classroom instruction with appropriate field exercise, and sixteen (16) hours of supervised on the job training.

At a minimum, all personnel will be trained to recognize on site hazards, the provisions of the SHASP, and the responsibilities of personnel.

All individuals entering the Contamination Reduction Zone (CRZ) and the Exclusion Zone will be required to present proof that they have the appropriate training and attend meetings as described below:

1) *40 Hour HAZWOPER*: Proof of attendance at a forty (40) hour Hazardous Waste Operations and Emergency Response (HAZWOPER) training course, with subsequent eight (8) hour annual refresher courses, will be required for any personnel engaged in activities routinely requiring Level C or higher protection.

2) *24 Hour HAZWOPER*: Proof of attendance at a twenty four (24) hour HAZWOPER training course, with subsequent eight (8) hour annual refresher courses, will be required for any personnel not engaged in invasive activities, or routinely requiring Level C or higher protection.

3) *8 Hour HAZWOPER*: Proof of attendance at an eight (8) hour HAZWOPER training course, with subsequent eight (8) hour annual refresher courses, will be required for any personnel not routinely required to enter the Contamination Reduction Zone or beyond.

4) *Supervisor Training*: Supervisors will be required to present proof of attendance at an eight (8) hour HAZWOPER Supervisor course. (Note: At this time, there is no requirement for supervisor annual refresher courses.)

5) *First Aid and Cardio-Pulmonary Resuscitation (CPR) Training*: The HSC will designate those individuals to be trained in first aid and CPR. It is expected that a select number of field team members will have this training. These courses will be consistent with the requirements of the American Red Cross Association, the American Heart Association, the Regional EMS Council or Medic First Aid Training Program of America.

A copy of the above CPR and first aid certifications will be available on site and in the individual's personnel file.

6) *Site-Specific Training*: Prior to any personnel commencing site work, they will be provided with training that will specifically address the activities, procedures, monitoring, and equipment to be used in their assignment. It will include site and facility layout, hazards, and emergency services at the site. It will detail all provisions contained in the SHASP. This training also will allow field workers to clarify anything they do not understand and to reinforce their responsibilities regarding safety for their particular activity.

7) *Safety Meetings*: Field team personnel will be given briefings by the SSO (or HSC) on a daily or as-needed basis to further assist site personnel in conducting their activities safely. It will be provided

when new operations are to be conducted, changes in work practices which must be implemented when new information is made available, or if site or environmental conditions change. Briefings also will be given to facilitate conformance with prescribed safety practices or when conformance with these practices is not being followed or if deficiencies are identified during safety audits.

8) *Advanced Training*: An advanced training course will be provided if any personnel will be expected to preform site work utilizing Level A protection. The course will provide training in the use of fully encapsulated suits and their associated problems. The Advanced Training course will comprise approximately eight (8) hours of classroom instruction and field exercise.

SECTION 4.0 MEDICAL MONITORING REQUIREMENTS

Consistent with OSHA's 29 CFR 1910.120 regulations covering Hazardous Waste Operations and Emergency Response, all personnel entering the Contamination Reduction Zone (CRZ) and the Exclusion Zone will be required to present proof of the following medical surveillance:

1) Statement of physical ability/limitations signed by a licensed physician within the last two years, and renewed as required.
2) Pulmonary function test, including Forced Expiratory Volume in one second (FEV1) and Forced Vital Capacity (FVC), within the last year, and renewed as required.
3) A medical data sheet. (See Figure 4.0-1.)

Figure 4.0-1
MEDICAL DATA SHEET

This brief Medical Data Sheet will be completed by all on-site personnel and will be kept in the Command Post during the conduct of on-site work. It is in no way a substitute for the medical surveillance program requirements. This data sheet will accompany any personnel when medical assistance is needed or if transportation to a hospital facility is required.

PROJECT:		
NAME:		**HOME PHONE: ( ) -**
ADDRESS:		
AGE:	**HEIGHT:**	**WEIGHT:**
PERSON TO CONTACT IN THE EVENT OF EMERGENCY:		
NAME:		**PHONE: ( ) -**
ALLERGIES:		
PARTICULAR SENSITIVITIES:		
DO YOU WEAR CONTACTS:		
PROVIDE A CHECKLIST OF PREVIOUS ILLNESS AND EXPOSURE TO HAZARDOUS CHEMICALS:		
WHAT MEDICATIONS ARE YOU PRESENTLY TAKING?		
DO YOU HAVE ANY PARTICULAR MEDICAL RESTRICTIONS?		
NAME OF PERSONAL PHYSICIAN:		
PHONE #:		

A copy of the above documents will be available to HSC in case of an emergency.

4) Complete blood chemistry.
5) Complete urine analysis.
6) Complete electrocardiogram.
7) Complete physical examination.
8) Complete medical history.
9) Metal screen (optional based on potential exposure).
10) Specific metabolites (optional based on potential exposure).

A copy of the above documents will be kept on file either by the employee or medical facility with ready access if medical treatment is required. Protection of employee privacy as provided by OSHA regulations will be followed.

SECTION 5.0 CHEMICAL/PHYSICAL/BIOLOGICAL HAZARDS

5.1 Exposure to Hazardous Chemicals

Chemicals can cause a variety of workplace hazards, which include flammable atmospheres, acute and chronically toxic atmospheres, oxygen-deficient atmospheres, and skin exposure to toxic liquids and solids. In addition, potentially violent physical hazards can result from chemical incompatibility and chemical instability. The actual level of the potential hazard depends upon the nature of the chemical, its physical form, its concentration, the environment in which it is present, and the operation performed at the site.

Chemical hazards are not only determined by the toxicity of a substance, but also how the employee will come in contact with it. The toxicity of a chemical is not synonymous with it being a health hazard. Toxicity is the capacity of a chemical to produce injury or harmful effects. Hazard is the possibility that exposure to a chemical will cause injury when it is encountered in the environment.

5.2 **Properties of Chemicals**

Chemical substances can be defined by their physical state, hazardous properties, and toxic mode of action. An understanding of these categories is necessary to properly assess the chemical hazard.

5.2.1   *Physical State*

Knowledge of the physical state of a chemical is necessary for the assessment of the level of a hazard. In particular, it is often necessary to distinguish between a solid and a gaseous contaminant, or to make distinctions based upon particle size. The following definitions are useful:

1. A **dust** is a solid particle produced by mechanical means (e.g., crushing, grinding, detonation). A relatively large particle size normally is assumed (e.g., quartz).

2. A **fume** is a solid particle formed through the condensation of material formerly in the gaseous state. For example, a metal fume is formed from the condensation of volatilized metal which results in a very small particle size. Hence, the potential for deep penetration into the respiratory system is always the case. Often oxidation accompanies the initial volatilization of the solid. Thus, welding fumes contain many metal oxides (e.g., lead oxide).

3. A **mist** is a suspension of liquid droplets in the air as the result of splashing, atomization, or condensation (i.e., fog). The terms mist and fog generally imply visible clouds or plumes. Droplet sizes generally are relatively large (e.g., sulfuric acid mist).

4. A **gas** is an airborne contaminant that normally exists in the gaseous state at "normal temperature and pressure" (25° C, 760 mm Hg) (e.g., chlorine).

5. A **vapor** is a gaseous airborne contaminant that normally exists in the liquid state at normal temperature and pressure (e.g., benzene).

5.2.2   *Hazardous Chemical Properties*

The physical state of a chemical will determine its hazardous properties. Once a chemical's physical state is determined, the substance can be classified by the hazard(s) it presents. A chemical is hazardous if, under specific circumstances, it causes injury to persons or damage to property because of its reactivity, instability, spontaneous decomposition, flammability, or volatility. Under this definition, chemical substances can be grouped into the following hazard classifications:

- *Explosives* can be gases, vapors, or dusts that reach a concentration high enough for a spark, flame, or the right temperature and pressure to enter into a combustion reaction so rapidly and violently as to cause an explosion.

  Explosions may arise spontaneously, but more often they are caused by site activities such as moving drums, accidentally mixing incompatible materials, or introducing ignition sources into explosive environments. It is important to anticipate and recognize potential explosive substances and situations, and to monitor the work site and eliminate the hazard. Explosive hazards can be minimized by structuring the work activities so vapor and gas build up is minimal. Chemical vapors should be monitored and kept below their Lower Explosive Limit (LEL). A chemical's LEL is that mixture of vapor and air that will combust when introduced to an ignition source.

- *Flammable* and *Combustible* Liquids are divided into two classifications by their flash point. Flammable liquids do not burn as liquids, but instead give off vapors that only ignite when a combustible mixture in air is obtained. The minimum temperature required to ignite a chemical vapor is called its flash point.

  Class I: Liquids with flash points below 140°F are called Flammable Liquids. These liquids ignite easily and pose an extreme fire hazard. Gasoline, which can vary greatly in composition, has a flash point of -45°, so a flammable atmosphere is possible in still air above liquid gasoline even in very cold weather.

  Class II: Liquids with flash points at or above 100°F are called Combustible Liquids. These liquids need elevated temperatures or sustained ignition sources to combust. Examples are kerosene, naphthalene, and creosote oil.

- *Corrosives* are any solid, liquid, gas, or vapor that burns, strongly irritates, or destructively attacks skin tissue. Severe chemical burns are caused by direct skin contact, inhalation, or ingestion. Corrosives must be stored and handled with great care, the use of impervious protective equipment is essential.

- *Oxidizers and Incompatible Chemicals* are chemical substances that will decompose readily at room temperature or under slight heating. Some chemicals and chemical combinations can produce deadly and often unexpected hazards, including explosions and the release of toxic or flammable air contaminants. Any study of potential hazards at a work site must include consideration of incompatible and unstable chemicals. The basic classifications follow:

  1. **Incompatible chemicals** can produce toxic or flammable reaction products upon combination, or they can explode or burn upon contact (e.g., nitric acid and hydrogen sulfide; perchloric acid and toluene).

  2. **Shock-sensitive chemicals** can explode if they are subjected to violent handling, or even to friction. Any dried material in a bottle that formerly contained liquid should be treated as a shock-sensitive chemical, unless the handler knows otherwise (e.g., acid crystals, peroxides of some ethers).

  3. **Water-reactive chemicals** can create the hazards described above when they contact water (e.g., metallic sodium, calcium carbide, anhydrous aluminum chloride).

  4. **Air-reactive chemicals** can create the hazards described above when they contact air (e.g., phosphorus is pyrophoric, sodium is pyrophoric in moist air).

In addition, some chemicals produce gases as they decompose, and the pressure in their containers can rise to dangerous levels. The unexpected explosion of old bottles can cause injury from glass fragments and chemical splashes.

Protection from these hazards requires knowledge of their possible presence and careful preparation for the work. No work with chemicals of any type should be performed without consultation with the SSO.

- *Asphyxiants* are gases and vapors that displace the necessary oxygen to sustain life, resulting in suffocation. Asphyxiants are divided into two classifications:

  1. **Simple asphyxiants** are physiologically inert gases, although they may pose a fire hazard. They asphyxiate by diluting atmospheric oxygen (21% naturally) below that required to maintain sufficient oxygen blood levels (19.5%). Atmospheres deficient in oxygen do not provide adequate warning properties and most asphyxiants are odorless. The worksite and all confined spaces should be monitored to determine oxygen levels. Common asphyxiants are methane, ethylene, nitrogen, and acetylene.

  2. **Chemical asphyxiants** prevent the uptake of oxygen by the blood through direct chemical action. These chemicals combined with the oxygen reactive sites of cells and prevent oxygen transport and interaction. Carbon monoxide is the most well known, but hydrogen cyanide and hydrogen sulfide are also severe chemical asphyxiants. These chemicals can cause asphyxiation despite the presences of adequate oxygen levels. Strict adherence to the recommended exposure limit to chemical asphyxiants is required.

- *Toxic chemicals* upon overexposure produce injurious or lethal systemic effects on a part of the body that may be distant from the point of initial contact. Injuries may be felt immediately or may take several years to manifest. Symptoms of toxic chemical overexposure may be obvious or insidious, and could result in the development of an occupational disease. The toxic effect of chemicals depend on several factors such as, chemical concentration, route of entry, duration of exposure, and personal factors like smoking and drinking habits, medication use, nutrition, age, and sex.

5.3 Chemical Exposure and Effects

The toxic action of a chemical substance can be divided into acute and chronic effects. In addition these categories can be used to distinguish the type of exposure to a given chemical.

Acute exposures and effects involve short-term high concentrations that immediately result in illness, irritation, or death. Acute exposures are usually associated with accidents. Such incidents involve a severe single exposure that is rapidly absorbed and effects one or more vital organs. Acute exposures are typically associated with deaths or complete recovery of effected individuals.

Chronic exposures are contrary to acute, and usually result in a permanent chronic illness. Chronic exposures are characterized by low levels of chemical exposure over long durations, usually a working lifetime. Organ damage is irreversible and disabling. Health effects such as cancer and respiratory disease are chronic occupational diseases.

A hazardous chemical might produce many types of health effects. Benzene at very high concentrations can rapidly produce narcosis and death, but at lower concentrations one is more concerned about toxicity to blood-forming organs. At very low concentrations, an increased risk of leukemia is the effect of concern. Thus, any classification of chemicals by their effect must consider the expected exposure level. A scheme for classification by effect is described below:

1. **Central nervous system depressants** produce narcosis and other effects that can increase the risk of accidents (e.g., dimethyl ether).

2. **Irritants** produce a vesicant effect upon the tissues that they contact. Generally the principal site of damage in the respiratory system is dependent upon solubility. An extremely soluble irritant attacks primarily the upper airways. Less soluble ones penetrate deeper into the lungs, where the consequences may be more severe. Less soluble irritants do not have good "warning properties" and they do not produce intolerable eye irritation or airway discomfort even at dangerous concentrations. Nitrogen dioxide, for example, is tolerable at levels that can produce fatal lung edema after the end of the shift (e.g., hydrochloric acid, vanadium pentoxide).

3. **Systemic poisons** primarily attack one or more organs or organ systems, producing various acute or chronic effects (e.g., mercury, lead oxide).

4. **Sensitizers** predispose susceptible individuals to serious allergic-like reactions upon subsequent exposure to very low concentrations (e.g., toluene diisocyanate, cotton dust).

5. **Carcinogens** cause a malignant growth of body tissue (e.g., benzene, asbestos).

6. **Pneumoconiosis-producing dusts** cause nonmalignant lung diseases as the result of long-term accumulation of material in the lungs (e.g., asbestos).

7. **"Nuisance" dusts** do not cause serious irreversible effects even upon frequent exposure to relatively high concentrations (e.g., gypsum).

5.3.1   *Routes of Chemical Exposure*

A hazardous chemical must enter the body before it can exert its toxic effect. Where absorption into the blood stream occurs, a toxicant may elicit general localized effects, or more likely, the critical injury will be a target organ or tissue remote from the site of entry. The following routes of chemical exposure are:

5.3.1.1   *Inhalation*

The lungs are extremely vulnerable to chemical agents. Even substances that do not directly affect the lungs may pass through lung tissue into the bloodstream, where they are transported to other vulnerable areas of the body. Some toxic chemicals present in the atmosphere may not be detected by human senses, i.e., they may be colorless, odorless, and their toxic effects may not produce any immediate symptoms. Respiratory protection is therefore extremely important if there is a possibility that the worksite atmosphere may contain such hazardous substances.

Chemicals can also enter the respiratory tract through punctured eardrums. Where this is a hazard, individuals with punctured eardrums should be medically evaluated specifically to determine if such a condition would place them at unacceptable risk and preclude their working at the task in question.

5.3.1.2 *Skin Absorption*

Direct contact of the skin and eyes by hazardous substances is another important route of exposure. Some chemicals directly injure the skin. Some pass through the skin into the bloodstream where they are transported to vulnerable organs. Skin absorption is enhanced by abrasions, cuts, heat, and moisture. Hot work environments increase the potential for exposure by this route.

Dermal absorption is easily minimized. Employees should avoid all skin contact with contaminated materials. If clothing or shoes become wet with contaminated water, they should be changed promptly. Any chemical deposited on the skin should be washed off immediately with soap and water. An employee so exposed should attempt to determine the nature of the chemical and the advisability of obtaining emergency medical services, if an extremely toxic substance is suspected.

A special case is **absorption through the eye.** Chemicals can dissolve in the moist surface of the eye and reach the blood in the shallow capillaries. Contact lenses can trap contaminants on the surface of the eye and increase the damage.

While absorption may be the major concern for many chemicals, others damage the skin upon contact and produce dermatitis or other lesions. The skin and the eyes must be protected from contact with chemicals.

5.3.1.3 *Ingestion*

Although ingestion should be the least significant route of exposure at a site, it is important to be aware of how this type of exposure can occur. Deliberate ingestion of chemicals is unlikely, however, personal habits such as chewing gum or tobacco, drinking, eating, smoking cigarettes, and applying cosmetics on site may provide a route of entry for chemicals. Good personal hygiene is necessary to prevent the transfer of chemicals from the hands to items that are placed in the mouth. Such items are not allowed in areas of potential contamination.

5.3.1.4 *Injection*

The last primary route of chemical exposure is injection, whereby chemicals are introduced into the body through puncture wounds (for example, by stepping or tripping and falling onto contaminated sharp objects). Wearing safety shoes, avoiding physical hazards, and taking common sense precautions are important protective measures against injection.

5.3.2 *Hazardous Chemical Exposure Limits*

Assessing the chemical hazard at a worksite requires identification and quantification of the airborne contaminant(s). Once a contaminant has been quantified its concentration must be compared to known exposure limits that have shown to cause no adverse health effects. An understanding of dose response, exposure limits, and agencies that issue toxicological information is necessary to conduct site activities in a safe manner.

5.3.2.1 *Background Understanding of Exposure Limits*

Toxicological information and subsequent exposure limits are based on the Dose-Response Relationship. This relationship applies in experimental studies and recognizes that there is a dose range for chemicals that begins with a threshold dose that exhibits a small non injurious response and ends with a dose that results in death of 100% of the exposed population.

Governmental agencies and professional associations review animal experimental studies, epidemiological studies, past industrial experiences, and chemical similarities to determine exposure limits. Most exposure limits are set 10 to 100 times below the threshold or "no effect" dose.

As industrial, experimental, and medical data is obtained on a chemical, its exposure limit may adjust to reflect the new findings. Therefore, an exposure limit should not be viewed as a black and white barrier, nor as a license to expose, but as a guideline to measure and modify safety procedures.

Exposure Limits and worksite chemical concentrations are expressed in terms of their airborne levels:

- ppm - Parts of a vapor or gas per million parts of contaminated air by volume at room temperature and pressure.

- mppcf - Millions of particles of a solid or aerosol per cubit foot of air.

- mg/m^3 - Milligrams of a contaminant per cubic meter of contaminated air.

In any assessment of an airborne chemical hazard, the concentration in the air is important. There are three ways of expressing concentration:

1. **Parts per million** by volume = million parts of total gas mixture or, 1 ppm of X = (1 ml of X)/(1,000,000 ml of total gas mixture) = (1 ml of X)/(1 m^3 of total gas mixture)

2. **Percent** by volume = hundred parts of total gas mixture or, 1% of X = (1 ml of X)/(100 ml of total gas mixture)

3. **Milligrams per cubic meter** = cubic meter of air or, 1 mg/m^3 = (1 mg of X)/(1 m^3 of air)

All three expressions of concentration can be used to quantify levels of gases or vapors, but *only mg/m^3 is applicable to dusts, fumes, and other contaminants that are not in the gaseous phase.* When the contaminant is a gas or vapor, the four units of measure have the following relationships:

1. 1% by volume = 10,000 ppm by volume.

2. Concentration in percent by volume = [(partial pressure)/(760 mm Hg)]-100, if a pressure of one atmosphere, or 760mm Hg is assumed.

3. Concentration in mg/m^3 = $\dfrac{\text{(Conc. in ppm)-(molecular weight)}}{24.45}$

4. Concentration in ppm = $\dfrac{\text{(Conc. in } mg/m^3\text{)-(24.45)}}{\text{molecular weight}}$,

    if "normal" temperature and pressure (25° C and 760 mm Hg), at which one mole of a gas or vapor has a volume of 24.45 L, is assumed.

If benzene is present at a concentration of 10 ppm, one can calculate readily that:

Concentration in mg/m^3 = (10-78)/(24.45) = 32 mg/m^3,

because the molecular weight of benzene is 78 grams/mole. If a work environment contains 40 mg/m^3 of ammonia, then

Concentration in ppm = (40-24.45)/(17) = 58 ppm.

Also, 800 ppm of carbon dioxide is 0.08% by volume.

5.3.2.2 *Publication of Exposure Limits*

Several governmental agencies and professional organizations have established or adopted chemical exposure limits. Some of these exposure limits are published as guidelines, others are federal or state enforced laws. Three major groups publish exposure limits. Only OSHA standards are enforced by law. However, in most cases ACGIH-TLVs are viewed as being more complete and in many cases lower than OSHA-PELs. NIOSH established the Recommended Exposure Limits (RELs) and Immediately Dangerous to Life and Health (IDLH) exposure limits.

5.3.2.2.1 *ACGIH-TLV*

The Threshold Limit Value (TLV) is recommended by the American Conference of Governmental Industrial Hygienists (ACGIH) and is a consensus review derived exposure guideline. The TLVs are not mandatory employee exposure guidelines. The ACGIH periodically publishes and updates TLVs and documentation on which the TLV for each substance is based. Three categories of Threshold Limit Values are specified as follows:

1. **Time-Weighted Average (TLV-TWA)** is the timed-weighted average concentration for a normal 8-hour workday or 40-hour work week, to which nearly all workers may be repeatedly exposed, day after day, without adverse effect.

2. **Short-Term Exposure Limit (TLV-STEL)** is the maximal concentration to which workers can be exposed for a period of up to 15 minutes continuously without suffering from any of the following:

    (a) Irritation

    (b) Chronic or irreversible tissue change

    (c) Narcosis of sufficient degree to increase accident proneness, impair self-rescue, or materially reduce work efficiently.

The STEL should be considered a maximal allowable concentration, or absolute ceiling, not to be exceeded at any time during the 15-minute excursion period. No more than four 15-minute exposure periods per day are permitted, with at least 60 minutes between those exposure period; also, provided that the daily TLV-TWA also is not exceeded.

None of the limits mentioned here, especially the TWA-STEL, should be used as engineering design criterion or considered as an emergency exposure level (EEL).

3. **Ceiling (TLV-C)** is the concentration that should not be exceeded even instantaneously.

For some substances, for example, irritant gas, only one category, the TLV-Ceiling, may be relevant. For other substances, either two or three categories may be relevant, depending upon their physiologic action. It is important to observe that if any one of these three TLVs is exceeded, a potential hazard from that substance is presumed to exist.

The amount by which threshold limits may be exceeded for short periods without injury to health depends upon a number of factors such as the nature of the contaminant, whether very high concentrations (even for short period) produce acute poisoning, whether the effects are cumulative, the frequency with which high concentrations occur, and the duration of such periods.

5.3.2.2.2   *OSHA-PEL*

The Permissible Exposure Limits (PELs) are established in the Occupational Safety and Health Administration (OSHA) Standards 29 CFR 1910.1000, Tables Z, Z_2, and Z_3. The PELs are required workplace standards enforced by law. These standards were derived from the federal standards and national consensus standards. Thus, many of the 1968 Threshold Limit Values (TLVs) established by the American Conference of Governmental Industrial Hygienists (ACGIH) became federal standards or permissible exposure limits (PELs). Also, certain workplace quality standards known as maximal acceptable concentrations of the American National Standards Institute (ANSI) were included in the Federal Standards. In adopting the Threshold

Limit Values of the American Conference of Governmental Industrial Hygienists, OSHA also adopted the concept of the time-weighted average concentration (TWA) for a workday.

5.3.2.2.3 *NIOSH-REL*

The Recommended Exposure Limits (RELs) are issued by the National Institute for Occupational Safety and Health (NIOSH) established by Public Law 91-596. NIOSH is a training, research and recommending body with responsibility to assist OSHA in the establishment of new PELs. RELs are not enforced by law, until OSHA adopts them as PELs. Few permanent PELs have been established from NIOSH-RELs because of the extremely thorough, yet cumbersome standard setting process.

5.3.2.2.4 *NIOSH-IDLH*

NIOSH and the Mining Enforcement and Safety Administration (MESA) promulgated 30 CFR, Part II, which is the respirator approval law. This is an enforceable law. 30 CFR, Part II.3t, defines exposure concentrations that are Immediately Dangerous to Life and Health (IDLH). IDLH are conditions which pose an immediate threat to life and health, or severe contaminant exposure, such as radioactive materials, which are likely to have adverse accumulative or delayed effects on health.

These values are considered maximum concentrations above which only extremely reliable breathing apparatus, providing maximum protection shall be permitted.

5.3.3 *Assessment Criteria for Chemical Hazards*

5.3.3.1 *Vapor Pressure*

Vapor pressure is an important physical property influencing the concentration of a chemical in a work environment. The vapor pressure of a chemical is the pressure that would be exerted by saturated vapor in equilibrium with a liquid surface. The vapor pressure of benzene is 100 mm Hg at 26° C, so saturated vapor at this temperature would contain concentration of benzene molecules sufficient to exert this pressure. Vapor pressure increases with increasing temperature.

Generally, vapor pressure is used to compare volatility of two chemicals. For example, benzene is quite volatile at 25° C, but mercury is far less volatile. Mercury's vapor pressure at 25° C is 0.002 mm Hg. One would not expect that a contaminant concentration would approach saturation in a normal work environment, but comparisons among chemicals often are useful to identify the extremely volatile ones. The chemicals need not be exclusively liquids. Solid materials that experience sublimation have vapor pressures.

Another property used to compare volatility of liquids is *evaporation rate*. This normally is defined as the time required for evaporation of test solvent divided by the time required for evaporation of a reference solvent (usually dimethyl ether) under the same conditions. Acetone, which has an evaporate rate of 1.9 is more volatile than ethyl benzene, for which the rate is 9.4. There are other ways to express absolute and relative rates of evaporation, so knowledge of the exact meaning of the values used is necessary to avoid improper application.

5.3.3.2   *Gas or Vapor Density*

Gas or vapor density can also be significant in a hazard assessment. When small amounts of a chemical are released from dispersed locations into circulating air, good mixing can be assumed. However, when large amounts of concentrated vapor are released into still air, stratification can exist at least temporarily. The density of a pure gas or vapor is proportional to its molecular weight (and inversely proportional to its temperature). The effective molecular weight of air is 29, so stratification can occur if a much heavier (benzene, 78) or much lighter (hydrogen, 2) contaminant is released under the unfavorable conditions described above. This could occur in trenches or basements into which gasoline vapor from contaminated groundwater enters, or in sewers, where a hydrogen gas layer can exist near the top of under-ground vaults. A temporary - but very dangerous - condition of stratification could exist in a poorly ventilated room into which a large amount of gas or vapor is released during an accident or other short episode. A test of the cleaner portion of these spaces could indicate a safe condition, when an extremely toxic flammable atmosphere existed above or below the tested layer.

5.3.3.3   *Order Threshold*

Odor Threshold is a chemical property that can be useful at times. Odor can serve as a good warning when the odor threshold is below or about equal to the exposure limit for the chemical. However, questions of safety should not be decided on the basis of odor alone. Olfactory abilities differ greatly among individuals, and the sense of smell rapidly becomes fatigued upon exposure to new stimulus.

5.3.4 *Material Safety Data Sheets*

When available, Material Safety Data Sheets (MSDS) can provide valuable information when handling a chemical substance. Since the establishment of the Hazardous Communication Standard (29 CFR 1910.1200), chemical manufacturers and distributors are required to provide MSDS and warning labels on their products. Obtaining a MSDS on a chemical substance may provide valuable information on the chemical and physical hazards the material presents.

The sections on a MSDS, and the information they can provide include:

- Chemical Identity and Manufacture Information
- Hazardous Ingredients and Exposure Limits
- Physical and Chemical Characteristics
- Fire and Explosion Hazard Data
- Reactivity and Stability Data
- Health Hazard and Medical Treatment Information
- Precautions and Protection for Safe Handling and Use
- Control Measures to Avoid Overexposure

The hazard information that MSDSs are intended to provide is numerous, however, many published MSDS are incomplete and lack accurate information to assess a chemical hazard. Therefore, MSDS should be used as a guide, along with more in depth information from other sources.

5.4 Physical Hazards

Discussions of the physical hazards and how these hazards are to be addressed are included in Section 12.0, Standard Operating Procedures. Because of the wide range of physical hazards that may be encountered on the site, those physical hazards specific to each delivery order (DO) will be addressed under the associated SHASP.

The physical hazards associated with any DO include potential for chemical reactions, physical obstacles, slip/trip/fall potential, limitations of PPE, heat stress, and unexploded ordnance (UXO). Before going to any site, the assessment team will review the conditions of that site with the Safety Office with regards to any unique hazards such as UXO or energetic materials. If the Safety Office advises that such hazards may be present, the HSC and SSO will determine what precautions are required and implement the necessary procedures. The SSO will be on alert for the detection of energetic and hazardous materials such as UXO that have a potential to be present at this site due to its historical use.

NOTE: Examples can be given of conditions that have been ruled out: This site does not include the removal or opening of any well heads/caps using flame- or spark-producing methods.

5.5 Exposure to Radioactive Substances

Radioactive substances that may be encountered at hazardous waste sites emit one or more of three types of harmful radiation:

- Alpha
- Beta
- Gamma

Radioactive materials emit energy which can damage living tissue. The exact mechanism of the manner in which ionizing radiation affects body cells and tissue is complex. At the risk of oversimplifying some basic physical principles and ignoring others, the purpose of this section is to inform site personnel when problems with radioactive substances exist and to know when to call on an Industrial Hygienist, Health Physicist, or radiation safety expert for help.

5.6 Hazards of Radioactive Substances

Radioactive materials can be subdivided into internal or external hazards. Alpha and Beta radiation have limited penetration ability and are considered to be internal hazards. Their harmful effects are exerted when materials emitting alpha or beta radiation are inhaled or ingested. Beta radiation is also an external hazard because it can produce damage when contacted with skin and is known as "beta burns."

Gamma radiation is an external hazard. Materials that emit gamma radiation can be located some distance from the body and still emit energy that can ionize tissue and cause damage.

Because radiation can cause serious and permanent damage, the use of monitoring, PPE, and scrupulous personal hygiene and decontamination is required when working with radioactive materials. The use of respirators and other protective equipment can help keep radiation-emitting materials from entering the body by inhalation, ingestion, injection, or skin absorption.

5.7 Monitoring Radioactive Substances

When radioactive materials are anticipated or discovered on a project site, a combination of area and personal monitoring will be initiated.

5.7.1 *Area Monitoring for Radioactive Substances*

Many types of meters are used to measure various kinds of ionizing radiation. These meters are useless unless they are accurately calibrated for the type of radiation they are designed to measure.

Meters with very thin windows in the probes can be used to check for alpha radiation. Geiger-Muller and ionization chamber-type instruments are used for measuring beta and gamma radiation.

These meters usually read out in REMs per hour or mREMs per hour. A REM is a unit of dose equivalent which takes into account the absorbed energy and the relative biological effect. Personal exposure limits are expressed in REM.

Areas of suspected or known radioactive materials will be monitored to determine the levels of radiation above background. (Background radiation from cosmic rays 0.02-0.05 mREM/hr.) At levels in excess of the standards, 2 mREM/hr, all site activity will cease until the site has been assessed by a health physicist.

5.7.2 *Personal Monitoring for Radioactive Substances*

Devices are available that will measure accumulated amounts (doses) of radiation. Film badges are used as dosimeters to record the amount of radiation received from beta or gamma radiation.

Film badges are worn by personnel continuously during each monitor period and, depending upon how they are worn, they will allow an estimate of an accumulated dose of radiation to the whole body or to just a part of the body, such as a hand or arm. NOTE: Alpha radiation cannot be measured with film badges because the alpha particles will not penetrate the paper which must be used over the film emulsion to exclude light.

In addition to the film badge, another device for measuring accumulated does of gamma radiation is the electrostatic dosimeter, a combination electroscope and ionization chamber. This type of dosimeter requires periodic charging with a battery to return the pointer on the scale to zero.

Personnel working with and around radioactive materials will be monitored with dosimeters and their accumulated dose will not exceed the standards set by Federal, state and local agencies, and outlined in Figure 5.7.2-1.

Figure 5.7.2-1 Radiation Exposure Limits	
Type of Exposure	**NRC 10 CFR 20**
A. Whole body: head and trunk; lens of the eyes; gonads; active blood forming organs	2 mREMs/hour 1.25 REMs/quarter 5 REMs/year Not to exceed B.
B. Cumulative lifetime limit	5 (N-18) REMs n = age in years
C. Hands and forearms; feet and ankles	18.75 REMs/quarter 75 REMs/year
D. Skin of the whole body	7.5 REMs/quarter 30 REMs/year

5.7.3   *Special Precautions When Working with Radioactive Substances*

Precautionary procedures on sites where radioactive materials are present will consist of:

- Area and personal monitoring
- Sample Monitoring
  - Respiratory
  - Skin Contact
- Caution signs and warning labels
- Decontamination
- Record Maintenance

Many of these precautions will be expanded on whenever a new task is added to the contract work.

5.8 Biological Hazards

The unanticipated uncovering of waste from hospitals and research facilities may contain disease-causing organisms that could infect site personnel. Like chemical hazards, etiologic agents may be dispersed in the environment via water and wind.

Other biological hazards that may be present at a hazardous waste site include poisonous plants, insects, animals and indigenous pathogens. Protective clothing and respiratory equipment can help reduce the chances of exposure. Thorough washing of any exposed body parts and equipment will help protect against infection.

Biohazard is a combination of the words "biological hazard" and refers to infectious agents which may present a potential risk to the health and well-being of man. Biohazards can affect man either directly through illness or indirectly through disruption of the environment. Infectious biological agents consist of five types of infection: bacterial, viral, rickettsial, and, to a lesser degree, fungal and parasitic infections.

Biohazards can be transmitted to a person through inhalation, injection, ingestion or physical contact. The combination of the number of organisms in the environment, the virulence of these organisms and the resistance of the individual ultimately determines whether or not the person will actually contract the disease. The effects of a biological agent are further compounded by the presence of concomitant physical and/or chemical stresses in the environment. For example, the incidence and severity of respiratory infections may be enhanced by the presence of irritant gases in the air. After exposure to nitrogen dioxide, animals have been found to show a great susceptibility to pneumonia. Thus, it is important to consider not only the biological agents which pose a hazard to the occupational worker, but also to realize that exposure to other environmental stresses may result in an additive or synergistic effect.

5.9 Biohazard Control Program

In the event that biohazardous materials (i.e., medical waste, slaughter house remains, and refuse) are uncovered, biohazard safety procedures should be initiated. The elements of the biological control program consist of:

- Medical surveillance
- Identification of biohazards
- Personal protective equipment
- Personal hygiene
- Decontamination

In addition to these procedures, all employees contacting biohazardous waste will immediately go through decontamination and scrupulous personal hygiene.

Decontamination of a biohazard will include the washing of protective equipment with a water and ammonia solution or similar disinfectant. All PPE and tools will be disinfected or disposed of according to the decontamination program. Decontamination solutions will also be disposed of properly.

Biohazards, and their area of contamination, will be identified by the presence of a Biohazard Label. This area or container will be demarcated and access disallowed. A suitable abatement of the situation will require input from the Project Manager, HSC, SSO and possible public agencies.

Special local conditions that produce an extra risk should be identified, such as:

Of particular concern at this site is the presence of Copperhead snakes. In order to minimize this hazard:

- On site personnel will always work on the buddy system.
- Whenever working in overgrown areas, make as much noise as possible. Snakes will avoid you if given the chance.
- Visually check any area where a snake may be resting prior to probing or touching with your hands.
- A snake bite will be viewed as a medical emergency. Decontamination steps will be minimized. First aid will be immediately administered. Medical attention will be immediately sought.

An additional biological concerns is the presence of ticks. In order to minimize this hazard:

- All onsite personnel will tape wrist and ankles.
- All onsite personnel will use coveralls when working in areas which may potentially be infested with ticks.
- Commercial insect repellants will be used provided that they will not interfere with sampling objectives.
- After working in an area which may be infested with ticks, visually check each other for ticks.
- If a tick has begun to attach itself to you, seek medical attention for its removal. Most of the "old wives' remedies" do not work and result in infection.

SECTION 6.0 HAZARD EVALUATION

Variables of Hazardous Waste Site Exposure

Complex, multisubstance environments such as those associated with hazardous waste sites pose significant challenges to accurately and safely assessing airborne contaminants. Several independent and uncontrollable variables, most notably temperature and weather conditions, can affect airborne concentrations. These factors must be considered when developing an air monitoring program when analyzing data. Some demonstrated variables include:

- *Temperature.* An increase in temperature increases the vapor pressure of most chemicals.
- *Windspeed.* An increase in wind speed can affect vapor concentrations near a free-standing liquid surface. Dusts and particulate-bound contaminants are also affected.
- *Rainfall.* Water from rainfall can essentially cap or plug vapor emission routes from open or closed containers, saturated soil, or lagoons, thereby reducing airborne emissions of certain substances.
- *Moisture.* Dusts, including finely divided hazardous solids, are highly sensitive to moisture content. This moisture content can vary significantly with respect to location and time and can also affect the accuracy of many sampling results.
- *Vapor emissions.* The physical displacement of saturated vapors can produce short-term, relatively high vapor concentrations. Continuing evaporation and/or diffusion may produce long-term low vapor concentrations and may involve large areas.
- *Work activities.* Work activities often require the mechanical disturbance of contaminated materials, which may change the concentration and composition of airborne contaminants.

The hazard evaluation for each task is dependent on the specific job functions. Certain assignments will have a predominantly chemical hazard, others will have a predominantly physical hazard, and others will have a combination of physical and chemical hazards.

In order to adequately address the hazard potential:

1) Each job function for a specific task will be identified.

2) The chemical hazard for that job function will then be assessed in terms of low, medium, and high.

    HIGH CHEMICAL HAZARD operations include:
    ·   Drum inspection/overpacking/sampling, etc. _____
    ·   Decon line technician, etc. _____

    MEDIUM CHEMICAL HAZARD operations include:
    ·   Environmental matrix sampling, etc. _____
    ·   Drilling operations, etc. _____

    LOW CHEMICAL HAZARD operations include:
    ·   Surveying, etc. _____
    ·   Employee interviews, etc. _____

3) The physical hazard for that job function will then be assessed in terms of low, medium, and high.

    HIGH PHYSICAL HAZARD operations include:
    ·   Confined space entry
    ·   Working around heavy equipment
    ·   Reconnaissance surveys

    MEDIUM PHYSICAL HAZARD operations include:
    ·   Working in protective equipment
    ·   Sample collection
    ·   Geophysical surveys

    LOW PHYSICAL HAZARD operations include:
    ·   Equipment operators
    ·   Support zone personnel
    ·   Clean area work

    On-the-ground personnel will have the highest exposure to physical and chemical hazards.

    Equipment operators, staging area personnel and supervisors will have low to moderate exposure to physical and chemical hazards.

4) In order to adequately address the varying potentials for exposure, Personnel Protective Equipment and Decontamination Procedures will be designated based upon work assignments.

SECTION 7.0 SITE ZONATION

The primary means of maintaining site control will be "designated work areas." The work areas serve to limit site access, contain gross contamination, provide site security, and place a buffer zone between the hazardous site and the adjacent community.

The designated work zones will be established and shown in Figure 7.0-1, Site Layout Map.

Exclusion Zone - The Exclusion Zone is defined as the area which is considered to be contaminated, potentially contaminated, or which could become contaminated in the event of an emergency. In addition, the Exclusion Zone may be designated dependent on the nature of the work taking place in it. No unauthorized persons shall be within this area. All persons within this area shall be wearing the designated personnel protective equipment for their job function.

Contamination Reduction Zone - The Contamination Reduction Zone (CRZ) should preferably be set upwind of the prevailing winds. Access control points to both the Exclusion Zone and the Support Zone are maintained here. This zone provides an area for the decontamination of personnel, equipment, and samples. It is established in an area assumed to be clean, but is assumed to be contaminated as soon as personnel or equipment are processed from the Exclusion Zone to the Support Zone. The Contamination Reduction Zone will contain the stations designated in Section 10.0, Decontamination and the emergency equipment designated in Section 12.0, Standard Operating Procedures.

Support Zone - The Support Zone is the area farthest away from the hazardous substances, known to be free of contamination. It is the area where the Command Post, support and storage trailers, and sanitary facilities are located.

Assembly Area - The Assembly Area is the area where site personnel assemble during a site evacuation.

Break Area - These areas are designated areas where site personnel can take short breaks. This area will be designated at the daily safety meeting and its location will be dependent on the prevailing wind direction and site activity.

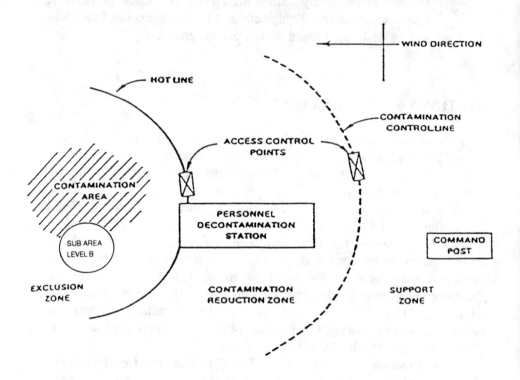

Figure 7.0-1. Site Layout Map

SECTION 8.0 PERSONNEL PROTECTIVE EQUIPMENT

This section describes the specific requirements for the various levels of protection required for each task.

8.1 Respiratory Protection Program

Respirators are one method of protecting personnel exposed to airborne contaminants at levels above established exposure limits. During field work, decisions on respiratory protection must be made quickly, so early preparation is essential.

No employee may use a respirator unless the following conditions are met:

- The user has been trained in the proper use of the device, and has been tested to ensure that the fit is acceptable. He is aware of its limitations, and he knows the procedure for testing the fit in the field before use.
- A determination has been made by a competent person that the device is appropriate for the intended application.
- A determination has been made by a physician that the user is medically fit to wear the respirator.
- The user is confident that the device is clean and that it has been maintained properly.

Respirator training may be included in the routine training for hazardous waste site workers, or it may be presented in a different session - even an informal one. In either case, documentation of the training must be filed with the HSC. The training must include information on the inspection of respirators and the limitations of respirators. If the respirator is one that operates with negative pressure inside the facepiece, then a successful fit test must be conducted by the HSC or by some other knowledgeable person. Documentation of the fit test must be filed with the HSC.

A medical determination of fitness to use a particular type of respirator normally will be included in the medical examination for hazardous waste site work. A record of this determination must be filed with HSC.

If respirators are assigned to individual workers for their exclusive use, then the user is responsible for cleaning the respirator, inspecting it, and ensuring that it is stored properly. In any case, the user must inspect the respirator and test its fit before each use. Respirators must be stored in clean locations where temperature extremes do not occur. The facepieces must not be deformed during storage.

Employees using respirators must be free of hair in areas where the respirator must form a seal on the face. Special glasses can be worn with a full-facepiece respirator. Contact lenses must not be worn in any area where respirators are considered necessary.

The Project Manager, Site Manager, and the HSC are responsible for enforcing these general requirements of the respiratory protection program. They are responsible for evaluating the effectiveness of the program and for correcting any noted deficiencies.

8.2 Respirator Selection

The selection of the appropriate respirator may be a complex task, which must be performed by someone knowledgeable of the environmental conditions at the work site and the capabilities of the various devices. The following questions are always to be considered.

- What contaminants are expected? What are the expected forms of the contaminants? (Are solid or vaporous contaminants expected?) (Are they hydrocarbons, metals, etc.?)
- What is the expected concentration? (Is the expected level far above the established exposure limit, or only slightly higher?)
- Could employees be exposed to contaminant levels that are immediately dangerous to life and health?
- Is the contaminant a strong irritant at relatively low levels?
- Do the anticipated conditions of use dictate some special type of equipment?

An important consideration in respirator selection is the *nominal "protection factor"* assigned to the various classes of devices. This factor is the nominal ratio of contaminant concentration outside the facepiece to that inside the facepiece.

Respirator Type	Protection Factor
Half-mask with filters	10
Full facepiece and filters	50
Powered air-purifying respirators	100
Continuous-flow supplied-air respirators with a full facepiece	100 - 2000
Full-facepiece supplied-air respirators operated in the pressure-demand mode	1000 - 2000
Full-facepiece self-contained breathing apparatus (SCBA) operated in the pressure-demand mode	1000 - 10,000

Devices with negative pressure inside the facepiece offer far less protection than those that maintain positive pressure. The integrity of the facepiece seal is much more important in the use of these negative-pressure devices, because leakage is inward. A full facepiece allows a much better seal than a half-mask facepiece. The pressure demand mode of operation offers the best protection since a slight positive pressure is maintained inside the facepiece.

If a condition immediately dangerous to life and health exists, then special provisions for escape are necessary. In most cases, such protection consists of a small bottle of air with associated apparatus, carried alone or worn in combination, with a primary protective device. If the failure of SCBA, or other primary respirator, could result in death or permanent injury, then an escape respirator must be a part of the protective ensemble. The bottle of auxiliary air is opened only if the primary device fails, and the auxiliary air is breathed through the SCBA facepiece during the brief interval required for escape. If an emergency could create a deadly atmosphere in an otherwise safe workplace, then employees working there without respirators (or with minimally protective respirators) must carry escape devices. This will be determined by the SSO and defined within the SHASP.

A full facepiece is necessary when eye exposure to the airborne contaminant would produce irritation - even when the concentration is sufficiently low to allow the use of a half-mask respirator to prevent excessive inhalation.

8.2.1   *Specific Respirator Types*

Two types of respirators are used most often: half-masked air-purifying respirators, and self-contained breathing apparatus operated in the pressure-demand mode. The former generally is appropriate for protection against lower contaminant concentrations - those less than ten times the established exposure limit. The latter is used when very high concentrations are expected, or when the airborne hazards are unknown. (Additional provisions for escape may be necessary for employees during use of either type of device, or under certain situations).

8.2.1.1   A half-mask air-purifying respirator with chemical cartridges is the device of choice for a wide range of situations. It operates with negative pressure inside the facepiece, so inward leakage can occur. For this reason, it must not be used if the concentration exceeds five to ten times the applicable limit (2 to 3 times the PEL, for example) is not detectable by odor or irritation, then the contaminant has poor warning properties, and the use of an air-purifying respirator requires special precautions. A half-mask respirator cannot be used if the contaminated atmosphere is irritating to the eyes. In this case, a full facepiece is needed. *An air-purifying respirator must never be used in an environment that is immediately dangerous to life and health or in one that could contain less than 19.5% oxygen.*

8.2.1.2   A Self-Contained Breathing Apparatus (SCBA) provides much greater protection, but is much more complicated. Proper selection, maintenance, and use are essential in the life-threatening environments in which a SCBA may be used. A SCBA must be used only by persons trained thoroughly in the operation of that specific model.

The pressure demand mode of operation provides the most protection. However, the slight positive pressure maintained continuously inside the facepiece causes the more rapid consumption of the air; the operating time for a new cylinder of air is relatively low. One receives less protection when the regulator is set for operation in the demand mode, but an air cylinder will last longer.

On some occasions, employees may use respirators to which air is supplied by a compressor or distant tanks of compressed air. If a compressor is used, then the SSO must ensure that it is designed for the provision of breathing air, and that the air meets the specifications detailed in 29 CFR 1910.134. Caution is required to ensure that the air drawn into the compressor is clean.

8.3 Personal Protective Equipment (PPE)

The purpose of PPE (suits, gloves, boots, earmuffs, hardhats, respirators, etc.) is to prevent illness or injury to the wearer by reducing contact with the hazardous material or environment to the extent that exposure remains within safe limits. Proper selection of PPE depends on the hazardous substance(s) or conditions present, the level of protection required, and the personal requirements of the wearer.

In many cases, PPE will be defined by a Site Safety Policy or outlined in the SHASP. In these cases, personnel are required to comply.

If an employee is on a job site where PPE requirements have not been defined, and the threat of personal injury is believed to exist, then that employee will obtain proper PPE or contact the SSO for PPE recommendations.

Certain general rules apply to job sites and the necessary personal protective equipment. These are:

- Hardhats shall be worn by all employees on sites where a hazard to head injury exists, such as: overhead work, work in and around pipes, confined spaces, moving objects, etc., or as required by the customer.
- Safety shoes shall be worn on all hazardous wastes sites and on jobs where the hazard to foot injury (i.e., heavy objects, punctures, etc.) exists, or as required by the customer.
    - Hazardous Waste Sites - Impermeable rubber boots with steel or safety plastic toe and shank are required. No tennis shoes or leather boots shall be worn. Leather safety shoes are allowed only in the Support Zone where there is no potential for contamination.
- Eye protection in the form of safety glasses, goggles, or a face shield shall be worn in areas where corrosives, liquids, vapors, and foreign bodies are present and the potential for splashing is possible. This includes all work with hazardous wastes; from site investigation to remediation.
- Gloves shall be worn when the hazard of hand injury exists, or work with corrosives or solvents is performed. The proper glove selection is important. Obtain proper glove selection from a chemical Material Safety Data Sheet or the SSO.
- Hearing Protection shall be worn by all personnel on job sites requiring such protection or when the employee feels the need for

hearing protection. The SSO can assist employees in defining the need and proper selection of hearing protection devices.

The use and selection of other forms of PPE (i.e., respirators, protective clothing) are detailed below. The use of PPE such as safety harnesses, slings, and proximity suits must be reviewed by the SSO and, if necessary, with the HSC and Site Manager.

Enforcement for the wearing of PPE is the responsibility of the SSO. Personnel must wear protective equipment when their work involves known or suspected airborne contamination, when airborne contaminants may be generated by site activities, or when skin contact with harmful substances may occur. Protective ensembles are classified in the following manner, according to the degree of protection afforded:

Level A - the highest level of respiratory, skin and eye protection.

Level B - the highest level of respiratory protection, but a lower level of skin protection.

Level C - a lower level of skin and respiratory protection than that specified by Level A. The criteria for using air-purifying respirators must be met.

Level D - no protection against chemical hazards. Level D specifies a "work uniform" for locations where chemical hazards are minimal.

The selection of the level of the protective ensemble depends upon the nature of the airborne chemical substances and their concentrations, as well as the potential for skin contact with chemicals during the course of the work. Skin contact could occur from splashes or from operations requiring that employees touch contaminated surfaces.

Skin exposure to airborne chemicals may present a significant hazard in some cases. Entry into confined spaces may require additional protection. The SSO may specify a protective ensemble that differs from those described above, if conditions warrant such a deviation.

8.4 Levels of Protection - Specific Requirements

8.4.1 *Level A - Selection Criteria.*

1. Available information indicates that likely or possible exposures warrant the highest level of respiratory, skin and eye protection. (Examples are fuming corrosives, cyanide compounds, potent

carcinogens, concentrated pesticides, infectious substances, and DDT Poison "A" materials. Fire, smoke, and other visible emissions almost always indicate a need for Level A.)

or

2. Substances with a high degree of hazard to the skin are present (or suspected) and skin contact is possible. (For example, moving drums of oleum, responding to accidents involving cyanide or arsenic, or excavating highly contaminated soil.)

or

3. Operations must be conducted in confined, poorly ventilated areas (confined spaces) until the absence of conditions requiring Level A protection is determined.

or

4. Readings on a flame ionization detector (FID) or a photoionization detector (PID) indicate concentrations of unidentified contaminants exceeding 500 ppm above background. (The SSO may approve a less cautious approach in cases involving known contaminants. Do not enter an area in which readings exceed 1000 ppm above background and the contaminants are unknown.)

8.4.2   *Level B - Selection Criteria*

1. Available information indicates that likely or possible exposures warrant the highest level of respiratory protection, but that the potential for harm from skin exposure is less than that requiring Level A. (An oxygen-deficient atmosphere, or one otherwise IDLH, would require Level B protection, if the chemical hazard to the skin were minimal. Level B often is appropriate for initial site reconnaissance.)

or

2. Readings on a flame ionization detector (FID) or a photoionization detector (PID) indicate concentrations of unidentified contaminants between 5 ppm and 500 ppm above background.

- The SSO may approve a less cautious approach in cases involving known contaminants.

8.4.3   *Level C - Selection Criteria*

1. Available information indicates that:

   a. An air-purifying respirator with a full face piece is adequate for protection against workplace concentrations of known contaminants, and
   b. The oxygen concentration in the workplace exceeds 19.5%, and
   c. The potential for harm from skin exposure is less than that requiring Level A.

   and

2. If contaminants are unknown, readings on a flame ionization detector (FID) or a photoionization detector (PID) indicate concentrations of below 5 ppm above background. (The SSO may approve a less cautious approach in cases involving known contaminants.)

8.4.4   *Level D - Selection Criteria:*

Excessive exposure to chemicals through the respiratory system, the skin, or the eyes is virtually impossible.

8.5 Levels of Protection - Upgrading and Downgrading

The decision on the appropriate level of protective clothing will be based upon the information discussed above - toxicity, concentration, potential for skin exposure to liquid or vapor, possible emergency conditions, etc. Caution dictates a very conservative approach when the nature of the contaminants is unknown, and additional precautions may be necessary when employees enter confined spaces or work in very hot environments.

When the conditions of exposure change, or when new information alters the hazard assessment, then a change in the level of protection may be indicated. The SSO and other responsible project personnel will conduct an ongoing evaluation on conditions of exposure, and monitor the suitability of the required level of protection. The HSC/SSO, in consultation with the

Project Manager, will specify a higher or lower level of protection whenever conditions change substantially. When these changes can be anticipated, the decision rationale will be written in the SHASP.

8.6 Repository Protection Requirements

Level A: Supplied air respirator (MSHA/NIOSH approved). Either positive pressure demand SCBA or positive pressure demand airline with 5 minute escape bottle, Max.300 feet of line, 45 # delivery pressure, and low air alarm. To be used in conjunction with impermeable barrier to prevent skin adsorption.

Level B: Supplied air respirator (MSHA/NIOSH approved). Either positive pressure demand SCBA or positive pressure demand airline with 5 minute escape bottle, Max.300 feet of line, 45 # delivery pressure, and low air alarm. To be used when skin adsorption is not a consideration.

Level C: Full face air purifying respirator, using either cartridge or canisters with acid gas/organic vapor/HEPA capabilities. To be used only when criteria for air purifying respirators are met. (i.e.: > 19.5% O_2 and < 5 ppm organic vapors).

Level D: No repository protection.

8.7 Protective Clothing

Protective clothing must meet the following requirements:

- Provide an impermeable barrier to the compounds of concern for a sufficient length of time to allow accomplishment of the task.
- Be able to withstand the mechanical abrasion which results in wear and tear and degradation of the protective clothing.
- Provide user with necessary dexterity and comfort to allow accomplishment of the task.

Chemically protective clothing will be assigned based on job function, the potential for exposure, durability requirements, and heat stress considerations.

Standard chemically protective clothing requirements are as follows:

Level 1: This level is of protection is to be used when there is a potential for being splashed with an unknown chemical.

- Bounty rubber apron or fully encapsulated suite.
- Chemical resistant Tyvek (Saran or polyethylene laminated)
- Cotton underalls.
- Neoprene boots with steel toe and shank.
- Butyl rubber outer gloves with neoprene and surgical inner glove.
- Cover boots and gloves.
- Hard hat with face shield.
- Hearing protection when required.

Level 2: This level is of protection is to be used when there is a low potential for being splashed with an chemicals having low dermal activity.

- PVC two piece suite.
- Chemical resistant Tyvek (Saran or polyethylene laminated)
- Cotton underalls.
- Neoprene boots with steel toe and shank.
- Butyl rubber outer gloves with neoprene and surgical inner glove.
- Cover boots and gloves.
- Hard hat with face shield.
- Hearing protection when required.

Level 3: This level is of protection is to be used when there is no potential for being splashed with an unknown chemicals, or chemicals which are known not to be a threat via the dermal route.

- Chemical resistant Tyvek (Spunwound)
- Cotton underalls.
- Neoprene boots with steel toe and shank.
- Playtex outer gloves with surgical inner glove.
- Cover boots and gloves.
- Hard hat with face shield.
- Hearing protection when required.

Level 4: This level is of protection is to be used when there is no potential for being splashed with an unknown chemicals.

- Cotton underalls.
- Neoprene boots with steel toe and shank.
- Cover boots and gloves.
- Hard hat with face shield.
- Hearing protection when required.

8.8 Personnel Protective Equipment by Job Function

Typical levels for personnel protective equipment are presented below. It should be noted that the Health and Safety Plan allows for upgrading or downgrading of levels of protection to conservatively preclude any potential for contamination while not sacrificing protection or efficiency

Job Function	Respiratory Protection	Protective Clothing
Surveyors	D (C available)	4 (3 available)
Well Measurement Personnel	D (C available)	4 (3 available)
Equipment Operators	D (C available)	4 (3 available)
EOD Personnel	C (B available)	3 (2 available)
Overpacking Ground Personnel	C (B available)	3 (2 available)
Drum Sampling Personnel	C (B available)	3 (2 available)
Reconnaissance Personnel	D (C available)	4 (3 available)
Decon Personnel	C (B available)	3 (2 available)
Oversight Personnel	D (C available)	4 (3 available)
Rescue Personnel	Next higher level than work team	

SECTION 9.0 PERSONNEL AND AMBIENT MONITORING

9.1 Air Monitoring

Airborne concentrations of chemical substances can be a significant hazard at hazardous waste sites. Therefore, identification and quantification of contaminants through proper air monitoring is essential. Reliable measurements of airborne contaminants are useful for:

- Selecting levels of PPE
- Delineating Hot Zone boundaries
- Assessing personnel's chemical exposures
- Determining the effectiveness of control measures

This section outlines the necessary information for the proper selection and use of air monitoring equipment. A complete understanding of air monitoring devices is necessary in order to accurately interpret instrument readings. Therefore, review of the SHASP section on monitoring is vital prior to conducting air sampling. SHASPs will provide the required air monitoring devices and action level readings that initiate administrative responses.

9.2 Selection of Air Monitoring Equipment

The selection of the air-sampling method and equipment depends on the physical and chemical characteristics of the air contaminant. In selecting sampling equipment, factors to be considered include the particulate sizes of dusts involved; and for gases and vapors, the density, solubility, vapor pressure, freezing point, and chemical stability. Other considerations include the presence of other substances that can interfere either with the collection or chemical analysis of the contaminant under investigation.

It may be necessary to collect samples by a number of different methods to determine the concentrations in a mixture of the contaminants. The factors to be considered in the proper choice of a particular measurement device are:

- Portability of instrument and ease of operation
- Sensitivity and accuracy of the instrument or procedure
- Reliability of instrument under various conditions of use
- Type of information required
- Availability of instrument

9.3 Types of Monitoring

9.3.1   *Equipment*

Air monitoring devices and sampling procedures can be divided into direct-reading or laboratory analysis methods. A combination of these two methods is usually practiced at hazardous waste sites.

9.3.1.1   *Direct Reading Instruments*

Direct-reading instruments may be used to rapidly detect flammable or explosive atmospheres, oxygen deficiency,certain gases and vapors, and ionizing radiation. They are the primary tools of initial site characterization. The information provided by direct-reading instruments can be used to institute appropriate protective measures (e.g., personal protective equipment, evacuation), to determine the most appropriate equipment for further monitoring, and to develop optimum sampling and analytical protocols.

All direct-reading instruments have inherent constraints in their ability to detect hazards:

- They usually detect and/or measure only specific classes of chemicals
- Generally, they are not designed to measure and/or detect airborne concentrations below 1 ppm.
- Many of the direct-reading instruments that have been designed to detect one particular substance also detect other substances (interference) and, consequently, may give false readings.

It is imperative that direct-reading instruments be operated, and their data interpreted, by qualified individuals who are thoroughly familiar with the particular device's latest operating instructions and calibration curves. At hazardous waste sites, where unknown and multiple contaminants are the rule rather than the exception, instrument readings should be interpreted conservatively. The following guidelines may facilitate accurate recording and interpretation:

- Calibrate instruments according to the manufacturer's instructions before and after every use.
- Develop chemical response curves if these are not provided by the instrument manufacturer.

- Remember that the instrument's readings have limited value where contaminants are unknown. When recording readings of unknown contaminants, report them as "needle deflection" or "positive instrument response" rather than specific concentrations (i.e., ppm). Conduct additional monitoring at any location where a positive response occurs.
- A reading of zero should be reported as "no instrument response" rather than "clean" because quantities of chemicals may be present that are not detectable by the instrument.
- The survey should be repeated with several detection systems to maximize the number of chemicals detected.

The flame ionization detector (FID) and the photoionization detector (PID) are commonly used at hazardous waste sites. These devices may be supplemental to other detection methods to detect inorganic toxic agents, such as hydrogen cyanide and hydrogen sulfide.

9.3.1.1.1   Oxygen Meter

The oxygen content in a confined space is of prime concern to anyone about to enter that space. Removal of oxygen by combustion, reduction reactions, or displacement by gases or vapors is a hazard which response personnel cannot detect. Consequently, remote measurements must be made before anyone enters a confined space.

Portable oxygen indicators are invaluable when responding to hazardous material spills or waste sites. Terrain variations in the land and unventilated rooms or areas may contain insufficient oxygen to support life. In addition, oxygen measurements are necessary when combustible gas indicator (CGI) measurements are made, since the oxygen level in the ambient air effects the accuracy of CGI's readout. When used properly the portable oxygen indicator will read the percent oxygen in the immediate atmosphere. The normal ambient oxygen concentration is 20.8%.

Most indicators have meters which display the oxygen content from 0-25%. There are also oxygen indicators available which measure concentration from 0-5% and 0-100%. The most useful range for response is the 0-25% oxygen content readout since decisions involving air-supplying respirators and the use of combustible indicators fall into this range.

Although several instruments can measure an oxygen-enriched atmosphere, greater than 21%, testing or other work should never be performed under such conditions because a spark, arc or flame could lead to fire or explosion.

9.3.1.1.2 *Combustible Gas Indicator*

Combustible gas indicator (CGI) readings are taken concurrently with O_2 level readings. It measures the concentration of a flammable vapor or gas in air, indicating the results as a percentage of the Lower Explosive Limit (LEL) of the calibration gas.

The LEL of a combustible gas or vapor is the lowest concentration by volume in air which will explode, ignite, or burn when there is an ignition source. The Upper Explosive Limit (UEL) is the maximum concentration. Above the UEL, there is insufficient oxygen to support combustion so ignition is impossible. Below the LEL, there is insufficient fuel to support ignition.

Most combustible gas indicators operate on the "hot wire" principle. In the combustion chamber is a platinum filament that is heated. The platinum filament is an integral part of a balanced resistor circuit called a Wheatstone Bridge. The hot filament combusts the gas on the immediate surface of the element, thus raising the temperature of the filament.

As the temperature of the filament increases so does its resistance. This change causes an imbalance in the Wheatstone Bridge. This is measured as the ratio of combustible vapor present compared to the total required to reach the LEL. For example, if the meter reads 0.5 (or 50, depending upon the readout), this means that 50% of the concentration of combustible gas needed to reach an unstable flammable or combustible situation is present. If the LEL for the gas is 5% then the meter indicates that a 2.5% concentration is present. Thus the typical meter readout indicates concentration up to the LEL of the gas.

If a concentration greater than LEL and lower than the UEL is present, then the meter needle will stay beyond the 1.0 (100%) level on the meter. This indicates that the ambient atmosphere is readily combustible. When the atmosphere has a gas concentration above the UEL the meter needle will rise above the 1.0 (100%) mark and then return to zero. This occurs because the gas mixture in the combustion cell is too rich to burn. This permits the filament to conduct a current just as if the atmosphere contained no combustibles at all.

As with any instrument based on an electrochemical reaction, all CGIs have several limitations:

- Sensitivity is a function of physical and chemical properties of the calibration gas versus those of the unknown contaminant. Most combustible gas indicators are calibrated to read accurately for methane or pentane, but not all combustible gases and vapors will give the same response as the calibration gas. Because of the variation in the relative response of the flammable substance in the atmosphere to the calibration gas (e.g., methane), the instrument may not give an accurate indication of the flammable hazard -- the reading (%LEL) may be higher or lower than the actual concentration.

· Leaded gasoline vapors, halogens, sulfur compounds, and silicones will foul the filament which decreases its sensitivity. Compounds containing silicone will destroy the platinum filament.

9.3.1.1.3   *Photoionization Detector*

The HNU is typical of field photoionization units now available. It consists of two modules connected via a single-power card.

· A readout unit consisting of a 4 1/2 inch analog meter, a rechargeable battery, and power supplies for operation of the amplifier and the UV lamp.

· A sensor unit consisting of the UV light source, pump ionization chamber, and a preamplifier.

An electrical pump pulls the gas sample past a UV source. Constituents of a sample are ionized, producing an instrument response, if their ionization potential (IP) is equal to or less than the ionizing energy supplied by the instrument UV lamp being utilized. The radiation produces an ion pair for each molecule of contaminant ionized. The free electrons produce a current directly proportional to the number of ions produced. The current is amplified, detected, and displayed on the meter.

The probes are available with the HNU, containing either an 11.7, a 10.2, or a 9.5-eV UV light source. Species that have IPs greater than the lamp rating will display a poor instrument response, or no response at all. Thus, employing the 11.7 eV lamp will ensure the greatest range of detectable species; however, it requires constant maintenance and frequent lamp replacement. For many applications, the 10.2-eV lamp/probe can be used. It offers relatively high radiation levels without frequent lamp replacement; and will detect many species. One notable exception is the chlorinated aliphatics.

Although the HNU photoionization unit is an excellent instrument for survey, there are very important limitations.

- The response to a gas or vapor may radically change when the gas or vapor is mixed with other materials. As an example, an HNU calibrated to ammonia and analyzing an atmosphere containing 100 ppm would indicate 100 on the meter. Likewise, a unit calibrated to benzene would record 100 in an atmosphere containing 100 ppm benzene. However, in an atmosphere containing 100 ppm of each, the unit could indicate considerably less or more than 200 ppm, depending on how it was calibrated.
- Radio frequency interference from pulsed DC or AC power lines, transformers, high voltage equipment and radio wave transmission may produce an error in response.
- The lamp window must be periodically cleaned to ensure ionization of the air contaminants.
- Although the HNU measures concentrations from about 1-2000 ppm, the response is not linear over this entire range. For example, the response to benzene is linear from about 0-600 ppm. This means the HNU reads a true concentration of benzene only between 0 and 600. Greater concentrations are read at a lower level than the true value.

The HNU can be used to help determine the health and safety protocols when evaluating a hazardous waste site or spill. However, the need to properly interpret the HNU's data and to understand the limitations of this instrument cannot be over emphasized. One particular important limitation is how the HNU responds toward mixtures of chemicals. If only one chemical species is present, the HNU can be set to quantitatively respond to that chemical. However, the HNU will not quantitatively respond to a mixture unless the IPs of all chemicals in the mixture are the same. This is because the HNU has a different sensitivity to compounds with different IP's. As a rule, the HNU is more sensitive to complex compounds and less sensitive to simpler ones.

9.3.1.1.4   *Flame Ionization Detector (FID)*

The FID uses ionization as the detection method, much the same as in the HNU, except that the ionization is caused by a hydrogen flame, rather than by a UV light. This flame has sufficient energy to ionize any organic species with an IP of 15.4 or less.

The OVA is a FID instrument that consists of two major parts:

·   A 9-pound package containing the sampling pump, battery pack, support electronics, flame ionization detector, hydrogen gas cylinder, and an optional gas chromatography (CG) column.
·   A hand-held meter-sampling probe assembly.

The OVA is generally calibrated to methane, but can be calibrated to the species of interest. The OVA can operate in two modes:

9.3.1.1.4.1   *Survey Mode*

During normal survey mode operation, a sample is drawn into the probe and transmitted to the detector chamber by an internal pumping system. When the sample reaches the FID it is ionized as described above and the resulting signal is translated on the meter for direct-reading concentration as total organic vapors or recorded as peak on a chart. The meter display is an integral part of the probe/readout assembly and has a scale from 0 to 10 which can be set to read 0-10, 0-100, or 0-1000 ppm v/v.

9.3.1.1.4.2   *Gas Chromatography Mode*

Gas Chromatography (GC) is a technique for separating components of a sample and qualitatively and quantitatively determining them. The sample to be separated is injected into a column packed with an inert solid, and carrier gas (hydrogen) flows through the column. As the carrier gas forces the sample through the column, the separate components of the sample are retained on the column for different periods of time. The amount of time a substance remains on the column, which is called its retention time, is a function of its affinity for the column material, column temperature, and flow rate of the carrier gas. Under preset instrument conditions, each component flows out of the column at a different but reproducible length of time. As the components flow out of the column, they flow into the detector. Since the output of the detector is connected to a strip chart recorder, separate peaks are recorded for each component. This readout is called a gas chromatogram. Since the retention times are reproducible, if the retention time of an unknown element agrees with the retention time of a known element recorded under the same set of analytical conditions, the unknown element is tentatively identified. In addition, the area under each peak is proportional to the concentration of the corresponding sample component. If these areas are compared to the areas of standards recorded under identical analytical conditions, the concentration of the sample components can be calculated. Note that the "base" of the peak can be made very narrow by varying the instrument conditions. Component concentration is proportional to peak height, which can be read directly off the chart.

9.3.1.1.5   *Infrared Spectrophotometer*

The infrared spectrophotometer is a compound specific instrument. Each compound being analyzed will absorb at a discrete infrared wavelength. The unit measures how much of the IR is absorbed and indicates in ppm or percent absorbed.

The Miran (acronym for miniature infrared analyzer) is a field IR spectrophotometer which uses a variable length gas cell to measure concentrations of vapors in ambient air.

Field analysis presents problems not normally encountered in spectrophotometry in the laboratory. Which lab instruments, the analyst can control the concentration of material entering the sample cell. To analyze uncontrollable gas the Miran must make repeated passes to achieve reliable results. Liquid or solid samples are preferable to gas samples because they possess more molecules than a gas of the same volume.

The Miran is designed for industrial hygiene work in occupational settings where known types of materials are generated and where 120-volt AC power is available. At hazardous waste sites neither condition is common, making Mirans of questionable value. They also have been recognized by any approving agencies as being safe for use in hazardous location. Basically, the Miran is designed for quantifying simple one- or two-component mixtures.

9.3.1.1.6   *Direct-Reading Colorimetric Indicator Tubes*

In evaluating hazardous waste sites, the need often arises to quickly measure a specific vapor or gas. Direct-reading colorimetric indicator tubes can successfully fill that need. They are usually calibrated in ppm or % concentration for easy interpretation. There are indicator tubes available for continuous sampling over a long period of time.

The interaction of two or more substances may result in chemical changes. This change may be as subtle as two clear liquids producing a third clear liquid, or as obvious as a colorless vapor and colored solid producing a differently colored substance. Detector tubes use this latter phenomenon to estimate the concentration of a gas or vapor in the air.

Colorimetric indicator tubes consist of a glass tube impregnated with an indicating chemical. The tube is connected to a piston cylinder- or bellows-type pump. A known volume of contaminated air is pulled at a predetermined rate through the tube. The contaminant reacts with the indicator chemical in the tube, producing a stain whose length is proportional to the contaminant's concentration. Detector tubes are normally species specific. In other words, there are different tubes for different gases (e.g., chlorine detector tube for chlorine gas, acrylonitrile tube for acrylonitrile gas, etc.). Some manufacturers do produce tubes for groups of gases (aromatic hydrocarbons, for example).

A preconditioning filter may precede an indicating chemical to:

· Remove contaminants (other than the one in question) that may interfere with the measurement.
· React with the contaminant to change it into a compound that reacts with the indicating chemical.
· Completely change a nonindicating contaminant into an indicating one.

Several different colorimetric indicating tubes may be able to measure the concentration of a particular gas or vapor, each operating on a different chemical principle and each affected in varying degrees by temperature, air volume pulled through the tube, and interfering gases or vapors. The "true" concentration versus the "measured" concentration may vary considerably among and between manufacturers. To limit these sources of error, to control the numerous types and manufacturers of tubes, and to provide a degree of confidence to users, the NIOSH Testing and Certification Branch has certified Dector Tube Units. The certified unit includes the aspirating pump, detector tube, and accessories. The certification implies that the unit must be accurate within + or - 35% at 1/2 the PEL and + or - 25% at 1 to 5 times the PEL. A list of certified units (by tube) can be found in the NIOSH detector tube Certified Equipment List. (Note: The NIOSH detector tube certification program has been discontinued.) To improve performance of all tubes, they should be:

· Refrigerated prior to use to maintain shelf life of approximately 2 years.
· Leak tested with the pump prior to sampling and volumetrically calibrated on a quarterly basis.

Undoubtedly the greatest source of error is how the operator "reads" the endpoint. The jagged edge where contaminant meets indicator chemical makes it difficult to get accurate results from this seemingly simple test.

9.4 Laboratory Analysis Methods

Direct-reading instruments rarely can distinguish and quantify specific substances. Their major advantage at hazardous waste sites is direct response which can be incorporated into an SHASP to initiate response team action.

Direct-reading and laboratory analysis methods are often used simultaneously at hazardous waste sites, because of their combined advantages. Also, mobile laboratories may be brought on site to shorten sample turn-around times.

Typically, the atmosphere is sampled at a hazardous materials site to identify and quantify any gases, vapors, or particulates present. Such information may be obtained by two methods:

9.4.1   Area sampling, which involves the placement of collection devices within designated areas and operating them over specific periods of time. Types of area-sampling would be:

- Monitoring for IDLH conditions
- General on-site monitoring to detect unexpected releases of chemicals
- Periodic monitoring when working conditions change
- Perimeter monitoring at fenceline to assess control measures

9.4.2 Personal sampling, which involves the collection of samples from within the breathing zone of an individual, sometimes by the individual wearing a sampling device. The selective monitoring of high-risk workers (i.e., those closest to the source of contaminant generation), is recommended. The approach is based on the rationale that the probability or significant exposure varies directly with the distance from the source.

Once the sampling method has been selected, the type of sample desired must be determined. Prevailing conditions, the scope of site operations, and the intended use of the resulting information dictate the type collected:

9.4.3 Instantaneous or grab-type samples, which are characteristically collected over brief time periods. They are useful in examining stable contaminant concentrations or peak levels of short duration. Instantaneous samples may require highly sensitive analytical methods due to the small sample volume collected.

9.4.4 Integrated samples. These are more typical of on-site measurements. They are collected when the sensitivity of an analytical method requires minimum sample periods or volumes, or when comparison must be made to an 8-hour, time-weighted average/Threshold Limit Value or other established standard.

Two types of sampling systems are used for the collection of integrated samples:

Active samplers which mechanically move contaminated air through a collection medium.

Passive samplers which rely on natural rather than mechanical forces to collect samples. Passive samplers are classified as either diffusion or permeation devices, according to their principle of operation.

9.4.4.1 *Active Samplers*

Active sampling systems, or "trains," mechanically collect samples on or into a selected medium. The medium is then analyzed in the laboratory to identify and quantify the contaminant(s) collected. Such a system typically consists of the following components:

- A sampling pump to mechanically induce air movement. The most practical electrical sampling pump is powered by rechargeable batteries and can operate continuously at constant flow rates for at least 6 to 8 hours. Typically, they are compact, portable, and quiet enough to be worn by individuals when monitoring personal exposures. Such a pump should contain a flow regulator to control the rate of movement and a flow monitor to indicate that rate.
- Flexible tubing to link the sampler to the pump.
- A sampler consisting of an appropriate sampling medium and a container designed for that medium. The sampler depends upon the contaminants(s) to be sampled and the selected sampling method.

Integrated samples are commonly collected over known time periods and at known fixed flow rates. Thus, sample train calibration and accurate time measurement are critical to active systems.

9.4.4.2 *Passive Dosimeters*

The key advantage of passive dosimeters is their simplicity. These small, light weight devices do not require a mechanical pump to move a contaminant through a collection medium. Thus, calibration and maintenance are reduced or eliminated, although the sampling period must still be accurately measured. Despite this obvious advantage, such sources of error as observer interpretation, and the effects of temperature and humidity hold true for both active and passive systems. Other sources of error unique to passive dosimeters arise from the need for minimum face velocities and the determination of contaminant diffusion coefficients.

The few passive dosimeters now available apply to gas and vapor contaminants only. These devices primarily function as personal exposure monitors, although they have some usefulness in area monitoring. Passive dosimeters are commonly divided into two groups, primarily on how they are designed and operated.

9.4.4.2.1 *Available Passive Dosimeters for Gases and Vapors Grouped by Principle of Operation*

Diffusion Devices	**Permeation Devices**
Ammonia	Chlorine
Carbon Monoxide	Hydrogen Sulfide
Ethylene Oxide	Vinyl Chloride
Formaldehyde	
Mercury	
Nitrogen	
Organic Vapor (General)	
Phosgene	
Sulfur Dioxide	

9.4.4.2.2 Diffusion samplers, which function by the passive movement of contaminant molecules through a concentration gradient created with a stagnant layer of air between the contaminated atmosphere and the indicator material. Some diffusion samplers may be read directly, as are colorimetric length-of-stain tubes, while others require laboratory analysis similar to that performed on solid sorbents:

9.4.4.2.3 Permeation dosimeters, which rely on the natural permeation of a contaminant through a membrane. The efficiency of these devices depends on finding a membrane that is easily permeated by the contaminant of interest and not by all others. Permeation dosimeters are, therefore, useful in picking out a single contaminant from a mixture of possible interfering contaminants. As with diffusion samplers, some passive samplers may be of the direct reading type while others may require laboratory analysis.

9.4.4.3 *Calibration*

Atmospheric sampling systems must be accurately calibrated to a specific flow rate if the resultant data are to be correctly interpreted. Flow rate calibration of the electrically powered pump in active systems is important to achieving the constant flow rates often specified in standard analytical methods. Passive sampling systems, however, because of their simplicity in design and principles of operation, require no formal calibration.

As a minimum, an active sampling system should be calibrated prior to use and following a prescribed sampling period. The overall frequency of calibration depends upon the general handling and use a sampling system receives. Pump mechanisms should be recalibrated after they have been repaired, when newly purchased, and following any suspected abuse.

As a rule, the sampling system as a whole should be calibrated to the desired flow rate rather than the pump alone. Only with all components connected can the system be adequately examined under field-like operating conditions. Once assembled, the flow rate of the sampling train can be measured on the calibrator in liters per minute (L/min). The general formula used for the calculation of a desired flow rate is as follows:

$$\text{Flow rate (L/min)} = \frac{\text{Liter}}{1000 \text{ milliliters}} \times \frac{\text{traveled by bubble (ml)}}{\text{Travel time of bubble(sec)}} \times \frac{60 \text{ Sec.}}{\text{minute}}$$

$$= \frac{\text{milliliters}}{\text{second}} \times \frac{60 \text{ seconds/minute}}{1000 \text{ milliliters/L}}$$

A system can be calibrated by any of several devices for measuring air flow, the most common is the bubble tube flow meter.

Soap bubble flow meter, is a primary standard and is used to calibrate the types of sampling pumps discussed earlier, as well as the manually operated pumps used for direct reading calorimetric tubes. This device typically consists of an inverted graduated burette connected by flexible tubing to the sampling train. Calibration is performed as follows: The open end of the burette is dipped into a soap solution creating a soap film bubble across the opening. The solution is removed, and the bubble is allowed to rise up through the burette. Travel time of the bubble between two graduated points on the burette is measured. The flow rate (measured in cc's/minutes) is varied by adjusting the pump flow regulator.

9.5 Air Monitoring Locations

Air monitoring will be conducted at various locations as follows:

· Work face
· Workers breathing zone
· Exclusion Zone, site perimeter and Support Zone.

These locations will be monitored at a frequency and duration which will preclude exposure.

9.6 Site Air Monitoring Systems

Air monitoring systems will include:
- LEL and Oxygen levels.
- PID and/or FID in survey mode.
- Direct reading or colorometric tubes where available.
- Particulate Monitors.

These instruments will be operated in accordance with the manufactures recommend operating procedures. Records of daily calibration will be kept by the SSO. Additional monitoring instruments may be added or deleted in response to the actual site conditions.

9.7 Action Levels for Worker Protection

Action levels for worker protection will be determined by air monitoring levels as shown in Table 9.7-1.

Table 9.7-1 Action Levels for Worker Protection		
Instrument	**Reading**	**Action Level**
Explosimeter	0 - 10% LEL	Continue work
	10 - 25% LEL	Monitor continuously. Note repository protection requirements
	+ 25% LEL	Evacuate area
Oxygen Meter	19.5 - 21.0%	Continue work
	< 19.5%	Level B. Note effect on LEL
FID/PID	0 - 0.2 ppm*	Level D**
	0.2 - 5.0 ppm*	Level C** +
	5.0 - 500ppm*	Level B**
Particulate Monitor	0 - 2.5mg/m³*	Level D**
	> 2.5mg/m³*	Level C**

*   Above background, in breathing zone, sustained for 5 minuets.
** This protection level is for unknown contaminates or for mixtures of contaminates where identification of the constituents is not practical.
\+   Must also meet Air Purifying Respirator Selection Criteria.

9.8 Action Levels for Environmental Protection

Action levels for environmental protection will be determined by air monitoring levels as follows:

- Downwind perimeter concentrations greater than background concentrations on any of the monitoring instruments will require immediate investigation of its source.
- Downwind perimeter concentrations greater than 1 ppm will require immediate stop work until prevailing winds preclude exposure to the adjacent community. If air contaminates can be identified, the state standards for air quality will be observed.

9.9 Personnel Air Sampling

Personnel air samples will be collected at regular intervals or in the event of an environmental release. Passive dosimeters will be used to collect organic vapor samples for analysis. Active samplers will be used for the collection of particulate samples. Target compounds will be selected based upon historical information and available analytical data.

9.10   Personnel biological monitoring

Biological monitoring will only be performed in the event of an overt exposure to an individual. Target compounds will be determined my the HSC and a physician, based upon the monitoring and air sampling results and the drum contents.

SECTION 10.0 DECONTAMINATION

10.1   Decontamination

Workplace chemicals present on clothing or tools must not be transported from the Exclusion Zone (or other dirty area) into the Support Zone (or other clean area). A decontamination protocol tailored to the specific operation is required to prevent this transfer. The exact methods of decontamination depend upon the nature of the contaminants, the extent of contamination, and the type of protective clothing used. Extensive contaminating of Level A garments would require much more cleaning than minimal contamination of Level C garments.

Decontamination consists of distinct steps, each of which is conducted at a designated station. As one proceeds along the path, from one step to the next, the level of contamination should diminish. Each decontamination station should be at least three feet from the adjacent ones. The following material describes all required steps for decontamination in the work place. However, abbreviated versions are allowed in some situations, including emergencies. In all cases, the SSO, the Site Manager and HSC - and possibly other specialists - will consult with the Program and Project Manager to determine the required steps and washing solutions appropriate for a given work site. These specific requirements will be detailed in the SHASP.

10.1.1 *Level A*

In the most extreme cases (full Level A garments and heavy contamination) there are nineteen stations or steps in the decontamination process. Steps 1 through 6 are in the Exclusion Zone, and the last two (18 and 19) are in the Clean Support Zone. The intervening steps are performed in the Contamination Reduction Zone.

If the worker intends to return to the Exclusion Zone after obtaining a new tank, then only gross decontamination is necessary. He proceeds through Step 8 to the Option Step 9, tank replacement, and returns to work. If conditions at the site are not severe, then outer gloves and boot covers may not be necessary, and Steps 2 through 6, 13, and 14 can be eliminated. The SSO will make all such determinations.

10.1.1.1 *Level A Decontamination Steps*

The nineteen steps of complete Level A decontamination are described below. (See Figure 10.1.1.1-1.)

Steps 1 through 8:   Gross Decontamination

1. Segregated Equipment Drop. Equipment is placed just inside the Contamination Reduction Zone on plastic sheets. Extremely contaminated items (e.g., shovels) are segregated from lightly contaminated ones (e.g., instruments).

Required apparatus: containers, plastic liners, plastic drop cloths.

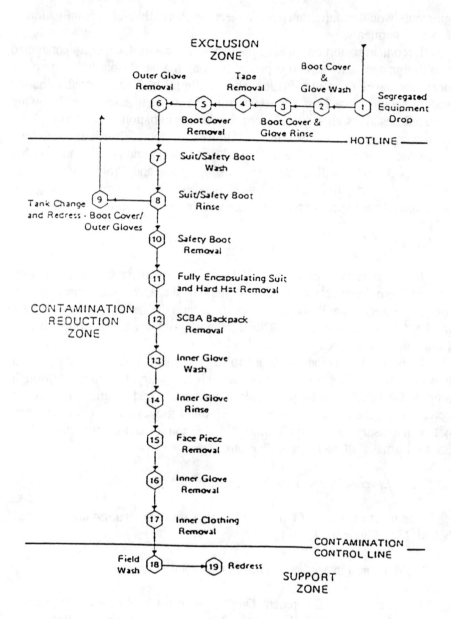

Figure 10.1.1.1-1. Level A Decontamination

2. Boot Cover and Glove Wash. Outer boot covers and gloves are washed with decontamination solution (detergent and water, in many cases) by means of long-handle, soft-bristle scrub brushes.

   Required apparatus: container (20-30 gal.), decontamination solution or water/detergent, long-handle brushes.

3. Boot Cover and Glove Rinse. Decontamination solution applied in Step 2 is rinsed with water. A high-pressure spray unit and long-handle, soft bristle scrub brush should be used.

   Required Apparatus: Container (30-50 gal.), high-pressure spray unit, long handle brushes.

4. Tape Removal. Tape around outer boots and gloves is removed and placed in a lined container.

   Required apparatus: container, plastic liners.

5. Boot Cover Removal. Boot covers are removed and placed in a lined container.

   Required apparatus: container (20-30 gal.), plastic liners, bench or stool.

6. Outer Glove Removal. Outer gloves are removed and placed in lined container.

   Required apparatus: container (20-30 gal.), plastic liners.

   The worker can now enter the Contamination Reduction Zone for further decontamination.

7. Suit and Safety Boot Wash. The protective suit and the safety boots are washed with decontaminating solution by means of long-handle, soft-bristle scrub brushes.

   Required apparatus: container (30-50 gal.), decontamination solution or water detergent, long handle brushes.

8.   Suit and Safety Boot Rinse. Decontamination solution applied in Step 7 is rinsed with water. A high-pressure spray unit and long-handle, soft-bristle scrub brushes should be used.

Required apparatus: container (30-50 gal.), high-pressure spray unit, long-handle brushes.

Step 9:   *Optional* Tank Change for Immediate Re-entry Only

9.   Tank Change. The Self-Contained Breathing Apparatus (SCBA) tank is exchanged for a full one. The worker receives new outer gloves and boots, which are sealed with new tape. He then returns to the Exclusion Zone.

Required apparatus: air tanks, tape, boot covers, gloves. (Note that the tanks must be stored in the Support Zone.

Steps 10 through 18: Final Decontamination (for those leaving the work area and entering the Support Zone) and redress.

10.   Safety Boot Removal. Safety boots are removed and placed in a lined container.

Required apparatus: container (30-50 gal.), plastic liners, bench or stool, boot jack.

11.   Suit and Hardhat Removal. The protective suit and the hardhat are removed and placed on a rack or a plastic sheet. An employee must be stationed here to provide assistance.

Required apparatus: rack, drop cloths, bench or stool.

12.   SCBA Backpack (Tank, Harness, Regulator, etc.) Removal. The hose is disconnected from the regulator valve, and the backpack - *but not the facepiece* - is removed and placed on a table.

Required apparatus: table

13. Inner Glove Wash. The inner gloves are washed with detergent and water or with some other decontaminating solution that does not harm the skin.

    Required apparatus: decontamination solution or water/detergent, basin or bucket, small table.

14. Inner Glove Rinse. Decontamination solution applied in Step 13 is rinsed with water.

    Required apparatus: water basin or bucket, small table.

15. Facepiece Removal. The facepiece is deposited in a lined container for subsequent decontamination. *The fingers should not touch the face.*

    Required apparatus: container (30-50 gal.), plastic liners.

16. Inner Glove Removal. Inner gloves are removed and placed in a lined container.

    Required apparatus: container (20-30 gal.), plastic liner.

17. Inner Clothing Removal. Inner clothing is removed and placed in a lined container.

    Required apparatus: container (30-50 gal.), plastic liners.

    The worker can new leave the CRZ.

18. Field Wash. Employees shower immediately if severe conditions at the site warrant this. Otherwise, they wash the face and hands immediately and shower later.

    Required apparatus: soap and water, table, basin, or bucket, towels, field shower (if necessary).

19. Redress. Employee dress in clothing appropriate for the Support Zone.

Required apparatus: tables, chairs, lockers, trailer or other protective structure (in inclement weather).

10.1.2   *Level B*

In the most extreme case (full Level B garments and heavy contamination) there are eighteen steps in the decontamination process. Steps 1 through 6 in the Exclusion Zone, and the last one (18) are in the Clean Support Zone. The intervening steps are performed in the Contamination Reduction Zone.

If the worker intends to return to the Exclusion Zone after obtaining a new tank, then only gross decontamination is necessary. He proceeds through Step 8 to the optional Step 9, tank replacement, and returns to work. If conditions at the site are not severe, then outer gloves and boot covers may not be necessary, and Steps 2 through 6, 13 and 14 can be eliminated. The SSO will make all such determinations.

10.1.2.1   *Level B Decontamination Steps*

The nineteen steps of complete Level B decontamination are described below.
See Figure 10.1.2.1- 1.

1.   Steps 1 through 8: Gross Decontamination

   1.-7.   These are the same as Steps 1-7 for Level A decontamination.

   The worker can new leave the Exclusion Zone and enter the CRZ for further decontamination.

8.   Suit/SCBA/Glove Rinse. Decontamination solution applied in Step 7 is rinsed with water. A high-pressure spray unit and long handle, soft-bristle scrub brush should be used.

   Required apparatus: container (30-50 gal.), high-pressure spray unit, long-handle brushes, sponges, small buckets.

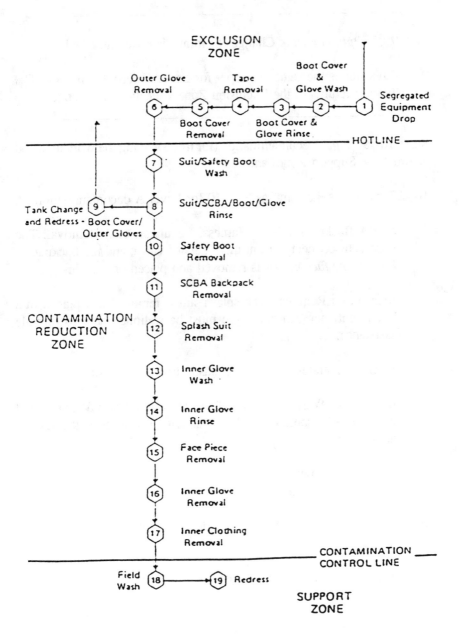

Figure 10.1.2.1- 1. Level B Decontamination

Step 9:   *Optional* Tank Change for Immediate Re-entry Only

9.   This step is the same as Step 9 for Level A decontamination. The worker returns to the Exclusion Zone after the tank change.

Steps 10-19: Final Decontamination (for those leaving the work area and entering the Support Zone) and redress.

10.   This step is the same as Step 10 for Level A decontamination.

11.   SCBA Backpack (Tank, Harness, Regulator, etc.) Removal. The hose is disconnected from the regulator valve, and the backpack - *but not the facepiece* - is removed and placed on a table.

12.   Splash Suit Removal. The splash suit is removed and placed in a lined container. An employee must be stationed here to provide assistance.

Retired apparatus: container, plastic liners, bench or stool.

13.   Inner Glove Wash. The inner gloves are washed with detergent and water or with some other decontaminating solution that does not harm the skin.

Required apparatus: decontaminating solution or water/detergent, basin or bucket, small table.

14.   Inner Glove Rinse. Decontamination solution applied in Step 12 is rinsed with water.

Required apparatus: water basin or bucket, small table.

15.   Facepiece Removal. The facepiece is deposited in a lined container for subsequent decontamination. The fingers should not touch the face.

Required apparatus: container (30-50 gal.), plastic liners.

16. Inner Glove Removal. Inner gloves are removed and placed in a lined container.

    Required apparatus: container (20-30 gal.), plastic liner.

17. Inner Clothing Removal. Inner clothing is removed and placed in a lined container.

    Required apparatus: container (30-50 gal.), plastic liners.

18. Field Wash. Employees shower immediately if severe conditions at the site warrant this. Otherwise, they wash the face and hands immediately and shower later.

    Required apparatus: soap and water, table, basin or bucket, towels, field shower (if necessary).

19. Redress. Employees dress in clothing appropriate for the Support Zone.

    Required apparatus: tables, chairs, lockers, clothes, trailer or other protective structure (in inclement weather).

10.1.3 *Level C*

In the most extreme cases (full Level C garments and heavy contamination), there are seventeen steps in the decontamination process. Steps 1 through 6 are in the Exclusion Zone, and the last two (Steps 17 and 18) are in the clean Support Zone.

If the worker intends to return to the Exclusion Zone after obtaining a new canister, then only gross decontamination is necessary. He proceeds through Step 8 to the Option Step 9 - canister or mask change, and returns to work. If conditions at the site are not severe, then outer gloves and boot covers may not be necessary, and Steps 2 through 6, 12, 13 and 15 can be eliminated. The SSO will make all such determinations.

10.1.3.1 *Level C - Decontamination Steps*

The seventeen steps of complete Level C decontamination are described below. See Figure 10.1.3.1-1.

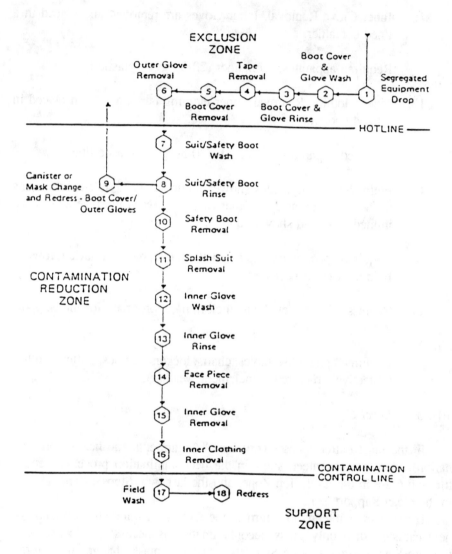

Figure 10.1.3.1-1. Level C Decontamination

1. Steps 1 through 6: Gross Decontamination

   1.-7.   These are the same as Steps 1-7 for Level A decontamination.

8. Suit/Safety Boot Rinse. Decontamination solution applied in Step 7 is rinsed with water. A high-pressure spray unit and long handle, soft bristle scrub brush should be used.

   Required apparatus: container (30-50 gallon), high-pressure spray unit, long-handle brushes, sponges, small buckets.

Step 9.   *Optional* Canister or Mask Change.

9. If the worker leaves Exclusion Zone to change canister (or mask), this is the last step in the decontamination procedure. Worker's canister is exchanged, new outer gloves and boot covers donned and joints tagged. Worker returns to duty.

Steps 10 through 18: Final Decontamination (for those leaving the work area and entering the Support Zone) and redress.

10. This step is the same as Step 10 in Level A decontamination.

11. Splash Suit Removal. With the assistance of helper, the splash suit is removed and placed in a lined container.

    Required apparatus: container (30-50 gallon), a bench or stool and plastic liner.

12. Inner Glove Wash. The inner gloves are washed with detergent and water or some other decontaminating solution that does not harm the skin.

    Required apparatus: decontamination solution or detergent and water basin or bucket.

13. Inner Glove Rinse. Decontamination solution applied in Step 12 is rinsed with water.

   Required apparatus: water basin or bucket, small table.

14. Faceplate Removal. The faceplate is deposited in a lined container for subsequent decontamination. The fingers should not touch the face.

   Required apparatus: container (30-50 gallon), plastic liner.

15. Inner Glove Removal. The inner gloves are removed and placed in a lined container.

   Required apparatus: container (30-50 gallon) plastic liner.

16. Inner Clothing Removal. The inner clothing is removed and placed in a lined container.

   Required apparatus: container (30-50 gallon), plastic liner.

   The worker can now leave the CRZ and enter the Support Zone.

17. Field Wash. Employees shower immediately if severe conditions at the site warrant this. Otherwise, they wash the face and hands immediately and shower later.

   Required apparatus: soap and water, table, basin or bucket, towels, field shower (if necessary).

18. Redress: Employees dress in clothing appropriate for the Support Zone.

   Required apparatus: tables, chairs, lockers, clothes, trailer or other protective structure (in inclement weather).

All personnel, equipment, drums, and samples exiting the Exclusion Zone must be thoroughly decontaminated.

Due to the potential for the drummed material to be impervious to the traditional soap and water decontamination solutions, a citric solution will be available as a decontamination solution. Citric will only be used if the traditional decontamination solutions prove to be ineffective.

Heavy equipment will be decontaminated using a steam cleaner.

All waste solutions and materials from the decontamination stations will collected, drummed, and disposed of along with the drums.

Certain equipment and sample containers can not be decontaminated due their delicate nature or the potential for contamination of the samples. In these cases, measures will be taken to protect the item from becoming contaminated by enclosing them in a disposable material.

SECTION 11.0 EMERGENCY AND CONTINGENCY PLAN

11.1   Emergency Response and Contingency Plan (ERCP)

Emergencies happen quickly and unexpectedly and require immediate assessment and response. Site emergencies vary in their complexity: from minor bumps and cuts to explosions that release toxic vapors throughout a community. Therefore, advanced planning for anticipated emergencies and a written contingency plan are essential to protect workers and the community. A specific ERCP will be developed for each project and will be included in the SHASP. Emergencies that require transport of personnel off-site will use the main gate unless specifically directed otherwise in the SHASP.

11.1.1   *Contingency Plan*

A Contingency Plan is a written document that sets forth policies, procedures, and outlines authority for responding to site emergencies. The Contingency Plan will be part of an SHASP and will anticipate the potential emergencies a the site and will integrate action of the local agencies, fire department, and medical care.

The Contingency Plan assigns the role of authority to the Site Manager and the SSO. These two individuals are responsible for directing emergency response operations,notifying on-site and off-site personnel, requesting aid from outside sources, and documenting the event.

11.1.1.1   *Contacting Off-Site Agencies*

The Contingency Plan will have arrangements with the local medical provider, police and fire department for support in the event of an emergency.

A list of phone numbers and directions to these agencies will be posted at the command center. All personnel will be informed of this list and the communication system. A map showing the location of the medical provider in relationship to the site will be included in the SHASP.

11.1.1.2 *Emergency Decontamination*

Decontamination of injured individuals may be eliminated depending on the severity of the injuries. Decontamination may aggravate the injury or delay life-saving treatment. If decontamination does not interfere with essential treatment, then it should be performed. If it cannot, cut the person out of his protective clothing or wrap them in blankets to limit contamination during transport.

11.1.2   *Emergency Response Action*

Emergency responses are the actions performed on site to control and eliminate an emergency situation. Emergency response action should only be attempted within the limits and training of the site personnel. The SSO must make the decision to attempt immediate control of a hazardous situation or to call in off-site assistance (i.e., fire department, bomb squad). If the control of a situation involves endangerment of untrained personnel, then off-site professionals should be called in. The sequence of emergency response operations consist of:

11.1.2.1 *Notification*

Alert personnel to emergency. Sound a site alarm to:

- Notify personnel
- Stop work activities if necessary
- Lower background noise in order to speed communication
- Begin emergency procedures

11.1.2.2 *Size-Up*

Available information about the incident and emergency response capabilities should be evaluated. The following information should be determined, to the extent possible:

- What happened:

  - Type of incident
  - Cause of Incident
  - Extent of chemical release and transport
  - Extent of damage to structures, equipment and terrain

- Casualties:

  - Victims (number, location, and condition).
  - Treatment required
  - Missing personnel

11.1.2.3 *Emergency Response Process*

- What could happen. Consider:

  - Types of chemicals on site.
  - Potential for fire, explosion, and release of hazardous substances
  - Location of all personnel on-site relative to hazardous areas. Potential for danger to off-site population or environment

- What can be done. Consider:

  - Equipment and personnel resources needed for victim rescue and hazard mitigation.
  - Number of trained and uninjured personnel available for response.
  - Resources available on-site.
  - Resources available from outside groups and agencies.
  - Time for outside resources to reach the site.
  - Hazards involved in rescue and response.

11.1.2.4 *Rescue/Response Action*

Based on the available information, the type of action required should be decided and the necessary steps implemented. Some actions may be done concurrently. No one should attempt emergency response or rescue until backup personnel and evacuation routes have been identified. Rescue/response actions may include:

- Enforce the buddy system: Allow no one to enter an Exclusion Zone or hazardous area without a partner. At all times, personnel in the Exclusion Zone should be in line-of-sight or communications contact with the SSO or designee.

- Survey casualties:

  - Locate all victims and assess their condition.
  - Determine resources needed for stabilization and transport.

- Assess existing and potential hazards to site personnel and to the off-site population. Determine:

  - Whether and how to respond.
  - The need for evacuation of site personnel and off-site population.
  - The resources needed for evacuation and response.

- Allocate resources. Allocate on-site personnel and equipment to implement rescue and response operations.

- Request aid. Contact the required off-site personnel or facilities, such as the ambulance, fire department, and police.

- Control. Bring the hazardous situation under complete or temporary control; use measures to prevent the spread of the emergency.

- Extricate. Remove or assist victims from the area.

- Decontaminate. Use established procedures to decontaminate uninjured personnel in the Contamination Reduction Zone. If the emergency makes this area unsafe, establish a new decontamination area at appropriate distance. Decontaminate victims before or after stabilization as their medical condition indicates.

- Stabilize. Administer any first aid procedures that are necessary before the victims can be moved. Stabilize or permanently fix the hazardous condition (e.g., repack; empty filled runoff dikes). Attend to what caused the emergency and anything (e.g., drums, tanks) damaged or endangered by the emergency.

- Transport. Take measures to minimize chemical contamination of the transport vehicle, ambulance and hospital personnel. Adequately protected rescuers should decontaminate the victims before transport. If this is not possible, cover the victims with adequate sheeting. Before transportation, determine the level of protection necessary for transport personnel. Provide them with disposable coveralls, disposable gloves, and supplied air, as necessary, for their protection. If appropriate, have response personnel accompany victims to the medical facility to advise on decontamination.

- Evacuate:

  - Move site personnel to a safe distance upwind of the incident.

  - Monitor the incident for significant changes. The hazards may diminish, permitting personnel to reenter the site, or increase thereby requiring public evacuation.

  - Inform public safety personnel when there is a potential or actual need to evacuate the off-site population. Do not attempt large-scale public evacuation. This is the responsibility of government authorities.

11.1.2.5 *Follow-up*

Before normal site activities are resumed, personnel must be fully prepared and equipped to handle another emergency.

- Notify appropriate government agencies as required. This will be performed by the Project Manager and the HSC.

- Restock all equipment and supplies. Replace or repair damaged equipment. Clean and refuel equipment for future use.

- Review and revise all aspects of the Emergency Response and Contingency Plan according to new site conditions and lessons learned from the situation. When reviewing the information, consider typical questions such as:

- Cause: What caused the emergency?
- Prevention: Was it preventable? If so, how?
- Procedures: Were inadequate or incorrect orders given or actions taken? Were these the result of bad judgment, wrong or insufficient information, or poor procedures? Can procedures or training be improved?
- Site profile: How does the incident affect the site profile? How are other site cleanup activities affected?
- Community: How is community safety affected?
- Liability: Who is liable for damage payments?

11.1.2.6 *Documentation*

The Site Manger, Program Manager, Project Manager, SSO and HSC will initiate an investigation of the incident. This is important in all cases, but especially so when the incident has resulted in personal injury, on-site property damage, or damage to the surrounding environment. Documentation may be used to help avert recurrences, as evidence in future legal action, for assessment of liability by insurance companies, and for review by government agencies. Methods of documenting can include a written transcript taken from tape recordings made during the emergency, or a bound file book (not a looseleaf book) with notes. The document must be:

- Accurate: All information must be recorded objectively.

- Authentic: A chain-of-custody procedure should be used. Each person making an entry must date and sign the document. Keep the number of documenters to a minimum to avoid confusion and because they may have to give testimony at hearings or in court. Nothing should be erased. If details change or revisions are needed, the person making the notation should mark a horizontal line through the old material and initial the change. At a minimum, the following should be included:

  - Chronological history of the incident
  - Facts about the incident and when they became available.
  - Title and names of personnel; composition of teams.
  - Actions: decisions made and by whom; orders given: to whom, by whom, and when; and actions taken: who did what, when, where and how.
  - Types of samples and test results; air monitoring results.

- Possible exposures of site personnel.
- History of all injuries or illnesses during or as a result of the emergency.

11.2   Overt Personnel Exposure

In the event of overt personnel exposure, the following procedures must be followed:

Skin Contact: Proceed through decontamination. Wash and rinse affected area for 15 minuets with copious amounts of soap and water. Eye wash located at CRZ & Support Zone. If necessary, seek medical attention.

Inhalation: Proceed through decontamination. Move to fresh air. If necessary, seek medical attention.

Ingestion: Proceed through decontamination. Seek medical attention.

Inoculation: Proceed through decontamination. Seek medical attention.

If medical attention is required, the SSO will:

1)   Designate the person to call for ambulance and notify the hospital using the following telephone numbers:

AMBULANCE   _____
PRIMARY HOSPITAL (or health clinic)   _____
SECONDARY HOSPITAL   _____
POISON CONTROL CENTER   **(800)882-9761**

2)   Provide medical data sheets to appropriate medical personnel as requested.

11.3   Overt Personnel Injury

In the event of overt personnel injury, the actions will be taken:

- Emergency first aid applied on-site as deemed necessary.

- Proceed through decontamination.
- If necessary, seek medical attention.

If medical attention is required, the SSO will:

1) Designate the person to call for ambulance and notify the hospital using the following telephone numbers:

AMBULANCE	_____
SAFETY (office of company or location)	_____
RESCUE (Fire Dept)	_____
PRIMARY HOSPITAL (or health clinic)	_____
SECONDARY HOSPITAL	_____
POISON CONTROL CENTER	**(800)882-9761**

2) Provide medical data sheets to appropriate medical personnel as requested.

11.4   Fire or Explosion

In the event of fire or explosion the following actions will be taken:

- Immediately evacuate site.
- Air horn will sound for 10 seconds.
- Assembly at assembly areas.

The SSO will:

1) Designate the person to call for fire, police, and other appropriate agencies using the following telephone numbers:

POLICE (or security)	_____
FIRE (Fire Dept)	_____
AMBULANCE	_____
SAFETY OFFICE	_____
(location) Environmental Services	

2) Account for all site personnel.

3) See that access for emergency equipment is provided and that all combustion sources are shut down.

11.5   **Environmental Incident**

In the event of environmental incident the following actions will be taken:

- Secure spread of contamination if possible.
- SSO will determine if site needs to be evacuated.

The SSO will:

1) Designate the person to call for fire, police, and other appropriate agencies using the following telephone numbers:

POLICE (or security)   _____
FIRE (Fire Dept)   _____
AMBULANCE   _____
SAFETY OFFICE   _____
(location) Environmental Services   _____

2) Account for all site personnel.

3) See that access for emergency equipment is provided and that spread of contamination is contained if possible.

11.6   **Adverse Weather**

In the event of adverse weather conditions the following procedure applies:

- The SSO will determine if work can continue, without sacrificing the health and safety of the workers, based upon the following factors:

  - Potential for heat stress.
  - Potential for cold stress.
  - Treacherous weather related working conditions.
  - Limited visibility.
  - Potential for electric storms.

11.7   **Emergency Telephone Numbers**

POLICE (or security)   _____
FIRE (Fire Dept)   _____
AMBULANCE   _____
SAFETY OFFICE   _____
(location) Environmental Services   _____
PRIMARY HOSPITAL (or health clinic)   _____
SECONDARY HOSPITAL   _____
POISON CONTROL CENTER   **(800)882-9761**
CLIENT CONTRACTING OFFICER   _____
PROJECT MANAGER   _____
HEALTH AND SAFETY COORDINATOR   _____
SITE SAFETY OFFICER   _____

11.8   **Hospital Route and Location**

Primary Hospital   Name, Address, Phone #
                            and Directions

Secondary Hospital   Name, Address, Phone #
                            and Directions

Example:

From the main gate: State Route 75 South, bear left onto
                            I-95 East. I-95 East to Exit 38 to
                            U.S. Route 46 East. Route 46 East
                            approximately 0.5 mile to West
                            Broadway. Turn left on West
                            Broadway. West Broadway 1 block,
                            turn left on Diamond Spring Road.
                            Diamond Spring Road approximate-
                            ly 0.3 mile to Pocono Road. Turn
                            right onto Pocono Road, approxi-
                            mately 0.7 mile to Hospital on left.

SECTION 12.0 STANDARD OPERATING PROCEDURES

12.1   General

The following standard operating procedures apply under this GHASP.

- Eating, drinking, and smoking are prohibited in the exclusion zone and the contamination reduction zone.
- Contact lenses shall not be worn in these zones.
- Work in pairs at all times. At a minimum maintain line of sight or adequate communications.
- Avoid, where possible, contact with contaminated objects.
- Do not climb over or under objects.
- Adhere to provisions of the SHASP.
- As new hazards are encountered, work procedures will be evaluated.
- Daily safety meetings will be conducted each day, and will discuss objectives and hazards expected to be encountered and their control measures, designation of break and assembly areas, and correction of any violations of the SHASP.
- Basic emergency and first aid equipment will be available at the Support Zone and the CRZ, as appropriate. It will include communications, first aid kit, emergency eye wash, fire extinguishers, and other safety related equipment
- A rescue team will be located in the CRZ and available for immediate deployment in the event of an emergency.
- Hand held walkie-talkies will be utilized by the field team for communications between downrange operations and the command post. Specific units will be approved by the HSC prior to on site use.
- Heat stress will be a major concern for personnel using PPE. Work rest regiments will be utilized to preclude the potential for heat stress. In addition, heart rates and weight loss will be monitored and used to monitor personnel.
- Practice contamination avoidance, on and off site.
- Apply immediate first aid to all cut, scratches,and abrasions. Decontamination procedures are required for minor injuries.
- Decontamination procedures are not required for life threatening situations. Cut the injured person out of their protective equipment, minimizing contamination, and transport to hospital.

- Be alert to your own physical condition. Watch your buddy for signs of fatigue, exposure, etc.
- No work will be conducted in the dark. A minimum of 5 foot candles will be required in all work areas.
- All provisions of 29 CFR 1926 and 1910 will be followed.
- Utilize seat belts, unless specifically exempted.

12.2   Fire Prevention

Personnel often work with and around flammable solvents and materials. Fire awareness and prevention, along with fire extinguisher training, are important for every individual to safely conduct site activities.

12.2.1   *General Fire Awareness*

Many gases and vapors form flammable mixtures with air. This means that the mixture will propagate a flame - perhaps very violently - away from a source of ignition. Two characteristics of flammable air contaminants are very important in assessing the risk.

1. **The lower explosive (or flammable) limit (LEL)** is the lowest vapor concentration in which flame propagation will occur.

2. **The flash point (FP)** is the lowest temperature at which a flammable mixture will exist in the air immediately above the surface of a pool of liquid.

A low value for flash point generally indicates a greater flammability hazard. A liquid with a flash point exceeding 100° (e.g., 180° F for phenol) would pose a flammability hazard only if the temperature of the liquid were elevated, and for this reason such chemicals usually are considered "combustible" rather than flammable.

The potential for danger from flammable atmospheres generally increases with decreasing LEL and FP and with increasing degree of confinement. Little flammability hazard could exist in an open field exposed to wind, but a more confined area could become much more hazardous. Also, the concentration of the liquid flammable species in the groundwater is very important, unless stratification occurs. A completely miscible contaminant present at a low level would present a low flammability hazard even in a confined area (but a severe toxicity hazard could exist). However, a thin layer of a flammable contaminant on groundwater could present an opportunity for the development of a flammable atmosphere in a basement, in a manhole, or even in a shallow excavation.

In addition to flammable atmospheres, the type of work performed at the site could be the source of a fire hazard. Some common causes of fire are electrical malfunctions, friction, open flames, sparks, hot surfaces, and smoking.

The SSO must inspect the job site for fire hazards prior to site activities. Also, the SSO must inspect electrical equipment, ensure grounding devices are in use, and enforce Standard Operating Procedures for Electrical Safety, Confined Spaces, and Chemical Hazards. These SOPs have provisions for fire prevention and awareness.

12.2.2   *Fire Prevention Plan*

Prior to site activities, the SSO must inform the employees of the fire emergency action plan. The plan will include:

- The fire hazards associated with the site activities.
- Fire alarm system
- Location and use of the portable fire extinguisher or fire prevention equipment.

12.2.2.1 *Portable Fire Extinguishers*

Approved portable fire extinguishers must be maintained in fully charged and operable condition at all times. Portable fire extinguishers must be visually inspected every day prior to site activities. On a hazardous waste site the fire extinguisher should be located in the contamination reduction zone.

Portable fire extinguishers are used as a first line defense on fires of a limited size. They are classified by the types of fires for which they are effective in extinguishing.

Class A - fires involving ordinary combustible material such as wood, paper, cloth, rubber, and many plastics. Extinguishment requires the heat-absorbing (cooling) effect of water or water solutions, the coating effects of certain dry chemicals which retard combustion, or the interrupting of the combustion chain reaction by halogenated agents.

Class A extinguishers are identified by a large A located inside a green triangle or pictures based on the international pictures system.

Class B - fires involving flammable or combustible liquids, flammable gases, greases, and similar materials. Extinguishment requires the excluding of air (oxygen), inhibiting the release of combustible vapors, or interrupting the combustion chain reaction.

Class B extinguishers are identified by a large B inside a red square or pictures based on the international picture system.

Class C - fires involving *live* electrical equipment. Because of the potential shock hazard, electrically nonconductive extinguishing agents must be used when combating fires in live electrical equipment. Extinguishment requirements are the same as for Class A or B fire depending upon the nature of the combustibles in the immediate area.

NOTE: When electrical equipment is de-energized, extinguishers for Class A, B or C fires may be used.

Class C extinguishers are identified by a large C inside a blue circle or pictures based on the international picture system.

Class D - fires involving certain combustible metals (such as magnesium, sodium, potassium, titanium, zirconium, lithium, etc.). Extinguishment requires a heat-absorbing medium that does not react with the burning metal.

Class D extinguishers are identified by a large D inside a yellow star or based on the international picture system.

Fire extinguishers are generally operated by pulling a locking pin, aiming the hose and squeezing the handle. Step by step instructions for operating an extinguisher are written on the name plate of each extinguisher.

12.3   Compressed Gas Cylinders

Compressed gas cylinders are present on hazardous waste sites as breathing air for supplied air respirators, welding gases, fire extinguishers, calibration gases, as well as possibly being unearthed during site remediation. When working with compressed gases it is important to be aware of the hazards involved with the chemical properties of the gas itself (i.e., flammable or toxic) as well as the physical state of the gas (i.e., high pressure or low temperature).

12.3.1   *Safe Handling of Compressed Gases*

The procedures adopted for the safe handling of compressed gases are mainly centered on containment of the material to prevent its escape to the atmosphere, and proper control of pressure and flow. All rules and regulations are directed toward these ends. Knowledge of emergency procedures is important to limit property damage and injury, but is usually necessary only because a basic rule of handling has been broken.

- Common OSHA Violations Involving Compressed Gases

  - Unsecured cylinders
  - Cylinders stored without protective caps.
  - Noncompatible gases (such as hydrogen and oxygen) stored together.
  - Cylinder valves open when cylinder is not in use (an attached regulator with a closed discharge valve is not sufficient).
  - Fire extinguishers not present during welding, burning, or brazing operations.
  - No safety showers and eyewash facility where corrosive gases are used.
  - No gas masks and/or self-contained breathing apparatus conveniently located near areas where toxic gases are used or stored.

12.3.2 *General Precautions*

Some general precautions for handling, storing, and using compressed gases follow:

1. Never drop cylinders or permit them to strike each other violently.
2. Cylinders may be stored in the open, but should be protected from the ground beneath to prevent rusting. Cylinders may be stored in the sun, except in localities where extreme temperatures prevail; in the case of certain gases, the supplier's recommendation for shading should be observed. If ice or snow accumulates on a cylinder, thaw at room temperature or with water at a temperature not exceeding 125° F.
3. The valve-position cap should be left on each cylinder until it has been secured against a wall or placed in a cylinder stand, and is ready to be used.
4. Avoid dragging, rolling, or sliding cylinders, even for a short distance. They should be moved by using a suitable hand truck.
5. Never tamper with safety devices on valves or cylinders.
6. Do not store full and empty cylinders together. Serious suck-back can occur when an empty cylinder is attached to a pressurized system.
7. No part of a cylinder should be subjected to a temperature higher than 125° F. A flame should never be permitted to come in contact with any part of a compressed gas cylinder.

8. Cylinders should not be subjected to artificially created low temperatures (minus 20° F or lower), since many types of steel will lose their ductility and impact strength at low temperatures. Special stainless steel cylinders are available for low temperature use.

9. Do not place cylinders where they may become part of an electric circuit.

10. Ground all cylinders, lines, and equipment used with flammable compressed gases.

11. Use compressed gases only in a well-ventilated area.

12. Check cylinders and all connections under pressure for leaks prior to using the contents.

13. When discharging gas into a liquid, a trap or suitable check valve should be used to prevent liquid from getting back into the cylinder or regulator.

14. When using compressed gas, wear appropriate protective equipment, such as safety goggles or face shield, rubber gloves and safety shoes.

15. When returning empty cylinders, close the valve before shipment, leaving some positive pressure in the cylinder. Replace any valve outlet and protective caps originally shipped with the cylinder. Mark or label the cylinder "empty" and store in a designated area for return to the supplier.

16. Before using cylinders, read all label information and data sheets associated with the gas being used. Observe all applicable safety practices.

17. Eye baths, safety showers, gas masks, respirators, and/or resuscitators should be located nearby but out of the immediate area that is likely to become contaminated in the event of a large release of gas.

18. Fire extinguishers, preferably of the dry chemical type, should be kept close at hand and should be checked periodically to ensure their proper operation.

Additional questions on gas cylinders should be directed towards the SSO, HSC, Project Manager or the gas supplier.

12.4   Electrical Safety

A variety of electrical hazards may be present on any work site. Overhead power lines, downed electrical wires, and buried cables pose a danger of shock or electrocution if workers contact them during site operations. Faulty electrical power tools, generators, and extension cords also pose shock hazards when not maintained and inspected. Finally, lightning is a hazard during outdoor operations, particularly for workers around drilling rigs and handling metal containers and equipment.

The following procedures and rules are to reduce and prevent electrical hazards at work sites.

12.4.1   *Utility Installations*

Prior to any excavation, trenching or drilling the Site Manager and SSO will determine that the area is free of underground utility lines by contacting utility suppliers, and if necessary having a representative on site. In addition, the customer will be advised of proposed work and provide drawings of all underground installations.

The SSO will note all overhead power lines and assure that drill rigs and other heavy equipment do not come within the following minimum clearances:

Power lines nominal system kv	Minimum required clearance
50 or under	10 feet (3.05 m)
69	12 feet (3.66 m)
115,161	15 feet (4.57 m)
230,285	20 feet (6.10 m)
345	25 feet (7.62 m)
500	35 feet (10.67 m)

Furthermore, operations adjacent to overhead lines shall not be initiated until coordinated with the utility supplier.

No work will be performed around downed electrical wire until they are determined to be de-energized by the utility supplier.

When underground installations are exposed during excavation, they shall be protected to avoid damage.

12.4.2   *Power Tools and Ground Fault Circuit Interrupters*

All electrical power tools and extension cords used at work sites will be UL approved and shall be grounded by a cord having an identified grounding conductor and multi-contact polarized plug-in receptacle.

All electrical extension cords used on work sites will be equipped with Ground Fault Circuit Interrupters (GFCI). GFCI are required in all circuits used for portable electrical tools. The GFCI will be UL listed and set to trip within 5 ma ± 1 ma as specified in UL Standard 943.

A Ground shall be provided for noncurrent carrying metallic parts of such equipment as generators and powered arc welders.

Power tools and extension cords will be visually inspected for damage and defects each day. Any equipment found defective must be taken out of service until repaired.

All power tools and wiring required to be explosion proof shall be maintained in that condition. There shall be no loose or missing screws, gaskets, thread connections, or other impairments to its tight condition.

12.4.3   *Grounding Fluid Transfers*

Transferring materials from one drum to another container by gravity, vacuum, or pump will require grounding both containers to each other to avoid the build up of a static charge.

Ground clamps and connecting cables will be kept in working condition and attachment to containers will be metal to metal.

See drum handling appendix for further information.

12.4.4   *Weather Conditions*

To eliminate the hazard of lightning electrocution, the weather conditions will be monitored and work suspended during electrical storms.

Electrical power tools will not be used in standing water. Trenches must be pumped free of standing water prior to work activities involving power tools.

12.5   *Trenching and Excavation*

Cave-ins are a serious hazard whenever people enter trenches or holes, or work near banks of loose earth. Many construction workers die each year when sides collapse and people are covered by earth. It can happen even in shallow trenches.

Employees must not enter trenches or excavations if major deviations from the following OSHA requirements are noted.

1.   If depth ≥ five feet, then walls and faces must be protected against cave-in by shoring and bracing or by sloping the sides to the angles of repose.

2.   Material removed from the excavation must be placed at least two feet away from the edge of the trench or hole. Other heavy material should not be placed within two feet of the edge either.

An inspection of the shoring and bracing to assess safety must be performed before trench entry. Materials of construction should be sound, and crossbraces should be horizontal. The vibration of heavy equipment can weaken even well built supports and make cave-in more likely. Also, rain and standing water can increase the risk.

Several other OSHA requirements exist, for example.

-    In trenches four or more feet deep, no more than 25 feet of lateral travel must be necessary to reach a ladder or other means of egress.
-    When excavations exceed 20 feet in depth, the support system must be designed by a "qualified person," such as an engineer.
-    Excavations and trenches must be inspected by a competent person daily and after rainfall.
-    Excavations and trenches must have barricades to prevent accidental falls into the openings.
-    Excavation must be preceded by a determination that no underground pipelines or wires are present. (Telephone numbers usually can be found in the Yellow Pages under "excavation.")
-    Supports must be removed safely (from the bottom to the top) upon completion of the project. If the soil is unstable, then braces and other components must be removed from above with ropes.

All OSHA requirements are to be reviewed for applicability. Additional requirements on entry into confined space and drilling safety may apply to a specific site or project. The Program Manager, Project Manager, HSC and SSO, will study these subject regulations to determine their applicability.

Entry into trenches in soil contaminated by chemicals can be particularly hazardous, because chemical vapors may concentrate and the trench sides could become unstable. During the collection of soil and water samples in trenches less than four feet in depth, an employee may enter the excavation, but the head must never cross the plane of the opening. If a sample is required from a trench exceeding four feet in depth, then an employee may enter only if the following precautions are taken in addition to those listed above:

-    Air monitoring is conducted if required by the SHASP.
-    The trench is terraced on both sides to ensure stability,

- Excavated earth is placed at least two feet away from the edge,
- Skin contact with soil or liquid is avoided, and
- Any applicable requirements of for entry into confined space, and drilling safety, are followed.

All trenches and excavations made by personnel for sample collection must be filled as soon as possible, to avoid accidents.

12.6   Entry Into Confined Spaces

Entry into confined spaces, and subsequent work in them, can be extremely dangerous. Many deaths of workers, and those attempting rescue, occur every year. Death can result from four causes:

- Oxygen deficient atmosphere,
- Flammable (or explosive) atmospheres.
- Toxic atmospheres, and
- Engulfment by liquid or solid material.

A confined space is one not intended for continuous occupancy in which at least one of these four conditions could exist at the time of entry or could develop during the period of work. Confined spaces often have limited means of entry and egress, and physical barriers hinder the rescue of an incapacitated employee (e.g., manholes and reaction vessels). However, these features are not common to all confined spaces, such as deep holes in contaminated soil. *Entry into a confined space occurs when the head crosses the plane of the opening.*

The term "confined space" should be defined broadly. This section applies to any entry into manholes or large tanks, as well as to entry into excavations in potentially contaminated soil. A basement in contact with potentially contaminated soil could also qualify as a confined space for the purposes of this section. The definition also includes rooms or buildings that could contain levels of airborne chemicals that are immediately hazardous to life and health. This section does not address all of the extreme hazards associated with entry into reaction vessels. The specific practices required will depend upon the nature of the contaminant, the characteristics of the work area, and the task performed.

Work in confined spaces can expose employees to a variety of hazardous conditions. An oxygen deficiency is possible in a manhole or a tank, but unlikely in a basement and virtually impossible in a shallow excavation. Ubiquitous ground contamination by a flammable liquid with a high vapor pressure can produce an explosive atmosphere in a manhole, a basement, or even a shallow excavation, but the probability would decrease with a decreasing degree of confinement. Similarly, extremely toxic vapors could exist in all three areas, if a toxic contaminant were present in the soil. Residual chemicals in a large tank easily could produce a flammable or extremely toxic atmosphere. An engulfment hazard would exist only if there were a potential for entrapment by the rapid entry of a liquid (water in a pipeline) or a solid (loose soil). *Unanticipated chemical hazards are always possible, especially in manholes, where toxic atmospheres unrelated to the ground contamination may exist.*

A room or building containing spilled chemicals could also qualify as a confined space, if a flammable or extremely toxic atmosphere were likely. Thus entry into a storage building containing deteriorated drums should be considered potentially hazardous. This section would apply both to brief initial entry as well as to prolonged periods of work in the space. Oxygen deficiency is extremely unlikely in a building, unless some large source of inert gas is present (e.g., a leaking cylinder of nitrogen).

12.6.1   *Elements of Confined Space Entry*

Work in confined spaces always requires ventilation and air sampling, as well as special provisions for communication and rescue. In addition, respiratory protection is required under any of the following conditions:

- The oxygen content is below 19.5%.
- The concentrations of toxic chemical contaminants exceed their applicable exposure limits.
- Unknown toxic chemicals could be present in the air.
- The SSO specifies respirators for some other reason.

Special precautions against fire and explosion are required whenever either of the following conditions exist:

- The flammable gas/vapor concentration exceeds 10% of the lower explosive limit (LEL).
- The oxygen concentration exceeds 21.5%.

12.6.1.1   *Air Sampling*

Air sampling is required before entry into a confined area and during the period of the employees' occupancy. The SSO must ensure that an instrument capable of detecting flammable and oxygen-deficient atmospheres is present whenever employees enter a confined space where these conditions could develop. If contamination by a specific toxic gas is considered possible, and an appropriate monitor is commercially available, then this device should be present also. Carbon monoxide and hydrogen sulfide are two gases for which monitors are available in combination with sensors that measure oxygen content and flammability. Indicator tubes may be used in some cases. The SSO must ensure that employees who will use monitoring equipment are familiar with proper operating procedures.

Good sampling technique can allow employees to detect dangerous conditions that they might otherwise overlook. This is particularly true in manholes and other enclosed spaces. The sampling probes should be inserted into the space through a slightly opened portal whenever possible, to avoid significant entry of outside air. Regions of the space that are farthest from the portal should be sampled first, whenever possible. It is necessary to test all areas (top, middle, bottom) of a confined space.

12.6.1.2 *Communication and Rescue*

Provisions for communication and rescue are essential. The SSO will ensure that those who enter the confined space will remain in communication with someone outside by voice, visible signal, or radio at all times. Suitably equipped standby personnel must be stationed nearby. They must be equipped to effect a rescue either by entering the space or by extracting incapacitated employees by means of an attached safety line.

Special provisions for rescue always are necessary when employees enter manholes, tanks, or spaces in which conditions favor the formation of toxic, flammable, or oxygen-deficient atmospheres. In manholes and other structures having restricted openings, employees must be equipped with safety lines, attached to a winch, designed to orient the body for easy extraction.

12.6.1.3 *Ventilation*

Employees always should look for opportunities to increase the rate of ventilation in confined spaces. Portals should be opened to their maximum extent before entry and during occupancy. Additional openings should be used to produce cross-drafts whenever this is possible.

Entry into manholes and extremely confined spaces may require forced ventilation before entry and during occupancy, as well as continuous monitoring of the air. In these cases, a blower and duct are used to introduce fresh air into the confined space and to force out potentially contaminated air.

12.6.1.4 *Isolation*

Isolation of a confined space is a process where the space is removed from service by:

- locking out electrical sources, preferably at disconnect switches remote from the equipment
- blanking and bleeding pneumatic and hydraulic lines
- disconnecting belt and chain drives, and mechanical linkages on shaft-driven equipment where possible, and
- securing mechanical moving parts within confined spaces with latches, chains, chock, blocks, or other devices.

12.6.1.5 *Respiratory Protection and Protective Clothing*

A major objective of a rigorous program on confined space entry is to ensure that contaminant levels remain as low as feasible - sufficiently low to avoid the necessity of respirator use. Respirators would be required, however, when the oxygen content could drop below 19.5%, or when established exposure limits could be exceeded.

If a toxic or oxygen-deficient atmosphere immediately hazardous to life and health could develop without warning, then an escape respirator would be required for employee protection during the brief interval necessary to evacuate the area. Such a respirator could consist of a small quantity of compressed air supplied through a hood, or a properly selected air-purifying respirator designed for emergency use only.

If the levels of toxic contaminants are above established safe limits, but below levels that are immediately dangerous to life and health, then respirators designed for routine use must be worn whenever employees work in the space. Such respirators could be used in addition to the escape devices described above, if the situation warranted this level of protection.

The atmosphere in a confined space may be immediately dangerous to life and health as a result of the entry of flammable gases or vapors in excessive amounts. Ventilation may not provide an adequate margin of safety in some cases. Such a condition would require the use of special non-sparking tools, low-voltage electrical devices, and other safety equipment. The SSO must be contacted in these cases to determine the necessary precautions.

12.6.2   *Recommendations for Safe Entry: A Checklist*

Use the following checklist to evaluate the confined space.

DO NOT ENTER A CONFINED SPACE UNTIL YOU HAVE CONSIDERED EVERY QUESTION, AND HAVE DETER-MINED THE SPACE TO BE SAFE.

<u>YES</u>   <u>NO</u>

____ ____   Is entry necessary?

TESTING

____ ____   Are the instruments used in atmospheric testing properly calibrated:

____ ____   Was the atmosphere in the confined space tested?

____ ____   Was oxygen at least 19.5% - not more than 23.5%?

____ ____   Were toxic, flammable, or oxygen-displacing gas-es/vapors present?

- Hydrogen Sulfide
- Carbon Monoxide
- Methane
- Carbon Dioxide
- Other (List)

_____

MONITORING

YES   NO

_____ _____   Will the atmosphere in the space be monitored while work is going on?

_____ _____   Continuously?

_____ _____   Periodically? (if yes, give interval:_____)

REMEMBER - Atmospheric changes occur due to the work procedure or the product stored. The atmosphere may be safe when you enter, but can change very quickly.

CLEANING

_____ _____   Has the space been cleaned before entry is made?

_____ _____   Was the space steamed?

_____ _____   If so, was it allowed to cool?

VENTILATION

_____ _____   Has the space been ventilated before entry?

_____ _____   Is the air intake for the ventilation system located in an area that is free of combustible dusts and vapors and toxic substances?

_____ _____   If atmosphere was found unacceptable and then ventilated, was it re-tested before entry?

ISOLATION

YES   NO

_____ _____   Has the space been isolated from other systems?

_____ _____   Has electrical equipment been locked out?

_____ _____   Have disconnects been used where possible?

YES   NO

____ ____ Has mechanical equipment been blocked, chocked, and disengaged where necessary?

____ ____ Have lines under pressure been blanked and bled?

CLOTHING/EQUIPMENT

____ ____ Is special clothing required (boots, chemical suits, glasses, etc.)?

(If so, specify: _____)

____ ____ Is special equipment required (e.g., rescue equipment, communications equipment, etc.)?

If so, specify: _____)

____ ____ Are special tools required (e.g., sparkproof)?

If so, specify: _____)

RESPIRATORY PROTECTION

____ ____ Are MSHA/NIOSH-approved respirators of the type required available at the worksite?

____ ____ Is respiratory protection required (e.g., air-purifying, supplied air, self-contained breathing apparatus, etc.)?

If so, specify: _____)

____ ____ Can you get through the opening with a respirator on? (If you don't know, find out before you try to enter).

TRAINING

YES   NO

____ ____ Have you been trained in proper use of a respirator?

____ ____ Have you received first aid/CPR training?

____ ____ Have you been trained in confined space entry and do you know what to look for?

STANDBY/RESCUE

____ ____ Will there be a standby person on the outside in constant visual or auditory communication with the person on the inside?

____ ____ Will the standby person be able to see and/or hear the person inside at all times?

____ ____ Has the standby person(s) been trained in rescue procedures?

____ ____ Will safety lines and harness be required to remove a person?

____ ____ Are company rescue procedures available to be followed in the event of an emergency?

____ ____ Are you familiar with emergency rescue procedures?

____ ____ Do you know who to notify and how in the event of an emergency?

PERMIT

(The permit is an authorization in writing that states that the space has been tested by a qualified person, that the space is safe for entry; what precautions, equipment, etc. are required; and what work is to be done).

YES   NO

____   ____   Has a confined space entry permit been issued?

____   ____   Does the permit include a list of emergency telephone numbers?

12.7   Noise Exposure

It is important that personnel recognize the situations that could cause excessive exposure and protect themselves appropriately if such a situation exists on a project.

12.7.1   *Definition of Noise*

Workplace noise is measured in units called dBA - decibels on the "A-weighted" scale. This measurement gives more weight to the sound pressures in the more damaging frequencies (around 2000 Hz) and less weight to the sound pressure in the frequencies outside this range. Some typical A-weighted sound pressure levels for various noise sources are shown below:

Noise Source	Sound Pressure Level (dBA)
Pneumatic Hammers	100
Backhoe	80
Heavy Truck	78
Typewriter	65
Conversational Speech	60

12.7.2   *Noise Standard*

The Permissible Exposure Limit (PEL) set by OSHA is a continuous exposure to 90 dBA over an 8-hour shift, or an exposure equivalent to this. Thus, an 8-hour exposure to 90 dBA is 100% of the OSHA limit. Obviously a higher fraction of the OSHA limit (> 100%) would be received if either the duration or the sound level exceeded 8 hours and 90 dBA, respectively. The following table demonstrates the relationship between continuous exposure level and permissible exposure time:

Continuous Sound Pressure Level (dBA)	Duration of	Fraction of Exposure (hr) OSHA Limit (%)	
105	1		100
100	2		100
95	4		100
90	8		100
85	16		100

A 5 dBA increase in the continuous sound level results in a 50% decrease in the permissible period of exposure. An unprotected person exposed to 100 dBA for 2 hours receives 100% of the limit during that brief period. No additional significant noise exposure would be permitted during the remainder of the shift.

It is instructive also to consider exposures to various continuous sound levels over an entire 8-hour shift. We have seen that such an 8-hour exposure to 90 dBA results in 100% of the OSHA limit. The information in the previous table permits the calculation of "doses" received by unprotected workers exposed to other sound levels during an 8 hour period.

This is presented below:

Continuous Sound Pressure Level (dBA)	Time Required to receive 100% of the PEL (hr)	Fraction of the the PEL Received in 8 hours (%)
105	1	800
100	2	400
95	4	200
90	8	100
85	16	50

12.7.3 *Hearing Conservation Amendment*

Note that an 8-hour exposure to 85 dBA, or its equivalent, is 50% of the PEL. This level of exposure is the OSHA Action Level. Exposure above this level is permissible in the workplace, but the employer must take certain actions to protect exposed employees from possible hearing loss. No unprotected employees may receive an exposure above 100% of the PEL.

Most exposures to loud noises are intermittent rather than continuous. Intermittent exposure to very loud noises does not necessarily result in a cumulative exposure that exceeds the PEL. The information presented above allows one to evaluate such situations. For example, a thirty-minute exposure to 100 dBA results in 25% of the OSHA limit, because a 2-hour exposure at this level produces 100%. If the exposure for the remaining 7 1/2 hours of the work day remained below 85 dBA, then there would be little cause for concern. A twenty-five-minute exposure to 105 dBA also would result in a 25% of the PEL. It is clear that one such exposure in a shift is acceptable, but several could lead to excessive exposure.

Employees who enter noisy environments should use ear plugs or ear muffs, even when their cumulative exposure for the day probably will not exceed the OSHA limit. These devices diminish the actual exposure level by at least 10 dBA, if they are used properly. Ear plugs must be inserted into the ear canal with care, and muffs must fit tightly around the ear. Employees should seek guidance from the Site Manager, HSC, or the SSO when they suspect that excessive noise exposures are possible.

12.8   Unexploded Ordnance (UXO)

If there is a potential for UXO at this site, the following procedures will be used to minimize the potential for accidental detonation in these areas:

1) Review all potential sites with the location Safety Office.
2) All sites will be cleared by certified explosive ordnance disposal (EOD) personnel prior to any site work.
3) Site communications (i.e., hand held radios, cellular telephones, etc.) will be approved by the Site Safety Office prior to any site work.
4) Any invasive operations penetrating to a depth greater than four (4) feet will be surveyed with a magnetometer at two (2) foot intervals below the four foot depth.
5) The buddy system will be used at all times when working at a potential UXO site.

12.9   Temperature Related Illness

Many workplace deaths due to heat stroke occur each year in warmer regions of the country, but there are no OSHA standards that explicitly address hot work environments. On a hazardous waste site, heat may present a hazard exceeding that of chemical exposure, because protective clothing hinders effective dissipation of accumulated heat by evaporation and convection. The prevention of illness and death due to heat stress is a responsibility of the SSO.

12.9.1   *Heat-Related Illnesses*

Excessive exposure to hot, humid work environments can cause several illnesses.

- **Heat cramps** are painful muscle spasms caused by the loss of salt from sweating during heavy work.
- **Heat exhaustion** often causes fatigue, nausea, and headache. The skin moist and pale. Victims should be taken to a cool place and given lightly salted liquids. Severe cases involving vomiting and loss of consciousness require medical treatment.
- **Heat stroke is a serious medical emergency** which frequently results in death. The victim usually experiences nausea, headache, and confusion before he collapses. His skin is hot, dry, and possibly discolored. **Immediate action** is necessary to lower the body temperature of the victim. Drenching the victim with cold water and fanning him vigorously is the best first aid. **An ambulance should be called immediately.**

In addition, excessive exposure to sunlight during outdoor work can increase the risk of **skin cancer.** People with fair skin burn easily and are affected the most. They should be especially careful during the summer months. Employees should use a sunscreen (#15 or greater) on the face, the arms, and the backs of the hands to prevent excessive exposure to sunlight. A hat and long sleeves also provide good protection.

12.9.1.1   *Basic Precautions*

The Program Manger will permit the employment of only **fit workers** for positions in which the potential for heat-related illness exists. In particular, obese individuals and those whose consumption of alcohol is excessive may not be employed in these jobs. In addition, many chronic diseases would disqualify an applicant. The Project Manager, Site Manager or HSC will inform the physician performing pre-employment or annual medical examinations whenever hot work environments are expected, and the examining physician will disqualify any applicant whose state of health increases the risk of heat-related illness. The symptoms of headache, nausea, vertigo, weakness, thirst and giddiness are common to heat exhaustion and the early stages of heat stroke.

The Project Manager and/or the Site Manager will allow the acclimatization of newly hired workers in hot jobs. New employees will not be assigned the normal work load during the first few days of employment. They should perform 50% of the normally expected work on the first day (lighter duty with more breaks). On each of the next five days, they should increase their output each day by an equal amount until 100% is reached on the sixth day. The Site Manager and the SSO will observe new employees closely to detect early signs of heat-related illness.

The SSO will ensure that workers understand the dangers of hot work environments and the necessary precautions. In addition, he will work with employees to reduce the risk through the following measures:

- Scheduling heavier work during the cooler part of the day.
- Encouraging employees and supervisors to organize tasks in a way that minimizes employee exposure to direct sunlight.
- Encouraging employees to be alert to the early signs of heat-related illness and to take breaks before problems begin. (One important sign of danger is a heart-rate at or approaching 100 beats/minute).
- Encouraging employees to drink water frequently to replace lost fluids. Drinks formulated to replace lost salts are desirable. Fluids will be readily available in break areas, and disposable cups will be provided.
- Enforcing a total ban on the consumption of alcoholic drinks during the work shift, and encouraging employees not to consume large amounts of alcohol on the evening before hot work. (Alcohol contributes to dehydration).

12.9.1.2   *Work/Rest Regimen*

The principle means of protecting workers from the excessive accumulation of heat is the use of a work/rest regimen through a cycle of periods of work and periods of rest. A prescribed portion of **each hour** is allocated to work, and the remainder of the 60-minute period is reserved for rest. The nature of the work and the environmental conditions both influence the work/rest regimen necessary in a given situation. The SSO is responsible, in consultation with the Site Manager, to establish the Work/Rest Regimen. The following conditions can serve as a useful reference point:

Work load:	light manual labor	Temperature:	85° F
Clothing:	cotton garments	Humidity:	high
Location:	indoors (shade)	Air movement:	very light

Work/rest regimen: About 45 minutes of work and about 15 minutes of rest each hour.

Very severe conditions actually reverse this distribution, while more favorable ones could eliminate the need for a cyclical rest period.

The SSO will consider the nature of each task, the temperature of the rest location, and the environmental conditions when determining a Work/Rest Regimen. He should consult the Project Manager and the HSC if questions arise or if extreme circumstances will be encountered by workers.

12.9.2 *Preventing Cold-Related Illness and Injury*

This section is intended to protect personnel for the severest effects of cold stress - hypothermia. Work in cold environments can be anticipated and measures taken to avoid hypothermia and prevent cold injury to body extremities. Other considerations to cold work environments are equipment problems, frozen decon solutions, and winter storms. These must be considered to prevent cold-related injury and stress at the job site.

12.9.2.1 *Types of Cold-Related Illness and Injury*

12.9.2.1.1 *Hypothermia*

Hypothermia results when the body loses heat faster than it can produce it. When this situation first occurs, blood vessels in the skin constrict in an attempt to conserve vital internal heat. Hands and feet are first affected. If the body continues to lose heat, involuntary shivers begin. This is the body's way of attempting to produce more heat, and it is usually the first warning sign of hypothermia. Further heat loss produces speech difficulty, forgetfulness, loss of manual dexterity, collapse, and finally death.

The temperature of the hands and feet can drop as much as 40°-50° F (23-38° C) below normal body temperature without permanent harm. A relatively small temperature drop in the body core (about 2.5° F or 1.5° C) produces shivering. As the body core temperature continues to drop, the brain becomes less efficient and the victim becomes confused and disoriented.

The body's sense of cold is a relative factor. The thermometer may read above 40° F (4.4° C) and the possibility of hypothermia might seem remote, but many cases of exposure have occurred in temperatures well above freezing. How cold the body gets depends on many factors, not just air temperature. Moisture on skin and clothes can conduct heat away from the body much faster than when the skin is dry.

12.9.2.1.2   *Frostbite*

Frostbite occurs when there is actual freezing of the tissues. Theoretically, the freezing point of the skin is about 30° F (-1° C); however, with increasing wind velocity, heat loss is greater and frostbite will occur more rapidly. Once started, freezing progresses rapidly. For example, if the wind velocity reaches 20 mph, exposed flesh may freeze within about one minute at 14° F (-10° C). Furthermore, if the skin comes in direct contact with objects whose surface temperature is below the freezing point, frostbite may develop at the point of contact in spite of warm environmental temperatures.

Air movement is more important in cold environments than in hot because the combined effect of wind and temperature can produce a condition called **windchill.** Windchill is heat loss from convection and is the greatest and most deceptive factor in loss of body heat. When the air is still and the temperature is 30° F (-1° C), the body will feel cool. Given the same temperature and a wind of 25 miles an hour (40 km/h) it will feel bitterly cold. In essence, the wind blows away the thin layer of air that acts as an insulator between the skin and the outside air temperature.

Efforts have been made to develop indices for evaluation cold environments. The windchill index is probably the best known and the most used of cold-stress indices. All of the cold stress indices have limitations as do those for heat stress, but under the right conditions, the information they yield can be helpful.

The windchill factor is the cooling effect of any combination of temperature and wind velocity or air movement. The windchill index should be consulted by everyone facing exposure to low temperatures and wind. Note that windchill "temperatures" have no significance other than indicating potential effect on the body. Although the windchill temperature may be below the freezing point of water, it will not freeze unless the air temperature is also below the freezing point.

The windchill index does not take into account that part of the body which is exposed to cold, the level of activity with its effect on body heat production, and the amount of clothing being worn.

12.9.2.2 *Control Measures*

The dead air space between the warm body and clothing and the outside air is essential. Clothing is worn to keep the body warmth in and the cold out. Usually, no one type of clothing is best for all weather conditions. Many layers of relatively light clothing with an outer shell of windproof material maintain body temperature much better than a single heavy outer garment worn over ordinary indoor clothing. The more air cells each of these clothing layers has, the more efficient it insulates against body heat loss. Make sure that clothing allows some venting of perspiration. Because wet skin will freeze more rapidly than dry skin, use all feasible means to keep as dry as possible. Make full use of windbreaks and avoid exposing skin to direct effects of the wind. Problems are created by the need to wear layers of special clothing that make the wearer very clumsy in performing many routine work procedures. Increased body dimensions must also be considered if tight spaces are encountered.

If exposed skin begins to sting or tingle, rub the area to stimulate circulation. However, if the exposed area is numb, do not rub it. Warm the affected parts in warm water (104°-113° F or 40°-45° C) or by other suitable means.

Thermal-type respirators are available for those bothered by breathing very cold air. At temperatures much lower than -49° F (-45° C), the lung tissue may start freezing unless the air is warmed before breathing. Because metal will conduct heat away from the body quite rapidly, be very careful of skin contact with metal objects such as tools, and, if possible, use tools that have nonmetallic handles, or are thermally insulated.

Heated warming shelters (tents, cabins, restrooms, etc.) should be made available nearby and the workers should be encouraged to use them at regular intervals, the frequency depending on the severity of the environmental exposure. The onset of heavy shivering, frostbite, the feeling of excessive fatigue, drowsiness, irritability, or euphoria, are indications for immediate return to the shelter. When entering the heated shelter the outer layer of clothing should be removed and the remainder of the clothing loosened to permit sweat evaporation or a change of dry clothing provided.

Dehydration occurs insidiously in cold environments and may increase susceptibility of the workers to cold injury. Warm sweet drinks and soups should be provided at work sites to provide caloric intake and fluid volume. The intake of coffee should be limited because of a diuretic and circulatory effect.

Despite the cold environmental conditions and the need for shelters, the decontamination of workers and equipment cannot be neglected. If possible, dry decontamination procedures should be used to avoid wet conditions in cold environments. Dry decon methods include sweeping, vacuuming or disposing of contaminated clothing and materials. If this is not possible then the Contamination Reduction Zone can be moved into a heated shelter (tent, cabin).

The SSO will consider the nature of the work task and the environmental conditions to determine Work/Rest Regimen and the need for shelters. He should consult with the Site Manager, Project Manager and the HSC if questions arise or if extreme circumstances are encountered on a job site.

12.10   Drilling Safety

Drilling into potentially contaminated soil can expose personnel both to chemicals and to the unusual hazards inherent in drilling operations. Similar dangers can exist when earth-moving equipment is used to excavate trenches for soil testing. Before any drilling or digging, the Site Manager will consult the Project Manager,and the HSC to discuss necessary precautions related to chemical exposure.

All reasonable measures will be taken to decrease the probability of drilling or digging in a spot where UXO, gas lines or electrical cables are buried. This must include a study of all available sources of relevant information on items buried on the site. It must include inquiries to those firms providing gas or electricity service and a review of any relevant documents in the possession of the Site Safety Office. (Sometimes information can be obtained by calling the number listed under "excavation" in the Yellow Pages of the telephone book.) The Site Manager will complete the Drilling Safety Checklist (Figure 12.10-1) before drilling begins and review the checklist with the SSO. The SSO will then retain control of the document.

The mechanical hazards of drilling and excavating can be significant. Employees should not wear clothing that can easily become entangled in moving parts. For example, neckties are always forbidden. (For the same reason, long hair must be held securely in place, close to the head.) Shoes with steel toes must be worn if there exists a potential for foot injury from dropped pipes or other heavy objects.

As discussed in the confined spaces section, entry into trenches for the collection of soil or water samples can be particularly hazardous, because chemical vapors may concentrate there and because the trench sides could become unstable. During sample collection from trenches less than four feet in depth, an employee may enter the excavation, but the head must never cross the plane of the opening. If a sample is required from a trench exceeding four feet in depth, then an employee may enter only if the following precautions are taken:

- The trench is terraced on both sides to ensure stability,
- Air monitoring is conducted if required by the SHASP,
- Excavated earth is placed at least two feet away from the edge,
- Skin contact with soil or liquid is avoided, and
- Any applicable requirements for entry into a confined space and trenching and excavation are followed.

All trenches must be filled as soon as the required samples are collected, to prevent accidents.

Chemical exposure can occur as the result of skin contact and the inhalation of dust or vapor. Work practices should minimize or eliminate exposure by these routes. Some health and safety plans will require respirators, routine air monitoring, and special protective clothing. If unexpected layers of solid or liquid chemicals are detected during drilling or excavation, then work must be halted until the situation can be evaluated more thoroughly.

FIGURE 12.10-1
(page 1 of 2)

<u>Drilling Safety Checklist</u>

(to be completed and signed to commencement of drilling)

Program Name	Location	Number of Holes

	Yes	No
1.0 Drilling Contract Signed and Approved	___	___

Contract Number _____

	Yes	No
1.1 Contract has adequate wording to protect company from liability. Program Manager has reviewed contract or consulted Legal to assure adequate liability protection.	___	___
1.2 Contract limits liability for:		
Consequential liability	___	___
Drilling damage to property	___	___
Environmental impairment resulting from drilling	___	___
2.0 SHASP prepared in advance and approved by Program Manager.	___	___
2.1 SHASP covers:		
Protective clothing	___	___
Respiratory protection	___	___
Safety of drillers	___	___

Figure 12.10-1
(Page 2 of 2)

<u>Yes</u>   <u>No</u>

3.0   As-built or equivalent drawings available
and reviews complete   ——

    3.1   Standard tank drawings available covering
dimensions, orientation and buried depths   ——   ——

    3.2   Utility lines shown and reviewed   ——   ——

    3.3   Drawings reviewed on site with client
representative prior to beginning operations   ——   ——

4.0   Pipeline location equipment available on site   ——   ——

    4.1   Equipment checked prior to field use   ——   ——

5.0   Hand augur pre-boring on industrial sites   ——   ——

    5.1   Will the hand augur holes be drilled to
appropriate depths   ——   ——

6.0   Client field representative signed form
approving field boring locations   ——   ——

7.0   Comments or explanations of problems encountered

_____

_____

_____

8.0   Authorized review and approval signature

_____

Site Manager

_____

Site Safety Officer

_____

Date

12.11   Seat Belts

All site personnel are required to wear a seat belt when operating or riding in a motor vehicle during working hours. This Standard Operating Procedure covers all vehicles and vans, rental cars, and personal vehicles used during normal or extended working hours.

No employee shall ride in a cargo van without occupying a firmly secured and stationary seat. Seat belts must be used by all employees.

12.12   First Aid

Planning and procedures are designed for emergency care at hazardous waste site. Planning is necessary to assure prompt and definite emergency care for injured and ill employees, and safe handing and transportation of injured and ill personnel.

Medical and first aid requirements are promulgated under the Occupational Safety and Health Act to provide emergency care to workers. The law requires an on site person to be adequately trained in first aid and first aid supplies readily available. In addition, where the eyes and body of a person may be exposed to corrosive materials, a suitable facility for quick drenching or flushing of the eyes and body shall be provided.

12.12.1   *Duties of First Aid Personnel*

The SSO, or his designated representative, will be trained in first aid and cardiopulmonary resuscitation (CPR). Documentation of this training shall be kept on site and also maintained by the individual. The duty of the first aid provider is to render only first aid as the situation demands until additional medical services are available.

12.12.2   *First Aid Supplies*

All work sites will have a first aid kit and eye wash station. These items will be maintained by the SSO and inspected prior to the initiation of site activities.

The Emergency Response and Contingency Plan outlines procedures for decontamination of injured personnel, and should be reviewed by the SSO.

12.12.3 *General First Aid Procedures*

First aid procedures should be administered by the SSO or his designated representative. General first aid procedures can be found on Material Safety Data Sheets and some product labels. The following are general guidelines and should not be viewed as complete, however, they may provide guidance in dealing with chemical exposures.

1. **Eye exposure.** If liquids get into the eyes, wash the eyes immediately with large amounts of cold water. Remove contact lenses if worn. Call a physician as soon as possible.

2. **Skin exposure.** If liquids gets on the skin, wash promptly using large quantities of water. If liquid soaks through clothing, remove the clothing promptly and wash the skin. If irritation persists, get medical attention.

3. **Breathing.** If a large amount of vapor is inhaled, move the exposed person to fresh air at once. If breathing has stopped, perform artificial respiration. Keep the affected person warm and at rest. Get medical attention immediately.

4. **Swallowing.** If a chemical is swallowed, do not cause the person to vomit. Get medical attention immediately.

5. **Rescue.** Move the affected person from the hazardous exposure. If the exposed person has been overcome, notify someone else and put into effect the established emergency rescue procedures. Do not become a casualty yourself. Understand the emergency rescue procedures and know the locations of the equipment before the need arises.

12.13 *Drum Inspection*

The appropriate procedure for handling drums depends on the drums contents. Prior to any handling, drums should be visually inspected to gain as much information as possible about their contents and conditions. The inspection should look for:

•   Symbols, words, or other markings on the drum indicating that its contents are hazardous, i.e., radioactive, explosive, toxic.

- Signs of deterioration such as corrosion, rust, and leaks.
- Signs that the drum is under pressure such as swelling or bulging.

As a precautionary measure, personnel should assume unlabeled drums contain hazardous materials until their contents are characterized. Drums may also be mislabeled and may not accurately describe its contents.

Monitoring instruments shall be used to monitor the area around the drum locations. When opening a drum monitoring instruments shall be used to measure the contamination levels at the opening and in the breathing zone of the workers.

A preliminary plan should be developed which specifies the extent of handling necessary, the personnel for the job, and the most appropriate procedures based on the hazards associated with the probable drum content as determined by visual inspection. This plan should be revised as new information is obtained during drum handling.

SECTION 13.0 MATERIAL SAFETY DATA SHEETS (MSDS)

Note: Attach each chemical MSDS sheet to the HASP as the chemicals are determined to be present on the site.

Appendix A
ABBREVIATIONS

alc	alcohol	eye	administration into eye (irritant)
amorph	amorphous		
anhyd	anhydrous	EYE	systemic eye effects
aq	aqueous	F	Fahrenheit
atm	atmosphere	fbr	fibroblasts
autoign temp	autoignition temperature	flamm	flammable
		flash p	flash point
bp	boiling point	fp	freezing point
BPR	blood pressure effects	GIT	gastrointestinal tract effects
b range	boiling range		
bz	benzene	g/L	grams per liter
C	Centigrade/Celsius	glac	glacial
carc(s)	carcinogen(s)	GLN	glandular effects
CARC	carcinogenic effects	gran	granular, granules
cc	cubic centimeter	hr	hour
CL	ceiling concentration	hexag	hexagonal
compd(s)	compound(s)	hmn	human
conc	concentration, concentrated	H_2	hydrogen
		htd	heated
contg	containing	htg	heating
corr	corrosive	ims	intramuscular
cryst	crystal(s), crystalline	incomp	incompatible
CUM	cumulative effects	inhal	inhalation
CVS	cardiovascular effects	insol	insoluble
d	density	intox	intoxication
D	day	ipr	intraperitoneal
dBA	decibel	irr	irritant, irritating, irritation
decomp	decomposition		
deliq	deliquescent	IR	infrared
dil	dilute	IRR	irritant effects (systemic)
eth	ether		
exper	experimental (animal)	itr	intratracheal
expl	explosive	iv	intravenous
expos	exposure	kg	kilogram
		L	liter

537

mem	membrane	PNS	peripheral nervous system effects
min	minimum		
µg, ug	microgram	ppb	parts per billion (v/V)
µmol, umol	micromole	pph	parts per hundred (v/V) (percent)
mg	milligram		
mg/m³	milligrams per cubic meter	ppm	parts per million (v/V)
		ppt	parts per trillion (v/V)
mg/L	milligrams per liter	PROP	properties
misc	miscible	psi	pounds per square inch
ml	milliliter		
MLD	mild irritation effects	PSY	psychotropic effects
mm	millimeter	PUL	pulmonary system effects
MMI	mucous membrane effects		
		rbt	rabbit
mo	month	refr	refractive
mod	moderately	resp	respiratory
MOD	moderate irritation effects	rhomb	rhombic
		S, sec	second(s)
mol	mole	scu	subcutaneous
mp	melting point	SEV	severe irritation effects
mR	milliroentgen		
mR/hr	milliroentgen per hour	SKN	systemic skin effects
MSK	musculoskeletal effects	slt	slight
		sltly	slightly
µ, u	micron	sol	soluble
mumem	mucous membrane	soln	solution
MUT	mutagen	solv(s)	solvent(s)
mw	molecular weight	spont	spontaneous(ly)
N	nitrogen	subl	sublimes
NEO	neoplastic effects	susp	suspected
nonflamm	nonflammable	SYS	systemic effects
NTP	National Toxicology Program	t_{re}	rectal temperature
		ta	ambient air temperature
o-	ortho		
ocu	ocular	ta adj	adjusted air temperature
p-	para		
par	parenteral	tech	technical
petr eth	petroleum ether	temp	temperature
pg	picogram	TER	teratogenic effects
pk	peak concentration	TFX	toxic effects
pmol	picomole	tox	toxic, toxicity

uel	upper explosive limits
unk	unknown
UNS	toxic effects unspecified in source
UV	ultraviolet
vap d	vapor density
vap press	vapor pressure
visc	viscosity
v/V	volume per volume
W	week(s)
Y	year(s)
>	greater than
<	less than
⇐	equal to or less than
⇒	equal to or greater than

Appendix B
ACRONYMS

ACGIH	American Conference of Governmental Industrial Hygienists
ALR	air-line respirator
ANSI	American National Standards Institute
APR	air-purifying respirators
ASTM	American Society for Testing and Materials
CA	carcinogen
CAA	Clean Air Act
CAS	Chemical Abstracts Service
CC	closed cup
CDC	Center for Disease Control
CELDS	Computer-Aided Environmental Legislative Data System
CEQ	Council on Environmental Quality
CERCLA	Comprehensive Environmental Response, Compensation, and Liability Act (also called Superfund)
CFR	Code of Federal Regulations
CGI	combustible gas indicator
CNS	central nervous system
COC	Cleveland Open Cup
CPC	chemical protective clothing
CPR	cardiopulmonary resuscitation
CRC	contamination reduction corridor
CRZ	contamination reduction zone
CWA	Clean Water Act
DOT	U.S. Department of Transportation
EKG	electrocardiogram
EPA	U.S. Environmental Protection Agency
ESCBA	escape-only self-contained breathing apparatus
ETA	equivocal tumorigenic agent
FEF	forced expiratory flow
FEMA	Federal Emergency Management Administration
FEV_1	forced expiratory volume in one second
FID	flame ionization detector
FIFRA	Federal Insecticide, Fungicide and Rodenticide Act
FIT	field investigation team
FRC	functional residual capacity

FVC	forced vital capacity
GC	gas chromatography
GI	gastrointestinal
GM	Geiger-Müller
HAZMAT	Hazardous Material Response Team
HAZWOPER	Hazardous Waste Operations and Emergency Response
HNU	name of company that manufactures a type of photoionizer used to detect organic gases and vapors
HR	hazard rating
HW	hazardous waste
IARO	International Agency for Research on Cancer
IDLH	immediately dangerous to life or health
ISO	International Organization for Standards
IUPAC	International Union for Pure and Applied Chemistry
LEL	lower explosive limit
LFL	lower flammable limit
MMEFR	maximal expiratory flow rate
MSDS	Material Safety Data Sheet
MSHA	Mine Safety and Health Administration
MVV	maximal voluntary ventilation
NCRP	North Carolina Research Park
NEPA	National Environmental Protection Agency
NFPA	National Fire Protection Agency
NIOSH	National Institute for Occupational Safety and Health
OC	open cup
OSHA	Occupational Safety and Health Administration
OVA	organic vapor analyzer
PCB	polychlorinated biphenyl
PDS	personnel decontamination station
PEL	permissible exposure limit or published exposure limit
PID	photoionization detector
PNA	polynuclear aromatic hydrocarbons
PPC	personal protective clothing
PPE	personal protective equipment
PVC	polyvinyl chloride
RCRA	Resource Conservation and Recovery Act
REL	recommended exposure limits
RV	residual volume
SARA	Superfund Amendments and Reauthorization Act
SCBA	self-contained breathing apparatus
SMAC 23	Sequential Multiple Analyzer Computer
SOP	standard operating procedure
SSO	site safety officer

STEL	short-term exposure limit
TAT	technical assistance team
TCC	taglibue closed cup
TD	toxic dose
THR	toxic and hazard review
TLC	total lung capacity
TLV	threshold limit value
TLV-C	threshold limit value-ceiling
TSCA	Toxic Substances Control Act
TSD	transportation, storage and delivery
TWO	time-weighted average
UEL	upper explosive limit
ULC	Underwriters Laboratory classification
USCG	U.S. Coast Guard

Ag_2O	silver oxide	IF_7	iodine heptafluoride
Al	aluminum	$KClO_3$	potassium chlorate
$AlCl_3$	aluminum chloride	K_2CrO_4	potassium chromate
BF_3	boron trifluoride	KHC	potassium carbide
B_2O_3	boron oxide	KOH	potassium hydroxide
BO_x	boron oxides	LiH	lithium hydride
Br_2	bromine gas	LiOH	lithium hydroxide
BrF_3	bromine trifluoride	$Mg(C_2H_5)_2$	magnesium ethyl
$CaCl_2$	calcium chloride	MgO	magnesia
$Ca(CN)_2$	calcium cyanide	Na_2C_2	sodium carbide
CaO_x	calcium oxides	$NaClO_3$	sodium perchlorate
$Ca(OCl)_2$	calcium oxychloride	NaK	sodium-potassium alloy
CCl_4	carbon tetrachloride	NaN_3	sodium nitride
CdO	cadmium oxide	$NaNO_3$	sodium nitrate
$Cd(OH)_2$	cadmium hydroxide	Na_2O	sodium oxide
C_6H_6	benzene	Na_2O_2	sodium peroxide
$CHCl_3$	chloroform	NaOBr	sodium oxybromide
CH_3OH	methanol	NaOCl	sodium oxychloride
Cl_2	chlorine gas	NaOH	sodium hydroxide
ClF_3	chlorine trifluoride	N_4PCP	sodium pentachlorophenate
ClO_2	chlorine oxide	NF_3	nitrogen fluoride
CN	cyanide	NH_3	ammonia
CO	carbon monoxide	NH_4^+	ammonium radical
CO_2	carbon dioxide	NH_4NO_3	ammonium nitrate
$COCl_2$	phosgene	NH_4OH	ammonium hydroxide
CoO_x	cobolt oxides	N_2O_4	nitrogen oxide
CrO_3	chromium trioxide	NO_x	nitrogen oxides
Cr_2O_3	chromium oxide	NOCl	nitrosyl chloride
CS_2	carbon bisulfide	O_2	oxygen gas
Cs_2O	cesium oxide	O_3	ozone
$CuFeS_2$	copper iron sulfide	OF_2	oxygen fluoride
EtOH	ethanol	OsO_4	osmium tetroxide
F_2	fluorine gas	PCl_3	phosphorus trichloride

Fe_2O_3	iron oxide	P_2O_3	phosphorus trioxide
F_2O_2	fluorine oxide	P_2O_5	phosphorus pentoxide
H_2	hydrogen gas	PO_x	phosphorus oxides
HCHO	formaldehyde	Rb_2C_2	rubidium carbide
HCl	hydrochloric acid	SCl_2	sulfur chloride
HF	hydrofluoric acid	SiO_2	silica
HgF_2	mercuric fluoride	SO_2	sulfur dioxide
HI	hydriodic acid	SO_x	sulfur oxides
HNO_3	nitric acid	2,3,7,8-TCDD	dioxin
H_2O	water	TeO	tellurium oxide
H_2O_2 or	hydrogen peroxide	$Tl(NO_3)_3$	thallium nitrate
HOOH			
HOAc	acetic acid	Tl_2O	thallous oxide
HOCl	hypochlorous acid	VO_x	vanadium oxides
H_2S	hydrogen sulfide	$ZnCl_2$	zinc chloride
H_2SO_4	sulfuric acid	$ZnCrO_4$	zinc chromate
H_2SO_3	sulfurous acid	$ZnCr_2O_7$	zinc dichromate
$H_2S_2O_3$	thiosulfuric acid	ZnO	zinc oxide

---

acetic acid	HOAc	magnesium ethyl	$Mg(C_2H_5)_2$
aluminum chloride	$AlCl_3$	mercuric fluoride	HgF_2
aluminum	Al	methanol	CH_3OH
ammonia	NH_3	nitric acid	HNO_3
ammonium hydroxide	NH_4OH	nitrogen oxides	NO_x
ammonium nitrate	NH_4NO_3	nitrogen fluoride	NF_3
ammonium radical	NH_4^+	nitrogen oxide	N_2O_4
benzene	C_6H_6	nitrosyl chloride	NOCl
boron oxides	BO_x	osmium tetroxide	OsO_4
boron oxide	B_2O_3	oxygen fluoride	OF_2
boron trifluoride	BF_3	oxygen gas	O_2
bromine gas	Br_2	ozone	O_3
bromine trifluoride	BrF_3	phosgene	$COCl_2$
cadmium oxide	CdO	phosphorus oxides	PO_x
cadmium hydroxide	$Cd(OH)_2$	phosphorus pentoxide	P_2O_5
calcium oxides	CaO_x	phosphorus trioxide	P_2O_3
calcium oxychloride	$Ca(OCl)_2$	phosphorus trichloride	PCl_3
calcium cyanide	$Ca(CN)_2$	potassium hydroxide	KOH
calcium chloride	$CaCl_2$	potassium chlorate	$KClO_3$

carbon monoxide	CO	potassium carbide	KHC
carbon bisulfide	CS_2	potassium chromate	K_2CrO_4
carbon tetrachloride	CCl_4	rubidium carbide	Rb_2C_2
carbon dioxide	CO_2	silica	SiO_2
cesium oxide	Cs_2O	silver oxide	Ag_2O
chlorine gas	Cl_2	sodium pentachlorophenate	N_4PCP
chlorine trifluoride	ClF_3	sodium nitride	NaN_3
chlorine oxide	ClO_2	sodium perchlorate	$NaClO_3$
chloroform	$CHCl_3$	sodium carbide	Na_2C_2
chromium trioxide	CrO_3	sodium oxide	Na_2O
chromium oxide	Cr_2O_3	sodium nitrate	$NaNO_3$
cobolt oxides	CoO_x	sodium hydroxide	$NaOH$
copper iron sulfide	$CuFeS_2$	sodium peroxide	Na_2O_2
cyanide	CN	sodium oxychloride	$NaOCl$
dioxin	2,3,7,8-TCDD	sodium oxybromide	$NaOBr$
ethanol	$EtOH$	sodium-potassium alloy	NaK
fluorine gas	F_2	sulfur dioxide	SO_2
fluorine oxide	F_2O_2	sulfur oxides	SO_x
formaldehyde	$HCHO$	sulfur chloride	SCl_2
hydriodic acid	HI	sulfuric acid	H_2SO_4
hydrochloric acid	HCl	sulfurous acid	H_2SO_3
hydrofluoric acid	HF	tellurium oxide	TeO
hydrogen gas	H_2	thallium nitrate	$Tl(NO_3)_3$
hydrogen peroxide	H_2O_2 or $HOOH$	thallous oxide	Tl_2O
hydrogen sulfide	H_2S	thiosulfuric acid	$H_2S_2O_3$
hypochlorous acid	$HOCl$	vanadium oxides	VO_x
iodine heptafluoride	IF_7	water	H_2O
iron oxide	Fe_2O_3	zinc oxide	ZnO
lithium hydride	LiH	zinc dichromate	$ZnCr_2O_7$
lithium hydroxide	$LiOH$	zinc chloride	$ZnCl_2$
magnesia	MgO	zinc chromate	$ZnCrO_4$

acute exposure Exposure to a substance in a short time span and generally at high concentrations.

alpha particle (alpha radiation) A positively charged particle having a mass and charge equal in magnitude to a helium nucleus (two protons & two neutrons). They are emitted by certain radioactive materials. They will travel only a few inches through the air before being stopped by air molecules. They are most dangerous when they are inhaled or ingested.

alpha radiation A type of ionizing radiation consisting of alpha particles, which are two protons and two neutrons bound together, with an electrical charge of +2. An alpha particle is equivalent to a helium nucleus.

autoreactive A compound that is reactive under normal conditions without initiation by heat or other compounds or change in conditions.

becquerel (Bq) A unit of activity equal to one nuclear transformation per second ($1 \text{ Bq} = 1\text{s}^{-1}$). The former special named unit of activity, the curie, is related to the becquerel according to $1 \text{ Ci} = 3.7 \times 10^{10} \text{ Bq}$.

beta particle (beta radiation) A charged particle emitted from the nucleus of an atom, with a mass and charge equal in magnitude to that of the electron. They are faster and lighter than an alpha particle.

breakthrough time The elapsed time between initial contact of the hazardous chemical with the outside surface of protective clothing material and the time at which the chemical can be detected at the inside surface of the material by means of the chosen analytic technique.

buddy system A system of organizing employees into work groups in such a manner that each employee is designated to be observed by at least one other employee in the group. The purpose of the buddy system is to provide rapid assistance to employees in the event of an emergency.

bulk container A cargo container, such as that attached to a tank truck or tank car, used for transporting substances in large quantities.

bung A cap or screw used to cover the small opening in the top of a metal drum or barrel.

canister A purifying device for an air-purifying respirator that is held in a harness attached tot he body or attached to the chin part of a face piece, is connected to the face piece by a breathing tube, and removes particulates or specific chemical gases or vapors from the ambient air as it is inhaled through the canister.

carboy A bottle or rectangular container for holding liquids with a capacity of approximately 5 to 15 gallons; made of glass, plastic, or metal and often cushioned in a protective container.

cartridge A purifying device for an air-purifying respirator that attaches directly to the face piece and removes particulates or specific chemical gases or vapors from the ambient air as it is inhaled through the cartridge.

chronic exposure Exposure to a substance over a long period of time, usually at low doses.

clean-up operation An operation where hazardous substances are removed, contained, incinerated, neutralized, stabilized, or in any other manner processed or handled with the ultimate goal of making the site safer for people or the environment.

closed-circuit SCBA A type of self-contained breathing apparatus (SCBA) that recycles exhaled air be removing carbon dioxide and replenishing oxygen. Also called a *rebreather SCBA*.

colorimetric tube An instrument for the chemical analysis of liquids by comparison of the color of the given liquid with standard colors.

CLO A unit of measure for CPC thermal heating values. Based on heat transfer rates through clothing at room temperature.

combustible Capable of burning.

contamination control line The boundary between the support zone and the contamination reduction zone.

contamination reduction corridor (CRC) The part of the contamination reduction zone where the personnel decontamination stations are located.

contamination reduction zone (CRZ) The area on a site where decontamination takes place, preventing cross-contamination from contaminated areas to clean areas.

continuous-flow respirator A respiratory protection device that maintains a constant flow of air into the face piece at all times. Airflow is independent of user respiration.

controlled area A defined area in which the occupational exposure of personnel to radiation or radioactive material is under the supervision of an individual in charge of radiation protection.

crazing The formation of minute cracks (as in the lens of a face piece).

cross-contamination The transfer of a chemical contaminant from one person, piece of equipment, or area to another that was previously not contaminated with that substance.

curie (Ci) See also Becquerel. (a) Formerly, a special unit of activity. One curie equals 3.7×10^{10} disintegrations per second exactly or $1\ Ci = 3.7 \times 10^{10}\ Bq$. (b) By Popular usage, the quantity of any radioactive material having an activity of one curie.

decay, radioactive A spontaneous nuclear transformation in which particles or gamma radiation is emitted, or x radiation is emitted following orbital electron capture, or the nucleus undergoes spontaneous fission.

decontamination The removal of hazardous substances from employees and their equipment to the extent necessary to preclude the occurrence of foreseeable adverse health effects.

decontamination line A specific sequence of decontamination stations within the contamination reduction zone for decontaminating personnel or equipment.

degradation A chemical reaction between chemical and structural materials (in, for example, protective clothing or equipment) that results in damage to the structural material.

demand respirator A respiratory protection device that supplies air or oxygen to the user in response to negative pressure created by inhalation.

dermal Pertaining to skin.

disinfection The application of a chemical that kills bacteria.

dose A general form denoting the quantity of radiation or energy absorbed. Most people receive between 150 and 200 millirems a year, and any level less than 5,000 millirems a year is considered low-level. Scientist have found that radiation doses of over 100,000 millirem will usually cause radiation sickness. Doses of over 500,000 millirems, if received in three days or less, will usually kill a person.

dosimeter An instrument for measuring doses of radioactivity or other chemical exposures based on collection media.

dress-out area A section of the support zone where personnel suit up for entry into the exclusion zone.

emergency response A response effort by employees from outside the immediate release area or by other designated responders (e.g., mutual-aid groups or local fire departments) to a situation that results, or is likely to result, in an uncontrolled release of a hazardous substance.

escape-only SCBA (ESCBA) A type of self-contained breathing apparatus (SCBA) that is approved for escape purposes only. It does not carry the safety features necessary for longer work periods.

etiologic agent A microorganism that may cause human disease.

exclusion zone The contaminated area of a site.

explosive A chemical that is capable of burning or bursting suddenly and violently.

facility Any site, area, building, structure, installation, equipment, pipe or pipeline (including any pipe into a sewer or publicly owned treatment works), well, pit, pond, lagoon, impoundment, ditch, storage container, motor vehicle, rolling stock, or aircraft where a hazardous substance has been deposited, stored, disposed of, or placed. Does not include any consumer product in consumer use or any waterborne vessel.

filter A purifying device for an air-purifying respirator that removes particulates and/or metal fumes from the ambient air as it is inhaled.

flammable Capable of being easily ignited or burning with extreme rapidity.

flammable gas Any compressed gas meeting the requirements for lower flammability limit, flammability limit range, flame projection, or flame propagation criteria as specified in 49 CFR 173.300(b).

flammable liquid Any liquid having a flash point below 100°F as determined by tests listed in 49 CFR 173.115(d). A *pyrophoric liquid* ignites spontaneously in dry or moist air at or above 130°F.

flammable solid Any solid material, other than an explosive, that can be ignited readily and when ignited burns so vigorously and persistently as to create a serious transportation hazard (49 CFR 173.150).

flash point The minimum temperature at which a liquid gives off enough vapors to form an ignitable mixture with the air near the surface of the liquid.

gamma radiation A type of ionizing radiation consisting of high-energy, short-wave length electromagnetic radiation. A type of radiation that is released in waves by unstable atoms when they stabilize. They are a very strong (range of energy from 10 keV to 9 MeV) type of electromagnetic wave. Gamma waves have no weight and travel even faster than alpha and beta radiation.

gamma-ray scintillation detector A gamma-ray detector consisting of a scintillation, such as sodium iodide, thallium-activated, NaI(Tl), and a photomultiplier tube housed in a light-tight container.

grappler An implement used to hold and manipulate objects from a distance.

hazardous materials response team (HAZMAT) An organized group of employees, designated by the employer, expected to handle and control actual or potential leaks or spills of hazardous substances requiring possible close approach to the substance.

hazardous substance Any substance designated by the following regulations: Sections 101(14) and 101(33) of CERCLA; 49 CFR 1172.101.

hazardous waste A waste or combination of wastes as defined in 40 CFR 171.6.

hazardous waste operation Any operation conducted within the scope of 40 CFR 261.3 or 40 CFR 171.6.

health hazard A chemical, mixture of chemicals, or pathogen for which there is statistically significant evidence based on at least one scientific study that acute or chronic health effects may occur in exposed employees.

health physics The science of radiation protection.

hot line The outer boundary of a site's exclusion zone.

immediately dangerous to life of health (IDLH) The maximum concentration from which one could escape within 30 minutes without any escape-impairing symptoms or any irreversible health effects.

incompatible Incapable of being combined without a dangerous effect (e.g., descriptive of two or more substances that produce an unfavorable chemical reaction if they come in contact).

injection The introduction of chemicals into the body through puncture wounds.

ionizing radiation High-energy radiation that causes irradiated substances to form ions, which are electrically charged particles.

LC_{50} Abbreviation for the median lethal concentration of a substances that will kill 50% of the animals exposed to that concentration.

LD_{50} Abbreviation for the median lethal dose of a substance that will kill 50% of the animals exposed to that dose.

manifest A list of cargo.

monitor, radiation A radiation detector the purpose of which is to measure the level of ionizing radiation (or quantity of radioactive material). It may also give quantitative information on dose or dose rate. The term is frequently prefixed with a word indicating the purpose of the monitor such as an area monitor, or air particle monitor.

monitoring, radiation (radiation protection) The continuing collection and assessment of the pertinent information to determine the adequacy of radiation protection practices and to indicate potentially significant changes in conditions or protection performance.

neutron A non-charged particle in the center of the atom. Together with the proton it forms the nucleus.

occupation dose (regulatory) Dose (or dose equivalent) resulting from exposure of an individual to radiation in a restricted area or in the course of employment in which the individual's duties involve exposure to radiation (see 10 CFR 20.3).

open-circuit SCBA A self-contained breathing apparatus (SCBA) in which the user exhales air directly into the atmosphere.

overpack 1. An oversized drum into which a leaking drum can be placed and sealed. 2. To overpack such a drum.

oxygen deficiency The concentration of oxygen by volume below which atmosphere-supplying respiratory equipment must be provided. It exists in atmospheres where the percentage of oxygen by volume is less than 19.5%.

palletize To place on a pallet or to transport or store by means of a pallet.

particulate Formed of separate, small, solid pieces.

penetration The chemical penetration of protective clothing through openings such as seams, buttonholes, zippers, or breathing air ports.

percutaneous Effected or performed through the skin.

permeation Seepage and sorption of a chemical through a material (e.g., the material making up protective clothing or equipment).

permissible exposure limit (PEL) The exposure, inhalation, or dermal permissible exposure limit specified in 29 CFR 1910, G and Z.

postemergency response That portion of an emergency response performed after the immediate threat of a release has been stabilized or eliminated and cleanup of the site has begun.

pressure-demand respirator A respiratory protection device that supplies air to the user and maintains a slight positive pressure in the face piece at all times. it supplies additional air in response to the negative pressure created by inhalation.

protection factor The ratio of the ambient concentration of an airborne substance to the concentration of the substance inside the respirator at the breathing zone of the wearer. The protection factor is a measure of the degree of protection the respirator offers.

published exposure limit (PEL) The recommended exposure limits published in *Recommendations of Occupational Health Standards* (NIOSH 1986).

qualified person A person with specific training, knowledge, and experience in the area for which he or she has the responsibility and the authority to control.

rad A former unit of absorbed dose 1 rad = 10^{-2} Gy = 10^{-2} J/kg {see gray (Gy)}.

radiation Energy in the form of electromagnetic waves.

radiation hazard A situation or condition that could result in deleterious effects attributable to deliberate, accidental, occupational, or natural exposure to radiation.

radiation protection All measures concerned with reducing deleterious effects of radiation to persons or materials (also called "radiological protection").

radioactive material A material of which one or more constituents exhibit radioactivity. NOTE: For special purposes such as regulation, this term may be restricted to radioactive material with an activity or a specific activity greater than a specified value.

reagent A substance used in a chemical reaction to detect, measure, examine, or produce other substances.

redress area A section of the exclusion zone where decontaminated personnel put on clothing for use in the support zone.

rem A former unit of dose equivalent. The dose equivalent in rems is numerically equal to the absorbed dose in rads multiplied by the quality factor, the distribution factor, and any other necessary modifying factors (originally derived from roentgen equivalent man).

restricted area Any area to which access is controlled for the protection of individuals from exposure to radiation and radioactive materials.

roentgen (R) - A unit of exposure; 1 R = 2.58 x 10^{-4} C/kg.

scintillation counter A counter in which the light flashes produced in a scintillation by ionizing radiation are converted into electrical pulses by a photomultiplier tube.

self-contained breathing apparatus (SCBA) A respiratory protection device that supplies clean air to the user from a compressed air source carried by the user.

sievert (Sv) The special name of the unit of dose equivalent. It is given numerically by 1 Sv = 1 J * kg^{-1} (= 100 rem).

site safety supervisor (SSO) the individual located on a hazardous waste site who is responsible to the employer and has the authority and knowledge necessary to implement the site safety and health plan and verify compliance with applicable safety and health requirements.

small-quantity generator A generator of hazardous wastes that in any calendar month generates no more than 2205 pounds (1000 kilograms) of hazardous wastes.

sorbent material A substance that takes up other materials either by absorption or adsorption.

staging area An area in which items are arranged in some order.

standard operating procedure (SOP) Established or prescribed tactical or administrative method to be followed routinely for the performance of a designated operation or in a designated situation.

Superfund A common name for the Comprehensive Environmental Response, Compensation and Liability Act (CERCLA) of 1980.

supplied-air respirator A respiratory protection device that supplies air to the user from a source that is not worn by the user but is connected to the user by a hose. Also called an *air-line respirator.*

support zone The uncontaminated area of a site where workers will not be exposed to hazardous conditions.

surfactant A decontamination agent that reduces adhesion forces between contaminants and the surfaces being cleaned.

swab A piece of cotton or gauze on the end of a slender stick used for obtaining a piece of tissue or secretion for bacteriologic examination.

swipe A patch of cloth or paper that is wiped over a surface and analyzed for the presence of a substance.

threshold The intensity or concentration below which a stimulus or substance produces a specified effect.

uncontrolled hazardous waste site An area where an accumulation of hazardous waste creates a threat to the health and safety of individuals, the environment, or both.

INDEX

557

Area sampling, 111, 143, 477-480
Asbestos, 439
Asphyxiants, 100, 437
Asthma, 185
Atmosphere classification, hazardous, 143-144
Atmospheric Research and EnvironmentalAssessment Laboratory (AREAL), 9
Atomic Energy Act (1954), 27

-B-

Banana oil, 232-233
Barriers, use of isolation and containment, 210
Becquerel, 395
Benzene, 94, 186, 438, 439
Beta particle/radiation, 395, 448
Biohazards/biological hazards, 450-452
BIOSIS PREVIEWS[R], 50
Birth defects, 92
Bloodborne Pathogen Rule, 66
Body motion, heat stress and, 280-281
Body reactions:to heat stress, 302-305; to toxic chemicals, 437-439
Botsball, 294-295
Bulk recontainerization, 157

-C-

CAB ABSTRACTS, 50
Canadian Environmental Protection Service, 368
Canadian Safety Association (CSA), 138, 147
CANCERLIT[R], 50
Carbon monoxide:confined spaces and, 516;
  respirator selection for, 223
Carcinogens, 91-92, 439
Cardio-pulmonary resuscitation (CPR) training, 430
Cardiovascular disease, 185
Carter, Jimmy, 2
CA SEARCH[R], 50
Catalytic combustion, 123-124
Cave-ins, 512-514

Centers for Disease Control and Prevention (CDC), 28
Central nervous system depressants, 438
Certification of air monitoring instruments:intrinsic safety testing, 145;
  labels, 153;
  performance testing, 146;
  programs, 146-147
Cesium, radioactive, 394
Chemical Control Corp., 1, 158
Chemical detector tubes, 111, 142
Chemical Information System (CIS), 46
Chemical Manufacturers Association, Inc., 161, 370
Chemical protective equipment (CPE): chemical hazards and selection of, 236-237;
  clothing included as, 220;
  performance and purchase considerations for, 249;
  sources of information on, 235, 248-249;
  test methods for, 246-248.
  See also Heat stress
Chemicals:assessment criteria for, 445-447;
  body reactions to toxic, 437-439;
  exposure limits, 441-445;
  hazardous properties of, 434-437;
  physical state of, 434;
  routes of exposure, 439-440;
  toxicity versus hazardous, 433
CHEMNAME[R], 51
Chlorine gas, respirator selection for, 223
Chronic health effects, 90, 114, 438
Cobalt, radioactive, 394
Colorimetric indicator tubes, 475-476
Combustible gas indicator (CGI), 141-142, 471-472
Compatibility testing:air reactivity testing, 166;
  background of, 157;
  common characteristics of, 160-161;
  explosive testing, 165-166;
  field analyses plan, 159-160;
  flammability, 168-170;
  guidelines, 157;

-I-

-U-